**Emergency Management of the Hi-Tech
Patient in Acute and Critical Care**

Emergency Management of the Hi-Tech Patient in Acute and Critical Care

Editors

Ioannis Koutroulis, MD, PhD, MBA
Attending Physician, Emergency Medicine
Children's National Hospital
Assistant Professor of Pediatrics, Emergency Medicine, Genomics and Precision Medicine
George Washington University School of Medicine and Health Sciences

Nicholas Tsarouhas, MD
Medical Director, CHOP Transport Team
Attending Physician, Emergency Medicine
Children's Hospital of Philadelphia
Professor of Clinical Pediatrics
Perelman School of Medicine at the University of Pennsylvania

Associate Editors

Richard J. Lin, MD
Attending Physician, Critical Care Medicine
Clinical Director, Progressive Care Unit
Associate Professor of Clinical Anesthesiology, Critical Care and Pediatrics, Perelman
School of Medicine at the University of Pennsylvania

Jill C. Posner, MD, MSCE, MSEd
Attending Physician, Emergency Medicine
Children's Hospital of Philadelphia
Professor of Clinical Pediatrics
Perelman School of Medicine at the University of Pennsylvania

Michael Seneff, MD
Director, Intensive Care Unit
Associate Professor of Anesthesiology and Critical Care Medicine
George Washington University Hospital
George Washington University School of Medicine and Health Sciences

Robert Shesser, MD
Professor and Chair
Department of Emergency Medicine
George Washington University School of Medicine and Health Sciences

WILEY Blackwell

Registered Office(s)
John Wiley & Sons Ltd, The Atrium, Southern Gate, Chichester, West Sussex, PO19 8SQ, UK

Editorial Office
9600 Garsington Road, Oxford, OX4 2DQ, UK

For details of our global editorial offices, customer services, and more information about Wiley products, visit us at www.wiley.com.

Wiley also publishes its books in a variety of electronic formats and by print-on-demand. Some content that appear in standard print versions of this book may not be available in other formats.

Library of Congress Cataloging-in-Publication Data

Names: Koutroulis, Ioannis, 1980– editor.
Title: Emergency management of the hi-tech patient in acute and critical care /
    senior editors, Ioannis Koutroulis, Nicholas Tsarouhas ; editors,
    Richard J. Lin, Jill C. Posner, Michael Seneff, Robert Shesser.
Description: Chichester, West Sussex ; Hoboken, New Jersey :
    Wiley-Blackwell, 2021. | Includes bibliographical references and index.
Identifiers: LCCN 2020028239 (print) | LCCN 2020028240 (ebook) | ISBN
    9781119262923 (cloth) | ISBN 9781119262954 (adobe pdf) | ISBN
    9781119262985 (epub)
Subjects: MESH: Emergency Treatment–instrumentation | Emergency
    Medicine–instrumentation | First Aid–instrumentation | Critical
    Care–methods
Classification: LCC RC86.8 (print) | LCC RC86.8 (ebook) | NLM WB 26 |
    DDC 616.02/5–dc23
LC record available at https://lccn.loc.gov/2020028239
LC ebook record available at https://lccn.loc.gov/2020028240

Cover Design: Wiley
Cover Image: © Donald Iain Smith/iStock/Getty Images

Set in 9.5/12.5pt STIXTwoText by SPi Global, Pondicherry, India
Printed and bound by CPI Group (UK) Ltd, Croydon, CR0 4YY

C066141_250421

Contents

List of Contributors

Chisom O.A. Agbim, MD, MSHS
Division of Emergency Medicine
Children's National Medical Center
Washington, DC
USA

Keith D. Baldwin, MD, MSPT, MPH
Department of Orthopedic Surgery
Perelman School of Medicine at the
University of Pennsylvania
Philadelphia, PA
USA
and
Department of Orthopedic Surgery
Children's Hospital of Philadelphia
Philadelphia, PA
USA

Marlet Bazemore, MD, MPH
Division of Ophthalmology
Children's National Hospital
Washington, DC, USA
and
George Washington University School of
Medicine and Health Sciences
Washington, DC, USA

Thane A. Blinman, MD, FACS
Division of General and Thoracic Surgery
Department of Surgery
Children's Hospital of Philadelphia
Philadelphia, PA, USA

and
Perelman School of Medicine at the
University of Pennsylvania
Philadelphia, PA, USA

Joseph J. Bolton, MBA, RRT-NPS
Department of Respiratory Care Services
Children's Hospital of Philadelphia
Philadelphia, PA
USA

Allison E. Boyd, MSN, CRNP
Division of Otolaryngology
Department of Surgery
Children's Hospital of Philadelphia
Philadelphia, PA
USA

Angela Burd, DNP, CPNP-AC
Hospital Medicine Division
Children's National Hospital
Washington, DC
USA

Guenevere V. Burke, MD
Department of Emergency Medicine
George Washington University School of
Medicine and Health Sciences
Washington, DC
USA

Adva Buzi, MD
Attending Physician
Division of Otolaryngology
Department of Surgery
Children's Hospital of Philadelphia
Philadelphia, PA
USA
and
Perelman School of Medicine at the
University of Pennsylvania
Philadelphia, PA
USA

Jerry Cabrera, RRT
Smith's Medical
Gary, IN
USA

Amy Caggiula, MD
Department of Emergency Medicine
George Washington University School of
Medicine and Health Sciences
Washington, DC
USA

Anne Marie Cahill, MBBch, BAO
Division of Interventional Radiology
Department of Radiology
Children's Hospital of Philadelphia
Philadelphia, PA, USA
and
Perelman School of Medicine at the
University of Pennsylvania
Philadelphia, PA
USA

Kelly Chiles, MD
Urology
Private Practice
Washington, DC
USA

Joy Collins, MD
Division of General and Thoracic Surgery
Department of Surgery
Children's Hospital of Philadelphia

Philadelphia, PA
USA
and
Perelman School of Medicine at the
University of Pennsylvania
Philadelphia, PA
USA

Daniel Dawson, RRT-NPS
Department of Respiratory Care Services
Children's Hospital of Philadelphia
Philadelphia, PA
USA

Eva Delgado, MD
Division of Emergency Medicine
Department of Pediatrics
Children's Hospital of Philadelphia
Philadelphia, PA, USA

Francesca Drake, RNFA, BSN, CNOR
Division of Plastic and
Reconstructive Surgery
Children's Hospital of Philadelphia
Philadelphia, PA
USA

Sarah Fesnak, MD
Division of Emergency Medicine
Department of Pediatrics
Children's Hospital of Philadelphia
Philadelphia, PA
USA
and
Perelman School of Medicine at the
University of Pennsylvania
Philadelphia, PA
USA

James B. Fink, PhD, RRT, FAARC, FCCP
Aerogen Pharma Corporation
San Mateo, CA, USA
and
Rush Medical School
Chicago, IL
USA

and
Texas State University
Round Rock, TX
USA

Tenagne Haile-Mariam, MD
Department of Emergency Medicine
George Washington University School
of Medicine and Health Sciences
Washington, DC
USA

Heather House, MD
Division of Emergency Medicine
Department of Pediatrics
Children's Hospital of Philadelphia
Philadelphia, PA
USA
and
Perelman School of Medicine at the
University of Pennsylvania
Philadelphia, PA
USA

Massoud Kazzi, MD
Department of Emergency Medicine
George Washington University School of
Medicine and Health Sciences
Washington, DC
USA
and
Critical Care Medicine
Washington Adventist Hospital
Takoma Park, MD
USA

Benjamin C. Kennedy, MD
Department of Neurosurgery
Perelman School of Medicine at the
University of Pennsylvania
Philadelphia, PA
USA
and
Division of Neurosurgery
Children's Hospital of Philadelphia
Philadelphia, PA
USA

Panagiotis Kratimenos, MD, PhD
Division of Neonatal-Perinatal Medicine
Children's National Hospital
Washington, DC, USA
and
George Washington University School of
Medicine and Health Sciences
Washington, DC, USA

Megan Lavoie , MD, FAAP
Division of Emergency Medicine
Department of Pediatrics
Children's Hospital of Philadelphia
Philadelphia, PA
USA
and
Perelman School of Medicine at the
University of Pennsylvania
Philadelphia, PA
USA

Jamie Lovell, MD
Division of Emergency Medicine
Department of Pediatrics
Cincinnati Children's Hospital
Medical Center
Cincinnati, OH
USA
and
University of Cincinnati College of
Medicine
Cincinnati, OH
USA

William P. Madigan, MD
Division of Ophthalmology
Children's National Hospital
Washington, DC, USA
and
Uniformed Services University of the
Health Sciences
Bethesda, MD, USA
and
George Washington University School of
Medicine and Health Sciences
Washington, DC, USA

Peter J. Madsen, MD
Division of Neurosurgery
Children's Hospital of Philadelphia
Philadelphia, PA, USA
and
Department of Neurosurgery
Perelman School of Medicine at the
University of Pennsylvania
Philadelphia, PA, USA

Meg Ann Maguire, MS, RN, CRNP, CPNP-PC
Division of Plastic and
Reconstructive Surgery
Children's Hospital of Philadelphia
Philadelphia, PA, USA

Peter Mattei, MD
Division of General, Thoracic and
Fetal Surgery
Children's Hospital of Philadelphia
Philadelphia, PA
USA
and
Perelman School of Medicine at the
University of Pennsylvania
Philadelphia, PA
USA

Oscar H. Mayer, MD
Division of Pulmonary and Sleep Medicine
Children's Hospital of Philadelphia
Philadelphia, PA
USA
and
Department of Pediatrics
Perelman School of Medicine at the
University of Pennsylvania
Philadelphia, PA
USA

Xenia Morgan, CRNP
Hemodialysis Unit
Division of Nephrology
Children's Hospital of Philadelphia
Philadelphia, PA
USA

Chariton Moschopoulos, MD
Division of Neurology
Boston Children's Hospital
Harvard Medical School
Boston, MA
USA

Anthony Mozzone, BA, CRT
Promptcare Respiratory
King of Prussia, PA
USA

*Natalie Napolitano, MPH, RRT, RRT-
NPS, FAARC*
Department of Respiratory Care Services
Children's Hospital of Philadelphia
Philadelphia, PA
USA

Courtney E. Nelson, MD
Division of Emergency Medicine
Department of Pediatrics
AI DuPont Hospital for Children
Wilmington, DE, USA
and
Sidney Kimmel Medical College at Thomas
Jefferson University
Philadelphia, PA, USA

Susan E. Nelson, MD, MPH
Department of Orthopedic Surgery
University of Rochester Medical Center
Rochester, NY
USA

Phuong D. Nguyen, MD
Division of Plastic and
Reconstructive Surgery
Children's Hospital of Philadelphia
Philadelphia, PA
USA

Amanda J. Nickel, MSc, RRT-NPS, RRT-ACCS
Department of Respiratory Care Services
Children's Hospital of Philadelphia
Philadelphia, PA
USA

Chima Oluigbo, MD
Department of Neurosurgery
Children's National Hospital
Washington, DC, USA
and
George Washington University School of
Medicine and Health Sciences
Washington, DC, USA

Michael J. O'Neal, MD
Department of Emergency Medicine
University of San Francisco
San Francisco, CA
USA

Michael Phillips, MD
Department of Urology
George Washington University School
of Medicine and Health Sciences
Washington, DC
USA

Pelton A. Phinizy, MD
Division of Pulmonary and Sleep Medicine
Children's Hospital of Philadelphia
Philadelphia, PA
USA
and
Department of Pediatrics
Perelman School of Medicine at the
University of Pennsylvania
Philadelphia, PA
USA

Desiree M. Seeyave, MB.BS
Department of Emergency Medicine &
Hospitalist Services
Children's Hospital of Georgia Emergency
Department
Augusta, GA
USA

Sameer Shakir, MD
Division of Plastic Surgery
Children's Hospital of Philadelphia
Philadelphia, PA
USA

Joanne Stow, MSN, APRN, PPCNP-BC, CORLN
Division of Otolaryngology
Department of Surgery
Children's Hospital of Philadelphia
Philadelphia, PA, USA

Ellen G. Szydlowski, MD
Division of Emergency Medicine
Department of Pediatrics
Children's Hospital of Philadelphia
Philadelphia, PA
USA
and
Perelman School of Medicine at the
University of Pennsylvania
Philadelphia, PA
USA

John F. Tamasitis, RRT-NPS
Children's Hospital Home Care
Children's Hospital of Philadelphia
King of Prussia, PA
USA

Andrew Tyler, MD, PhD
Department of Orthopedic Surgery
Vanderbilt University Medical Center
Nashville, TN
USA

R. Jason VonDerHaar, MD
Department of Surgery
Indiana University Health
Indianapolis, IN
USA
and
University of Indiana School of Medicine
Indianapolis, IN
USA

Katie Wagner, BS
George Washington University School
of Medicine and Health Sciences
Washington, DC
USA

Carmelle Wallace, MD, MPH
Division of Emergency Medicine
Department of Pediatrics
University of Alabama at Birmingham
Birmingham, AL
USA

Anna Weiss, MD, MSEd
Division of Emergency Medicine
Department of Pediatrics
Children's Hospital of Philadelphia
Philadelphia, PA
USA
and
Perelman School of Medicine at the
University of Pennsylvania
Philadelphia, PA
USA

Kimberly Windt, MSN, RN, CNN
Hemodialysis Unit
Division of Nephrology
Children's Hospital of Philadelphia
Philadelphia, PA
USA

Liza C. Wu, MD
Department of Surgery
Hospital of the University of Pennsylvania
and the Children's Hospital of Philadelphia
Philadelphia, PA, USA
and
Division of Plastic Surgery
Perelman School of Medicine at the
University of Pennsylvania
Philadelphia, PA
USA

David Yamane, MD
Department of Emergency Medicine
George Washington University Hospital
and
Department of Anesthesia and Critical
Care Medicine
George Washington University Hospital
Washington, DC
USA

Preface

The idea of writing this book was born in early 2016; we knew that the road would be bumpy yet exciting! We are thrilled to introduce the first edition of our manual to assist health care providers in managing our very unique patients with various hardware devices. These "hi-tech" devices help our patients breathe, walk, hear, and do a host of other essential activities of daily living. Importantly, when these patients seek emergency care due to device malfunction, infections, or other complications, it is crucial that the medical provider know how to manage both the patient and the device.

It is often challenging for the emergency/critical care clinician to troubleshoot and, sometimes, even identify the problems with many of these hi-tech devices. Moreover, specialized consultation is not always readily available. It is quite challenging for providers to recall complex diagnostic and therapeutic algorithms for patients with specialized equipment, thus increasing the risk for morbidity and mortality. This guide provides a stepwise approach to acute presentations of patients with clinical hardware, focusing on specific instructions for initial evaluation and management. Our intent is that this endeavor will assist health care providers in both community settings and academic centers in the treatment of complex patients with "hi-tech" equipment.

It is our sincere hope that this book will improve the quality of care to our unique patient population who utilize specialized hardware. Our goal is to provide our readers with an overview of the basic approach to clinical scenarios of device malfunction and related complications of the most commonly used medical devices. However, as it was impossible to include all devices in this book, the practitioner should make every effort to ensure they have the most accurate information for each patient's hardware.

We want to thank our fellow editors, authors, and contributors, who gave their time selflessly so that we could produce this book. Also, we would like to thank our teachers, mentors, and colleagues, from whom we learn every day. Most importantly, the real source of our inspiration, our patients and their families, deserve our eternal heartfelt gratitude.

Ioannis and Nick

Acknowledgments

I would like to thank Nick and all the editors of the book, as, without them, this effort would not have been possible. Nick's support was really amazing, and his help with some of the problems we faced during the creation of the book really made a difference. As a great clinician, researcher, and educator, Nick's contribution was vital for the whole project. Jill, Mike, Rich, and Rob went above and beyond to have all the chapters completed on time and make sure the content was appropriate. Thank you all!

I want to dedicate this book to my mother who, despite all the difficulties, never left my side. She has been my inspiration all these years. Also, to Dr. Levinsky, who discussed the initial idea for the book with me. And finally, to all the people in my life who made a difference, thank you!

Ioannis Koutroulis

I'd like to first acknowledge, Ioannis, the creator of the book and our persevering leader. Through thick and thin, Ioannis remained upbeat and encouraging. Ioannis stayed enthusiastic, despite delays as a result of our heavy administrative and clinical workloads due to sustained high volumes and acuities in our emergency departments (EDs), inpatient areas, and intensive care units. With an eternally positive attitude, he even respectfully pushed us through a pandemic toward the completion of the "Hi-Tech Book" project. Thank you, Ioannis! My most genuine love and appreciation goes to my family – wife Debbie, my son Christopher, and my daughter Nicole. The importance of their continual support of my long ED shifts, constant meetings, and endless "homework" cannot be understated. They have forever tolerated "Daddy" in his study ... reading, writing, typing, answering pages, making phone calls, etc. Finally, a special thank you to my mother who, with little education and even less money, somehow managed to raise three pretty good kids. Love you, mom.

Nick Tsarouhas

To my parents, who raised me to believe I can do anything.
To my mentors, who have showed me the way.
To my patients, who have inspired and humbled me.
And to my husband and daughters, my loves and light.

Jill C. Posner

Section I

Gastro-intestinal Devices

1

Using and Troubleshooting Enteral Feeding Devices

Courtney E. Nelson[1,2] and Thane A. Blinman[3,4]

[1] Division of Emergency Medicine, Department of Pediatrics, Al DuPont Hospital for Children, Wilmington, DE, USA
[2] Sidney Kimmel Medical College at Thomas Jefferson University, Philadelphia, PA, USA
[3] Division of General and Thoracic Surgery, Department of Surgery, Children's Hospital of Philadelphia, Philadelphia, PA, USA
[4] Perelman School of Medicine at the University of Pennsylvania, Philadelphia, PA, USA

Introduction

Enteral feeding devices deliver nutrition directly to the stomach and/or small intestine for patients with anatomic or physiological feeding impairments. Common indications for enteral feeding devices include feeding and swallowing dysfunction, severe gastroesophageal reflux, malnutrition, neurological disorders, and prolonged ventilation. Given the breadth of indications for enteral feeding devices, a clinician in any setting, and particularly those in the emergency department, is likely to encounter these devices on a daily basis. These are simple devices with a simple purpose, but their dysfunction is highly disruptive and worrisome to patients and their caregivers. This chapter will teach you how to manage the simplicity of a working enteral feeding device and navigate the intricacies of an unruly device.

Equipment/Device

Enteral feeding devices can be categorized into temporary and long-term devices. Furthermore, the name for each device comes from its origin (nose, mouth, or stomach) and terminus (stomach or small intestine) (Table 1.1). Nasal and oral tubes are temporary and work well for patients with transient feeding difficulties. Gastrostomy tubes (G-tube) and jejunostomy tubes (J-tube) are ideal for more long-term or permanent enteral nutrition. Enteral feeding devices are sized in French (Fr) units, which is the outer diameter of the tube in millimeters multiplied by three. A 9 Fr tube, for example, has an outer diameter of 3 mm. Tube lengths are usually given in centimeters and vary widely from very short low profile "button" type tubes to very long naso-jejunal (NJ) tubes.

Emergency Management of the Hi-Tech Patient in Acute and Critical Care, First Edition. Edited by Ioannis Koutroulis, Nicholas Tsarouhas, Richard J. Lin, Jill C. Posner, Michael Seneff, and Robert Shesser.
© 2021 John Wiley & Sons Ltd. Published 2021 by John Wiley & Sons Ltd.

Table 1.1 Enteric feeding devices.

Origin	Destination	Tube	Abbreviated	Placement
Temporary feeding devices				
Nose (naso-)	Stomach (gastric)	Naso-gastric	NG	Bedside
	Duodenum	Naso-duodenal	ND	
	Jejunum	Naso-jejunal	NJ	
Mouth (oro-)		Oro-gastric	OG	Bedside
Long-term feeding devices				
Percutaneous	Stomach	Gastric[a]	G-tube	Surgically or endoscopically
	Jejunum	Gastro-jejunostomy	GJ	Fluoroscopically
		Jejunostomy	J-tube	Fluoroscopically

[a] Commonly, these tubes are called "PEG tubes"; however, a percutaneous endoscopic gastrostomy is a procedure and not a specific tube.

Temporary Feeding Devices

Naso-gastric (NG), naso-duodenal (ND), NJ, and oro-gastric (OG) feeding tubes are used for short-term enteral feeding, defined as that less than 12 weeks. OG tubes are reserved for patients in the intensive care unit and rarely seen in the emergency department. Temporary feeding tubes are typically constructed from polyurethane or silicone-based polymers, both of which are flexible, reasonably durable, minimally reactive biologically, and, for most, immunologically inert. Polyurethane tubing has the added benefit of being made with a water-activated lubricant to ease insertion and increased durability. Depending on the manufacturer, NG, NJ, ND, and OG tubing may come with weighted tips, radiopaque indicators, stylets, and/or magnets to help with placement. Common pediatric tube size for feeding is a 6–8 Fr and for adults a 12–14 Fr.

Gastric Decompression Devices

Similar to the temporary feeding devices, there are NG and OG tubes used for decompression and lavage. These devices are larger than feeding tubes: 8–10 Fr for children and 12–14 Fr for adults. Decompression devices are divided into single and double lumen tubes. Single lumen tubes, such as the Levin tube, are used more frequently in the emergency department or intensive care unit for intermittent decompression. Single lumen tubes should not be placed on continuous suction because they can adhere to the stomach wall and cause tissue damage. A double lumen tube is the preferred decompression device because it has both a large lumen for suction or irrigation and a small lumen (typically blue in color) that vents the large lumen. This small lumen serves as a pop-off valve for the device to prevent excessive suctioning. There are two common types of double lumen tubes: Salem sumps and Replogle tubes. Salem sumps are preferred in an emergency setting because they have several suction holes along the side of the tubing for rapid efficient suctioning, whereas Replogle tubes have suction holes only at the most distal end of the tube.

When using a double lumen tube, it is critical that the small lumen be kept to room air to adequately vent the large lumen. It should not be clamped, used for suction, or used for irrigation. Finally, the proximal end of a double lumen decompression device must be kept above waist-height, otherwise the gastric contents may reflux into the small lumen.

Long-term Feeding Devices

G-tubes are used for long-term or permanent enteric feeding. G-tubes are divided into standard adjustable length tubes and low-profile (i.e. button) tubes. When caring for a patient with a long-term feeding device, it is imperative that you know the type of tube the patient has, how the tube was placed, and how to use the tube in order to adequately care for your patient.

Basic G-tube Anatomy

G-tubes are made of silicone, polyurethane, or, rarely, latex rubber to provide the flexibility and durability needed for long-term feeding. They serve as a direct pathway to the gut. G-tubes are made up of one to three ports on the most proximal end, followed by a tube or shaft that carries nutrition to the gastrointestinal (GI) tract, and then a balloon or nonballoon retention device on the distal end (Figure 1.1). In some tubes, there are separate feeding and medication ports. Only in balloon G-tubes is there a port that is used to expand the retention balloon. In addition, standard G-tubes have an external retention device with air vents and feet that hold it 1–2 mm above the skin surface to prevent skin breakdown and keep the stoma site clean and dry.

There are advantages and disadvantages to balloon and nonballoon G-tubes. The benefit of balloon G-tubes is that they can be replaced at home; however, they are not as well tolerated as nonballoon retention devices because of the size of the balloon. Furthermore, balloon retention devices need to be changed more frequently than nonballoon G-tubes (every three months compared to every six months, respectively). The main disadvantage of nonballoon G-tubes is that every tube change has to be done by a medical professional.

Standard G-Tube

Standard G-tubes are adjustable length tubes that have an external bolster, which sits on the skin and can be moved up and down to adequately secure the tube in a patient of any size (Figure 1.1 a and b). These are particularly helpful in patients with increased soft tissue or in patients with a projected weight gain where a low-profile tube with a fixed shaft length may not fit properly. Standard G-tubes can be placed surgically or endoscopically.

Standard G-tubes are placed surgically using the Stamm procedure or via a laparoscopic approach. You will know your patient had the Stamm procedure if he or she has a 6–8 cm midline incision on examination. During the procedure, the surgeon dissects down to the anterior wall of the stomach. The G-tube is placed directly into the stomach via an anterior

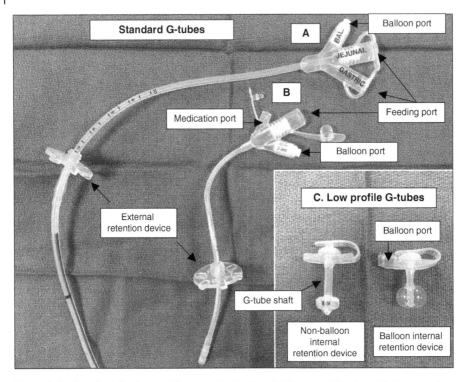

Figure 1.1 Standard G-tubes and low-profile G-tubes. (a) Standard GJ tube with three ports: balloon port, jejunal port, and gastric port. (b) Standard G-tube with three ports: medication port, gastric port, and balloon port. (c) Low-profile tubes with both nonballoon and balloon retention devices.

incision. The balloon is inflated and used to pull the stomach against the inner abdominal wall to determine the best location for the percutaneous exit of the tubing. Once this incision is made, the tubing is pulled through the abdominal wall and the tube is anchored in place with sutures. A standard G-tube placed surgically will have a well-healed tract within four weeks.

Standard G-tubes are placed endoscopically by using the percutaneous endoscopic gastrostomy(PEG) technique. Of note, the term "PEG" is used inaccurately in medical vernacular to refer to all kinds of G-tubes, but a PEG is actually the procedure and not a type of tube. During a PEG procedure, an endoscope is used to transilluminate the stomach and identify the stoma site. A needle is then inserted through the skin into the stomach with a guidewire that is pulled up through the esophagus and out of the mouth. This guidewire is then used to guide the G-tube into the stomach. A small incision is made, and the G-tube is pulled through the stomach and abdominal walls and secured in place by the internal and external bolsters alone.

There are two main advantages to a surgically placed G-tube compared to a PEG procedure. First, a mature tract forms in 4 weeks with a laparoscopic procedure compared to 6–12 weeks with a PEG procedure. Second, a surgically placed G-tube provides direct visualization of the anatomy, whereas, with an endoscopically placed G-tube, there is always the risk of a bowel perforation if a portion of bowel is caught between the abdominal wall and the gastric wall during G-tube placement.

Low-Profile G-Tube

Low-profile G-tubes have a port that sits flush with the skin surface (Figure 1.1c). They are more easily hidden than the standard G-tubes simply by the nature of their size, and patients tend to prefer them for this reason. In addition, the smooth surface of a G-tube port site without tubing is less prone to accidental dislodgement compared to standard G-tubes. However, there are drawbacks to a low-profile tube. First, external tubing has to be attached in order to deliver a feed, which creates one additional step and an additional piece of equipment that can malfunction. Second, low-profile tubes cannot be adjusted to accommodate increased abdominal wall thickness and must be replaced with a tube that has a longer shaft length when there are signs of abdominal wall compression.

Although they were not designed to be placed primarily, low-profile G-tubes can be placed laparoscopically. In pediatric surgical practice, the laparoscopic primary G-button gastrostomy is now widely performed. In this approach, one trocar is placed through the umbilicus and another through a small incision in the left upper quadrant. A stitch is placed in the anterior wall of the stomach and passed through the trocar in the left upper quadrant. Once the suture material is outside the abdomen, the trocar is removed and the anterior wall is pulled through the initial trocar site. The stomach and abdominal walls are sutured together. The gastrostomy is made in the portion of stomach wall that is exposed. The appropriate button is then placed in the gastrostomy and sutured in place. Similar to a surgically placed standard G-tube, a low-profile G-tube tract matures in four weeks.

Jejunal Tubes

NJ, gastro-jejunal (GJ), and J-tubes are ideal for patients with gastric dysmotility, severe gastroesophageal reflux, recurrent emesis, and those at risk for pulmonary aspiration. The jejunum is fed continuously and at a lower rate compared to bolus feeds given through a G-tube. Whereas the NJ and J-tubes provide direct access to the jejunum, GJ tubes are a hybrid with both gastric and jejunal ports. The gastric port is used for medications or venting the stomach, while the jejunal port is used for continuous enteral nutrition. J-tubes are secured to the abdominal wall with an internal retention device in the jejunum, while GJ tubes have an internal retention device within the gastric cavity and a jejunal extension that passes through the G-tube and bypasses the stomach. Jejunal extensions carry the added risk of tube migration, volvulus around the extension tubing, and higher rates of tube clogging secondary to smaller tube size. Percutaneous J-tubes are rarely used because of the thinness of the jejunal wall and increased risk of complications.

NJ and GJ tube placement requires fluoroscopic or endoscopic guidance for placement. Percutaneous J-tubes are placed surgically.

Indications

Enteral feeding devices are indicated when a patient has a functional GI tract but cannot safely or adequately feed by mouth. This includes patients with a swallowing dysfunction or neurologic disorder. Similarly, patients on a ventilator or those with severe reflux require enteral feeding to prevent aspiration. Finally, patients with inadequate nutrition or in a hypermetabolic state (i.e. cardiac disease, renal disease, or pulmonary disease) may not be able to meet their nutritional demands with oral feeding alone and require enteral feeding as supplementation. The indication for enteral nutrition and duration of feeding needed determine the type of tube recommended. Contraindications specific to each feeding device are listed in Table 1.2.

Management

Routine Care

Enteral feeding devices require daily care to ensure the tube is patent and to protect the surrounding skin from irritation. All feeding devices need to be flushed with room temperature water following each feed or medication administration to prevent clogging. The tubes should also be monitored for tube deterioration that indicates the tube needs to be changed: discoloration, foul smell, and tube deformity. NG and OG tubes need to be monitored for pressure necrosis at the point of insertion and retaped as needed. Similarly, G-tubes and GJ tubes can cause pressure ulcers if the tissue between the internal and external retention devices is compressed too tightly. Standard G-tubes should be turned regularly and evaluated to ensure the external retention device sits 1–2 mm above the skin surface without creating a dimple in the skin. Finally, internal balloon retention devices should be checked regularly to confirm the appropriate amount of fluid is in the balloon to prevent tube dislodgement.

Routine Replacement

Temporary Tubes

NG and OG tubes can be placed and replaced by home nursing or properly trained family members (Table 1.3). NG/OG tubes should be replaced approximately every 7–10 days.

Table 1.2 Enteric feeding device contraindications.

NG/OG feeding tubes	G-tubes	J-tubes
• Maxillofacial disorders • Esophageal or oropharyngeal tumors or trauma • Laryngectomy • Confirmed skull or cervical spine injury above C4 • Clotting dysfunction • Ingestion of corrosive substance	• Severe gastroesophageal reflux • Gastric dysmotility • Gastric outlet obstruction	• Ascites • Crohn's disease • Immunosuppression

Discuss with appropriate consulting service prior to NG/OG placement

Table 1.3 NG tube insertion.

Supplies

- Nasogastric tube
- Sterile water
- 50 mL catheter tip syringe
- Tape to secure tubing

Stepwise procedure

1) Position patient sitting upright with neck midline; avoid hyperextension.
2) Lubricate the NG tip with sterile water. Avoid jelly as it will affect the pH.
3) Direct the tube into one of the nostrils and, keeping the tube horizontal, aim the tube directly posterior. Ask the patient to swallow, as this will help guide the tube into the esophagus by closing the epiglottis.
4) Once the tube passes through the nasopharynx, have the patient lean forward and bend his/her chin while continuing to swallow which will further push the tube down the esophagus.
5) Continue to pass the tube until you reach the predetermined tube depth.
6) Stop and remove the tube if the patient has any signs of respiratory distress.
7) Attach a 50 ml syringe and aspirate contents to the tube.
8) Test aspirate on pH paper, any value below 4.0 is considered gastric contents.
9) Secure the tube by taping to the nose and face.

Properly sizing the tubing is necessary prior to placement. When choosing a tube size, most feedings can be given with a 6 or 8 Fr tube in pediatric patients and a 12–14 Fr tube in adult patients. Appropriate tube insertion depth is classically measured by taking the feeding tube and measuring from the tip of the nose to the ear lobe and finally to the xyphoid. Several pediatric studies have found that this measurement may underestimate tube depth and result in tubes that terminate in the distal esophagus and pose an aspiration risk. Therefore, in pediatric patients, a better measurement is either using published age-related height-based measurements or by measuring from the tip of the nose to the ear lobe and then to the midpoint between the xyphoid and umbilicus. For OG tubes, the measurement should start at the mouth. Once the appropriate tube size and depth of insertion are determined, the same steps may be followed for either NG or OG tube placement, substituting the nasal passages for the oropharynx in the place of OG placement (Table 1.3). Finally, NG/OG tube placement is an uncomfortable procedure, and patients should be treated with topical lidocaine either as 4% lidocaine spray, 2% lidocaine jelly, or nebulized 4% lidocaine prior to the procedure.

NG/OG tube placement can be verified by the aspiration of gastric contents with a pH < 4.0. However, be aware that medications can change the gastric pH, and in a patient with reflux, an esophageal aspirate may have the same pH as a gastric aspirate. Likewise, the aspiration of "gastric fluid" does not confirm gastric placement alone because there is fluid within the bronchial tree and distal esophagus that resembles gastric fluid. In addition, lack of fluid aspirate can lead to falsely believing the tube is not in the stomach when the tube collapses or is above the fluid level. Finally, auscultation is an unreliable method of determining NG/OG tube placement because the sound of an NG tube in the thorax may transmit to the upper abdomen. **X-ray confirmation remains the gold standard for NG/OG tube placement in both adult and pediatric patients.**

Bedside placement of ND and NJ feeding tubes is still controversial; however, there are increasingly more studies supporting this practice. Most research has focused on the placement of ND tubes. ND tube placement is similar to NG tube placement; however, the patient is kept in the right-lateral decubitus position. Several adjunctive measures have been described including the use of promotility agents and gas insufflation to promote tube position past the pylorus. Of note, these techniques are better described in the adult patients and less so in pediatric patients. All post-pyloric feeding tubes should be confirmed with an X-ray prior to use.

G-tubes and GJ tubes

G-tubes may be replaced by a caregiver following the first tube change and at least four weeks from initial tube placement (Table 1.4). Typically, a gastrostomy tube is changed every three to four months. G-tube replacement should be confirmed with the aspiration of gastric contents and/or pH testing. The gold standard for G-tube confirmation is a fluoroscopic dye study whereby dye is injected through the G-tube port and a radiograph is taken to verify dye positioning in the stomach. If there is any trauma to the G-tube site or if the tube is considered an immature tube (<4 weeks from placement), aspiration of gastric

Table 1.4 Gastrostomy-tube replacement.

Supplies

- G-tube low profile button with extension tubing

  Or

- Traditional G-tube
- Luer slip tip syringe to inflate balloon
- Larger catheter tip syringe to prime and flush tubing

  Optional:

- G-tube port stylet

Stepwise procedure

1) Deflate the G-tube gastric balloon with a 10 ml syringe.
2) Gently remove the G-tube by holding the port site and steadily pulling it back.
3) Keep stoma patent with a Foley catheter (do not exceed the G-tube size).
4) Remove the G-tube from packaging and check balloon by filling it with tap water (do not fill with normal saline as this will degrade balloon and do not use air as it will not provide adequate tension on the balloon).
5) Deflate balloon prior to tube insertion.
6) Insert the G-tube stylet, if one is provided.
7) Lubricate the tube with sterile jelly (do not use petroleum jelly as it will degrade tubing).
8) Direct the G-tube into the stoma and apply steady pressure.
9) Stop and reposition if you meet resistance.
10) Once the G-tube external base is resting on the skin surface, inflate the balloon.
11) Confirm positioning by pulling gently on the port site.

contents and pH testing are inadequate, and the tube site should be verified with a fluoro-scopic dye study.

GJ tube must be placed by interventional radiology under fluoroscopy to ensure proper placement for both the initial placement and any subsequent tube replacement. GJ tubes are replaced every six months.

Complications/Emergencies

Tube Dislodgment

Tube dislodgment is a common emergency department chief complaint in both adults and children. This can occur because of coughing, gagging, pulling on the tubing, or getting the tubing caught around an object. In all cases, stop the feeding and inquire how long the patient can maintain his or her blood sugar without feeding. Hypoglycemia is a common complication for patients who are accustomed to receiving continuous feeds, and an infusion of dextrose-containing IV fluids is commonly needed while awaiting feeding tube replacement. Replacement follows an algorithm based on the type of enteric feeding device and the duration since its initial placement (Figure 1.2). Unfortunately, tube replacement is not without risk, and the astute provider must be aware of clinical signs of an improperly positioned tube and how to best verify tube placement.

NG tube replacement is a simple procedure, and some patients may even replace their own NG tubes nightly; however, it is not without risk. Complication rates range from 1 to 2% in adults and up to 20–40% in pediatric patients, with higher rates seen in neonatal patients. Complications with improper NG tube placement include pneumonia if the tube is placed in the lungs and peritonitis if the tube perforates the bowel. Given this high complication rate, all NG tube replacements in the emergency department setting should be confirmed with a radiograph. Auscultation, enzyme testing, and pH testing are unreliable.

G-tube placement is an equally common emergency department procedure, and complication rates range from 0.6 to 20%, with higher rates seen in immature tubes and tubes with traumatic dislodgement. The definition of an immature tube is debated in the literature. Most studies define immature tubes as those less than four to six weeks from placement; however, some studies define immature tubes as those less than six months from placement. There is an inverse relationship between the age of the tube, and, therefore, G-tube tract healing, and the complication rate. In addition, patients who are symptomatic postreplacement are more likely to have a G-tube complication. Complications include gastric outlet obstruction and intraperitoneal tube placement.

All G-tube replacements can be completed at the bedside; however, the person performing the procedure and the method of checking placement are dependent on the age of the tube and the patient's presenting symptoms. The first tube change postoperatively is the most critical and should be completed by the subspecialty service responsible for the tube's placement. In addition, any stoma site with significant trauma or stoma that is difficult to identify should be evaluated by general surgery. Uncomplicated mature G-tubes can be replaced at the bedside by the emergency department team, and placement should be confirmed with gastric aspirate and pH testing alone. For patients with immature tracts,

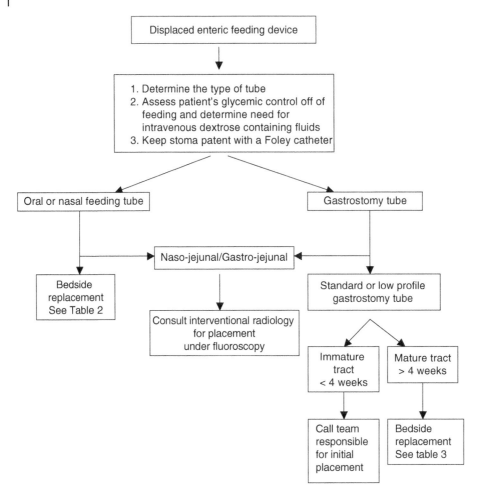

Figure 1.2 Algorithm of the displaced enteric feeding device.

trauma to the stoma site, or symptoms following G-tube replacement, contrast-enhanced radiograph is needed to confirm G-tube placement prior to use. Extravasation of contrast dye on imaging and failure to fill the stomach indicates that the tube is improperly positioned.

All transgastric jejunal tubes must be replaced by interventional radiology under fluoroscopic guidance.

Peristomal Skin Irritation

Patients can present with G-tube erythema for a variety of reasons. While the presence of skin irritation can be highly distressing to patients and caregivers, the cause is commonly nonurgent. However, it is vital that providers have a healthy differential in order to distinguish severe causes of peristomal irritation from those that are less severe.

Peristomal Leakage

Peristomal leakage of gastric contents is seen with most G-tubes. Diabetes, malnutrition, and poor wound healing can increase the likelihood and amount of leakage secondary to poor approximation of skin tissue around the tubing. In addition, a tightly secured retention device, noted by dimpling of the skin, can cause an inflammatory reaction and lead to increased leakage of gastric contents.

Skin irritation from peristomal leakage can be distinguished from infection by the color, which is a faint pink instead of the deep red color of cellulitis (Figure 1.3a). Likewise, the skin is not tender. Finally, crusting around the tube site, that is, dried formula and gastric juices, should easily wipe away.

Treatment options for peristomal leakage include skin barrier creams such as zinc oxide and antacid treatment to decrease the acidity of the gastric contents. If the stoma appears too large for the tubing, do not increase the size of the tube. A larger stoma site is not because the patient grew or gained weight. The stoma size increases secondary to repetitive trauma from the tube moving within the stoma. Increasing the tube size will only stretch the stoma further and lead to greater leakage of gastric contents. **Do not make this common mistake.** Instead, remove the tube and allow the stoma to shrink in size over the next several hours. A stoma can close within as little as 24 hours, so a smaller catheter should be left in place to maintain patency of the stoma. Once the stoma has decreased to the appropriate size, place the original sized G-tube into the site.

Stomal Cellulitis

Stomal cellulitis is distinguished from skin irritation by the deeper red color and spreading erythema around a G-tube site with significant pain to touch (Figure 1.3b). Patients with poor wound healing and an immunocompromised state are at increased risk for cellulitis. Pathogens are typically skin flora including beta-hemolytic streptococci and *Staphylococcus aureus*.

(a) (b) (c)

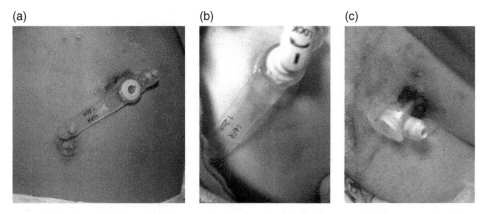

Figure 1.3 (a) Peristomal leakage notable for dried crusted skin without surrounding erythema. (b) Peristomal cellulitis distinguished from simple leakage by the deeper erythematous skin extending from the G-tube site. (c) Peristomal candidiasis distinguished from cellulitis by its satellite lesions.

In a well-appearing child with otherwise no systemic symptoms, a first-generation cephalosporin is adequate to treat streptococcal infection. If a patient is a known methicillin-resistant *S. aureus* carrier or appears ill, coverage should include agents that treat methicillin-resistant *Staphylococcus aureus* (MRSA) based on local antibiograms. The tube does not need to be removed in the setting of stomal cellulitis. If there is fluctuance around the tube, an ultrasound should be obtained to evaluate for a peristomal abscess. Peristomal abscesses will require bedside incision and drainage and broad-spectrum antibiotic coverage.

Stomal Candidiasis

Stomal candidiasis is much less common than bacterial infections of the stoma. Patients with candidiasis should be well appearing and have typical satellite lesions around the stomal site (Figure 1.3c). Similar to other forms of candidiasis, treatment with topical antifungal agents alone (nystatin or clotrimazole) is sufficient.

Necrotizing Fasciitis

Necrotizing fasciitis of the stoma is an exceedingly rare but life-threatening complication. The patient will have erythematous, edematous, and tender skin with bullae. The lesion will rapidly expand, and the patient will look toxic. Similar to all infections, those patients with poor wound healing, diabetes, and malnutrition are at greatest risk. Necrotizing fasciitis is a surgical emergency that requires immediate surgical evaluation, wound debridement, and intravenous antibiotic treatment.

Stomal Bleeding

Bleeding at the stomal site is one of three things: hypergranulation tissue, mucosal irritation with or without prolapse, and upper GI bleeding. Distinguishing between the three is important because, while, to the patient they may all be an emergency, the severity and treatment are dramatically different.

A granuloma is a well-circumscribed, pearly piece of tissue adherent to the stoma (Figure 1.4a). It presents as chronic, low-grade bleeding. Its cause is unknown, but it is thought to arise from repetitive trauma from the G-tube rubbing against the stoma. Hypergranulation tissue is of low risk but causes significant distress among patients and caregivers. Treatment is largely topical, including 0.1% triamcinolone cream, commercially available granuloma-reducing agents, and salt packing. These agents are not without risk; specifically, triamcinolone can cause skin thinning, systemic absorption, and may precipitate a fungal infection. Silver nitrate application, kenalog injections, electrocautery, and G-tube site revision are used in more persistent cases.

Another cause of chronic mild stomal bleeding is mucosal irritation. This too is caused by repetitive movement of the tube within the stoma and can be quickly resolved with properly sizing the tube. In addition, gauze and tape can be used to better secure the tube in position.

Finally, acute stomal bleeding is either prolapsed stomal tissue or upper GI bleeding. Prolapsed gastric tissue has a deeper red color compared to the color of a granuloma, and it is acute not chronic (Figure 1.4b). This distinction is important because silver nitrate would injure the gastric mucosa and should not be used in the setting of gastric tissue

(a) (b)

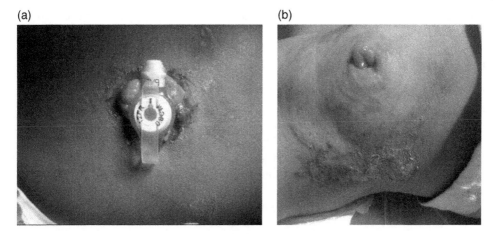

Figure 1.4 (a) Granuloma notable for its pearly color and irregular shape. (b) Prolapse distinguished from granuloma by the deeper erythema and more uniform shape.

prolapse. Prolapse can be treated with the application of salt or sugar to shrink the gastric tissue and then firm and steady pressure to direct the tissue back into the stomal site. If this is unsuccessful, general surgery should be consulted. Significant stomal site bleeding without prolapsed tissue, skin irritation, or granuloma development is upper GI bleeding, until proven otherwise, and should be evaluated by endoscopy.

Clogged Tubing

A clogged feeding tube is one of the most common causes for enteric feeding device malfunction. Residue from medications and formula build up over time and ultimately can lead to complete occlusion of the tube lumen. Resins and bulking agents are contraindicated through any enteric feeding device as they both can lead to obstruction of the tubing. Likewise, all medications and formula administrations should be followed by a 20 ml flush to prevent blockage.

The management of a clogged feeding tube depends on the type of tubing. An NG or OG tube should simply be replaced. Likewise, a G-tube in a well-healed tract with no trauma should also be replaced if simple declogging measures do not remove the obstruction. Every effort should be made to release the obstruction for GJ and NJ tubes, as the placement of both of these requires fluoroscopic guidance.

Most feeding tube obstructions can be flushed with a 60 ml syringe. First, try pumping air into the tubing to break apart the clot. If that does not work, the best irrigant is warm water. Carbonated beverages and colas have been studied and are inferior. Finally, if warm water does not remove the obstruction, then a mixture of pancreatic enzymes dissolved in a bicarbonate solution can be used. The mixture is left in the feeding tubing for two to three minutes, and then flushed through with warm water. One option is to mix a pancrelipase tablet with 650 mg of bicarbonate in 10 ml of water. If neither of these treatments is successful, a contrast-enhanced radiograph should be ordered to confirm tube placement, and alternative diagnoses such as buried bumper or G-tube displacement should be considered.

Ulceration

Ulcerations from enteric feeding devices can be at the proximal and distal ends of the tubing. For both NG and G-tubes, the pressure of the device against the nasal ala and abdominal wall, respectively, can lead to local superficial bleeding. Bleeding that comes directly from a tube aspirate is more indicative of GI tract bleeding. In the case of an NG tube, the tubing can irritate the lining of the esophagus and develop into esophageal ulceration. For a G-tube, the pressure of the internal retention device against the stomach lining can form an ulcer. Superficial ulcerations can be treated with tube repositioning, but internal ulcerations require tube removal to allow for healing.

Peritonitis

Peritonitis in a patient with an enteric feeding device is caused by an improperly placed tube, until proven otherwise. In the case of NG tube placement, the tube perforates the bowel wall; and in the case of G-tube placement, the tube can be improperly placed in the peritoneum. Patients may initially be asymptomatic but will progress to diffuse abdominal tenderness, rebound, and sepsis. All NG tubes should have radiographic confirmation of their placement. For G-tubes, patients with immature tracts, trauma to the tract, or any difficulty placing the G-tube should have a contrast-enhanced radiograph to confirm tube placement. Some argue that if a patient is observed receiving a feeding without difficulty, the tube is likely properly positioned. However, patients with multiple comorbidities may not be able to show discomfort. One must have a heightened level of suspicion and err on the side of caution when confirming NG and G-tube replacements because while complications are rare, they can be life-threatening.

Gastric Outlet Obstruction

Gastric outlet obstruction is a significant complication, but the insightful physician will be able to identify the problem and treat it within moments. Obstruction is caused by the retention balloon blocking the pylorus either because the tube migrated to the pylorus in the case of a standard G-tube or because the balloon is overfilled in the case of a low-profile button. Patients will present with abdominal pain, nausea, feeding intolerance, and nonbilious emesis. A contrast-enhanced radiographic study that shows dye filling the small intestine but sparing the stomach confirms the diagnosis (Figure 1.5). Treatment is relatively anticlimactic and includes deflating the internal balloon, repositioning it away from the pylorus and reinflating it or simply reducing the amount of fluid in the retention balloon itself.

Buried Bumper Syndrome

Buried bumper syndrome (BBS) is a rare but life-threatening complication of children with G-tubes. BBS is defined as the presence of an embedded internal fixation device into the gastric mucosa of the abdominal wall. This is typically caused by securing the external retention device too tightly to the skin surface and thus narrowing the space between the internal and

Figure 1.5 Radiograph of a G-tube dye study shows dye within the small intestine only. This image is consistent with a gastric outlet obstruction whereby the balloon is located in the pylorus blocking dye from filling the stomach.

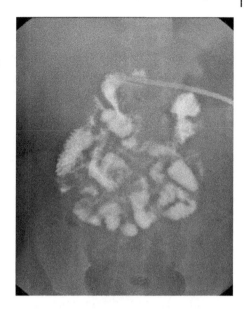

external retention devices and pressing the internal device into the gastric mucosa. Rates of BBS in adults average 1% but can be as high as 5% in pediatric patients. This is seen with both internal balloons and rigid retention devices, but it is more common with the latter. Risk factors for BBS include pediatric age, jejunal extension from the G-tube, multiple G-tube placements, and improper home care. Pediatric patients are at a higher risk because of their expected weight gain and compression against the external bolster. Those with GJ tubes are at higher risk because the weight of jejunal extensions is thought to pull the internal bolsters out of their perpendicular placement and cause unequal pressure on the stomach wall. Finally, repeat G-tube replacements can increase the inflammatory reaction in the stomach wall and thus encourage tissue growth around the internal retention device.

Patients can be asymptomatic and simply present with inability to feed through the tube. The classic triad for BBS is inability to insert the G-tube further into the stomach, loss of tube patency (unable to feed or draw back from tubing), and leakage around the tube site. BBS can be complicated by GI bleeding, perforation, and peritonitis, which can be fatal.

BBS is diagnosed by endoscopy. However, abdominal ultrasound and computerized tomography (CT) scan can help identify bumper location if it is not apparent on endoscopy. Depending on the extent of the internal bumper's migration through the gastric mucosa, the bumper may be removed either endoscopically or surgically. Bumpers that have passed through the lamina muscularis propria and are located between the stomach and abdominal wall will need surgical removal.

Intussusception

Intussusception is a well-described complication of patients with jejunal feeding devices (NJ, GJ, and J-tubes). Intussusception is defined as one part of the small intestine invaginating or folding into the adjacent portion of small bowel. Complications arise from the pressure placed on the outer layer of small bowel tissue as the inner layer presses against it, thereby decreasing blood flow to the tissue. The pathogenesis of intussusception requires a lead point to pull one section of small bowel into the other. Contrary to classic intussusception where the lead point is either gastric lymphatic tissue or cancerous material, in patients with an enteric feeding device, the extension tubing in the jejunum serves as the lead point.

Patients with intussusception typically present with abdominal pain, bilious emesis, and/or hematemesis. Because of the many comorbidities of patients with enteric feeding devices, the patient may appear asymptomatic. One must have a heightened clinical suspicion. Diagnosis is made by contrast-enhanced radiography, ultrasound, endoscopy, upper GI, or abdominal CT scan. Tube-related intussusceptions resolve with tube removal.

Colocutaneous Fistula

Colocutaenous fistula formation is a complication only seen with the percutaneous approaches to gastrostomy. A colocuteneous fistula is caused by trapping a loop of bowel between the abdominal wall and the stomach wall and piercing the G-tube through all three tissue layers. While, in some cases, patients present with colonic obstruction, this complication may not be detected until the first tube change at which point the tube is replaced into the colonic wall but does not make it to the stomach wall. The feeds are started directly into the colon, and the patient develops diarrhea and dehydration. Treatment includes removing the G-tube and surgical closure of the fistula.

Consultation

Surgical consultation is needed for surgical emergencies: intussusception, BBS, colocutaneous fistula, peritonitis, and necrotizing fasciitis. Immature tube dislodgement will require replacement by the team responsible for its initial placement, but the emergency department team can initially manage all mature tracts. Consultation is needed if there is significant trauma to the tract, the tube is improperly positioned on dye study, or the patient is unable to tolerate feeds following tube replacement. GJ and J-tube replacements will typically need interventional radiology consultation. Stomal site bleeding, leakage, or infection may be initially managed by the emergency department and seen in subspecialty clinic for further care. Similarly, gastric outlet obstruction can first be treated with tube repositioning by the emergency department team, but if the obstruction does not resolve, surgical consultation is needed.

Further Reading

1 Pearce, C.B. and Duncan, H.D. (2002). Enteral feeding: nasogastric, nasojejunal, percutaneous endoscopic gastrostomy, or jejunostomy: its indications and limitations. *Postgrad. Med. J.* 78: 198–204.

2 Prabhakaran, S., Doraiswamy, V.A., Nagaraja, V. et al. (2012). Nasoenteric tube complications. *Scand. J. Surg.* 101: 147–155.

3 Taheri, M.R., Singh, H., and Duerken, D.R. (2011). Peritonitis after gastrostomy tube replacement: a case series and review of literature. *J. Parenter. Enteral Nutr.* 35: 56–60.

4 Ibegbu, E., Relan, M., and Vega, K.J. (2007). Retrograde jejunoduodenogastric intussusception due to a replacement percutaneous gastrostomy tube presenting as upper gastrointestinal bleeding. *World J. Gastroenterol.* 13: 5285–5284.

5 Jamil, Y., Idris, M., Kashif, N. et al. (2012). Jejunoduodenogastric intussusception secondary to percutaneous gastrostomy tube in an adult patient. *Jpn. J. Radiol.* 30: 277–280.

6 Cyrany, J., Rejchrt, S., Kopacova, M., and Bures, J. (2016). Buried bumper syndrome: a complication of percutaneous endoscopic gastrostomy. *World J. Gastroenterol.* 22: 618–627.

7 Stewart, C.E., Mutalib, M., Pradhan, A. et al. (2016). Buried bumper syndrome in children: incidence and risk factors. *Eur. J. Gastroenterol. Hepatol.* 29: 181–184.

8 Goldin, A.B., Heiss, K.F., Hall, M. et al. (2016). Emergency department visits and readmissions among children after gastrostomy tube placement. *J. Pediatr.* 174: 139–145.

9 Powers, J., Chance, R., Bortenschalger, L. et al. (2003). Bedside placement of small-bowel feeding tubes in the intensive care unit. *Crit. Care Nurse* 23: 16–24.

10 Tiancha, H., Jiyong, J., and Min, Y. (2015). How to promote bedside placement of postpyloric feeding tube: a network meta-analysis of randomized controlled trials. *J. Parenter. Enteral Nutr.* 39: 521–530.

11 Gallagher, E.J. (2004). Nasogastric tubes: hard to swallow. *Ann. Emerg. Med.* 44: 138–141.

12 Cirgin Ellett, M.L.C., Cohen, M.D., Perkins, S.M. et al. (2012). Comparing methods of determining insertion length for placing gastric tubes in children 1 month to 17 years of age. *J. Spec. Pediatr. Nurs.* 17: 19–32.

13 Stepter, C.R. (2012). Maintaining placement of temporary enteral feeding tubes in adults: a critical appraisal of the evidence. *Medsurg Nurs.* 21: 61–69.

14 Irving, S.Y., Lyman, B., Northington, L. et al. (2014). Nasogastric tube placement and verification in children: review of the current literature. *Crit. Care Nurse* 34: 67–78.

15 Cirgin Ellett, M.L.C., Cohen, M.D., Croffie, J.M.B. et al. (2014). Comparing bedside methods of determining placement of gastric tubes in children. *J. Spec. Pediatr. Nurs.* 19: 68–79.

16 Otjen, J.P., Iyer, R.S., Phillips, G.S., and Parisi, M.T. (2012). Usual and unusual causes of pediatric gastric outlet obstruction. *Pediatr. Radiol.* 42: 728–737.

17 Campwala, I., Perrone, E., Yanni, G. et al. (2015). Complications of gastrojejunal feeding tubes in children. *J. Surg. Res.* 199: 67–71.

18 Zamora, I.J., Fallon, S.C., Orth, R.C. et al. (2014). Overuse of fluoroscopic gastrostomy studies in a children's hospital. *J. Surg. Res.* 190: 598–603.

19 Guana, R., LOnati, L., Barletti, C. et al. (2014). Gastrostomy intraperitoneal bumper: migration in a three-year-old child: a rare complication following gastrostomy tube replacement. *Case Rep. Gastroenterol.* 8: 381–386.

20 Saavedra, H., Losek, J.D., Shanley, L., and Titus, M.O. (2009). Gastrostomy tube related complaints in the pediatric emergency department: identifying opportunities for improvement. *Pediatr. Emerg. Care* 25: 728–732.

21 Jacobson, G., Brokish, P.A., and Wrenn, K. (2009). Percutaneous feeding tube replacement in the ED-are confirmatory x-rays necessary? *Am. J. Emerg. Med.* 27: 519–524.

22 Showalter, C.D., Kerrey, B., Spellman-Kennebeck, S., and Timm, N. (2012). Gastrostomy tube replacement in a pediatric ED: frequency of complications and impact of confirmatory imaging. *Am. J. Emerg. Med.* 30: 1501–1506.

23 Wu, T.H., Lin, C.W., and Yin, W.Y. (2006). Jejunojejunal intussusception following jejunostomy. *J. Formos. Med. Assoc.* 105: 355–358.

24 Hughes, U.M., Connolly, B.L., Chair, P.G., and Muraca, S. (2000). Further report of small-bowel intussusceptions related to gastrojejunostomy tubes. *Pediatr. Radiol.* 30: 614–617.

2

Gastrointestinal Diversions

Colostomies, Ileostomies, Mucous Fistulas, and Spit Fistulas

Ellen G. Szydlowski[1,2] and Peter Mattei[1,3]

[1] *Perelman School of Medicine at the University of Pennsylvania, Philadelphia, PA, USA*
[2] *Division of Emergency Medicine, Department of Pediatrics, Children's Hospital of Philadelphia, Philadelphia, PA, USA*
[3] *Division of General, Thoracic and Fetal Surgery, Children's Hospital of Philadelphia, Philadelphia, PA, USA*

Introduction

Patients may require a gastrointestinal (GI) diversion for several reasons, including congenital causes and acquired lesions. The most common type of GI diversion is the ostomy where a purposeful anastomosis is created between a segment of the GI tract and the external skin. An ostomy can be established almost anywhere along the GI tract, including the large intestine (colostomy), distal small intestine (ileostomy), and the esophagus (esophagostomy or spit fistula). These GI diversions may be temporary or permanent, and the emergency department (ED) physician should be comfortable with the evaluation and management of the different types of ostomies and their potential complications.

Equipment/Device

The type of ostomy is classified according to the segment of the GI tract utilized to create the ostomy and the method of surgical construction. Depending on the manner of the disease or the site of the obstruction, the surgeon will determine the optimal location to establish the ostomy.

An ileostomy is created when it is necessary to bypass the entire colon and rectum. In general, patients with ileostomies have watery frequent stooling patterns since they do not possess large bowel function. It is usually created within the rectus sheath, in the infraumbilical fat pad, and can be temporary or permanent. In a diverting loop ileostomy, a loop of terminal ileum is brought out through the abdominal wall, opened, and sutured to the dermis. This is the most common type of temporary diversion ostomy and is used in patients who are considered high risk for anastomotic breakdown. A mucous fistula, which will be described in more detail in the next paragraph, can also be created within the

Emergency Management of the Hi-Tech Patient in Acute and Critical Care, First Edition. Edited by Ioannis Koutroulis, Nicholas Tsarouhas, Richard J. Lin, Jill C. Posner, Michael Seneff, and Robert Shesser.
© 2021 John Wiley & Sons Ltd. Published 2021 by John Wiley & Sons Ltd.

construct of a loop ileostomy. An end-ileostomy is an ostomy in which the ileum is delivered through the interior abdominal wall and sutured in place with everting sutures to create an end stoma.

A colostomy is created when it is necessary to bypass or remove the distal colon, rectum, or anus. As with other ostomies, they can be temporary or permanent and can be created in the loop or end fashion. In general, loop ostomies are easier to reverse and are more frequently used when a temporary ostomy is required. Patients with colostomies usually have semi-formed stools because the absorptive and storage function of the large bowel is preserved. A mucous fistula is sometimes created during an end-colostomy. Usually, the distal end of the colon is oversewn or stapled and left in the abdominal cavity as a nonfunctional stump. However, in cases where there is a high likelihood of breakdown of the stump, which can then lead to abdominal sepsis, or if the anus is strictured to a degree that does not allow rectal mucous to drain freely, it can be secured in place adjacent to colostomy as a mucous fistula in the subcutaneous tissue but not matured out to the skin. The mucous fistula does not pass stool but does allow passage of mucous or gas from the nonfunctioning portion of the distal colon or rectum.

The spit fistula is rarely used anymore, but may be created in the setting of an esophagectomy where part of the esophagus is excised, such as in esophageal cancer, swallowing disorders, and trauma. If an anastomotic leak occurs, an ostomy can be created that will allow drainage to be diverted outside the body to the lower neck or clavicle region.

Indications

GI diversions may be necessary for a variety of reasons, both congenital and acquired. Common congenital anomalies requiring ostomy placement include Hirschsprung's disease and imperforate anus. Acquired lesions may include ulcerative colitis, Crohn's disease, necrotizing enterocolitis, obstruction, decompression, trauma, and malignancy. An ostomy may be temporary or permanent depending on the likelihood that a restorative procedure will be possible. Most temporary ostomies are reversed within three to six months of placement.

Management

Stomatherapists are an excellent resource for families and physicians when managing ostomies. However, patients will still present to the ED with ostomy-related complications, and all ED physicians should be familiar with the types of GI diversions and their complications.

Pouches are used to collect the ostomy effluent, contain odor, and protect the peristomal skin. There are one- and two-piece pouch systems available, and they come in both reusable and disposable varieties. Patients typically empty the pouch when it is one-third full and change pouches 1–2 times a week.

Diet is also important in the routine management of ostomies. Patients may prefer to modify their diet to avoid gas-producing foods and must be cognizant of the amount of fluid they must intake to compensate for the volume lost through the effluent, which is determined by location of the stoma relative to the ileocecal valve.

Complications/Emergencies

Overall, complication rates following stoma formation have been reported between 21 and 70%. The incidence is the highest in the first five years postoperatively, but the complication risk is lifelong and can be associated with significant morbidity. Early stomal complications occur within three months of placement and include stomal necrosis, bleeding, and retraction. Late stomal complications usually present in permanent ostomies and can include parastomal hernia, prolapse, and stenosis. Cutaneous complications can occur at any time, and ileostomies can also be associated with metabolic derangements due to their large output.

Early Stomal Complications

Stomal necrosis can be seen in up to 14% of cases, most often in the immediate postoperative period. It is usually due to venous congestion or arterial insufficiency. If the necrosis involves only the superficial few millimeters of the stoma, then observation will usually be successful; however, if it extends deep to the fascial planes, then an urgent revision is warranted. The ED physician can determine the extent of necrosis by inserting a lubricated test tube in the stoma and with a flashlight or using a lighted anoscope.

Major bleeding from the stoma is uncommon. Minor bleeding can be from the initial surgery or over from vigorous stomal cleansing. Pressure, handheld cautery, or silver nitrate is usually sufficient to manage minor bleeding episodes. Topical hemostatic agents are sometimes helpful adjuncts. Finally, a well-placed figure-of-eight stitch of monofilament suture on a noncutting needle can stop bleeding from an isolated bleeding vessel on the surface of the stoma, which is insensate.

Stomal retraction is defined as any stoma that is 0.5 cm or more below the skin surface, is noticed within six weeks of stoma formation, and requires surgical intervention. It can occur from excessive tension on the bowel and occurs more often with ileostomies and in obese patients. Stomal retraction can cause leakage, difficulty with pouch adherence, and skin irritation. Supportive care includes using a convex pouching system and belt and binder; however, many require revision.

Late Stomal Complications

Parastomal hernias are more common with colostomies and have a reported incidence of up to 48%. Other risk factors include obesity, poor abdominal muscle tone, chronic cough, and placement of the stoma outside the rectus muscle. Parasternal hernias are usually asymptomatic, but, as the size increases, it can impede adherence of the ostomy pouch. Strangulation and obstruction are rare but serious complications, and it is important for the ED physician to be comfortable determining if a hernia is incarcerated. Any hernia that cannot be manually reduced, is extremely painful, or appears dusky requires urgent

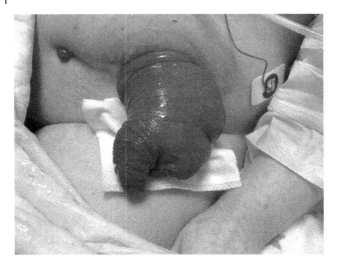

Figure 2.1 Stomal prolapse. (*Source:* Photos courtesy Judith Stellar)

surgical consultation. Symptoms of obstruction, including vomiting, abdominal distention, and decreased ostomy output, require two-view abdominal x-rays. Elective surgical revision is performed for definitive management of parastomal hernias; however, there is a high recurrence rate. Nonoperative management includes abdominal support belts and education regarding avoidance of heavy lifting or other maneuvers that may increase intra-abdominal pressure.

Stomal prolapse occurs when a proximal segment of the bowel intussuscepts and protrudes through the stoma (Figure 2.1). The incidence of prolapse is 7–26% and is more common with loop transverse colostomy and end descending colostomies. The majority of prolapses are not of clinical significance but can be distressing to patients and make appliance placement difficult. Small, uncomplicated prolapses can be manually reduced by the ED physician at the bedside. Sedation may be necessary depending on the size of the prolapse and the discomfort of the patient. Before reduction is attempted, the edema of the prolapse may be reduced by applying cool compresses or osmotic agents such as honey or sugar for approximately 30 minutes. The prolapse is then lubricated with a water-soluble lubricant, and with gloved hands, circumferential pressure is applied on the prolapsed mucosa. Placing a finger in the center of the prolapse may help guide the reversal process. After the prolapse is reduced, an abdominal binder should be placed, and the patient should be instructed to avoid lifting or other activities that increase intra-abdominal pressure and should follow up with their ostomy team as an outpatient. Complicated prolapses, prolapses causing ischemic changes or severe mucosal irritation and bleeding, and those that are unable to be reduced by the ED physician usually require surgery.

Stomal stenosis is a less common complication of ostomies with an incidence of 2–15% and more often seen in patients with Crohn's disease. Symptoms of stomal stenosis include noisy stoma when flatus is passed, reduced output, diarrhea, or cramping abdominal pain followed by explosive output. Severe stenosis may present with obstruction. The ED physician may assess for mild stenosis by digital exam or attempting to pass a catheter.

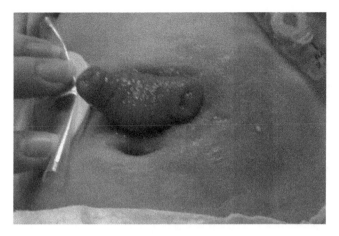

Figure 2.2 Irritant dermatitis. (*Source:* Photo courtesy of Judith Stellar)

Cutaneous Complications

Dermatitis is common among patients with GI diversions and usually caused by the chronic effect of the proteolytic enzymes and high alkaline content of the stool and other drainage on the peristomal skin. The degree of irritation can range from mild dermatitis to severely denuded skin along the inferior aspect of the stoma (Figure 2.2). Fungal infections due to *Candida albicans* frequently accompany the dermatitis since the warm moist environment makes an ideal location for fungal infections. In these cases, the skin is often raised and erythematous with well-circumscribed papules or satellite lesions. Application of clotrimazole or miconazole nitrate 2% powder is often sufficient for treating candidal infections. Mixing an antifungal powder with a small amount of water and then painting it onto the skin can enhance the adherence of the pouch. Contact dermatitis due to an allergic reaction from the stoma products or tape can also present with mild to severe skin breakdown; however, the hallmark of allergic dermatitis is the precise outline of the rash that matches the stoma product. Avoidance of the appliance and application of topical steroid cream and oral antihistamines are often helpful. Cellulitis can occur in the setting of severe excoriations and may require systemic antibiotics. The rash associated with cellulitis is usually more tender, warm, and indurated than in typical forms of irritant or allergic dermatitis.

Metabolic Derangements

Patients with ileostomies are at higher risk for metabolic derangements due to the larger volume of effluent that is produced daily. The normal adult output is 500–1300 ml/day, which may be increased in the setting of obstruction, infectious enteritis, bacterial overgrowth, and dietary indiscretion such as diets high in sugar, salt, and fat. High stoma output can lead to hyponatremia, hypokalemia, and hypomagnesaemia. If more than 60–100 cm of the terminal ileum is resected, malabsorption of fat and vitamin B12 can occur. The initial evaluation for high stoma output includes obtaining a set of electrolytes such as magnesium and phosphorous; a complete blood count to assess for anemia; a two-view abdominal x-ray; stool studies for *Clostridium difficile*, ova and parasite and bacterial culture; and obtaining a detailed diet history. Management of high stoma output includes identifying and treating the underlying cause. Patients with Crohn's disease may present with increased output as a sign of an acute flare, and gastroenterology consultation should be obtained for these patients. If the electrolytes are normal, and the patient is well hydrated and hemodynamically stable with a benign abdominal exam, the patient may be discharged home with instructions to increase their fiber intake and decrease their intake of sugar, salt, and fat. For patients with metabolic derangements, dehydration, or other concerns, intravenous fluids, electrolyte replacement, and bowel rest are the initial steps. Once the patient is stabilized, long-term management of high stoma output may include antidiarrheal agents including loperamide, oral fluid restriction, dietary salt supplementation, H_2 antagonists, and proton pump inhibitors. Patients with ileostomies are also predisposed to kidney stone formation due to their state of chronic mild dehydration and acidic urine.

Consultation

ED physicians can manage many of the complications from GI diversions such as small parastomal hernias, uncomplicated prolapses, and dermatitis. Cases of early postoperative complications and any concern of ischemia require immediate surgical consultation.

Further Reading

1 Bafford, A.C. and Irani, J.L. (2013). Management and complications of stomas. *Surg. Clin. N. Am.* 93: 145–166.

2 Fine, J.A., Cronan, K.M., and Posner, J.C. (2010). Approach to the care of the technology-assisted child. In: *Textbook of Pediatric Emergency Medicine*, 6e (eds. G.R. Fleisher and S. Ludwig), 1510–1513. Philadelphia, PA: Lippincott, Williams and Wilkins.

3 Landman RG. Routine care of patients with an ileostomy or colostomy and management of ostomy complications (ed. Weiser M). UpToDate, 2016.

4 Martin, S.T. and Vogel, J.D. (2012). Intestinal stomas. Indications, management, and complications. *Adv. Surg.* 46: 19–49.

5 Shabbir, J. and Britton, D.C. (2010). Stoma complications: a literature overview. *Colorectal Dis.* 12: 958–964.

3

Management of the Bariatric Surgery Patient in the Emergency Department

Megan Lavoie[1,2] and Joy Collins[1,3]

[1] *Perelman School of Medicine at the University of Pennsylvania, Philadelphia, PA, USA*
[2] *Division of Emergency Medicine, Department of Pediatrics, Children's Hospital of Philadelphia, Philadelphia, PA, USA*
[3] *Division of General and Thoracic Surgery, Department of Surgery, Children's Hospital of Philadelphia, Philadelphia, PA, USA*

Introduction

Obesity, defined as $BMI > 35 \, kg/m^2$, is becoming increasingly prevalent in the US and globally. According to the most recent Centers for Disease Control and Prevention (CDC) data, in the US, >35% of adults in the US are obese and close to 20% of children meet the definition of obesity or severe obesity ($BMI > 40 \, kg/m^2$). Obesity brings with it significant physical and psychosocial comorbidities that carry a large health burden: type 2 diabetes mellitus, hypertension, obstructive sleep apnea, dyslipidemia, nonalcoholic steatohepatitis, and orthopedic complications, among others, have been seen in severely obese adolescents as well as in adults. Medical and psychological management alone is often not adequate to achieve significant, sustainable weight loss. Surgical weight loss techniques are increasingly being offered to severely obese patients experiencing comorbid conditions. According to the American Society of Metabolism and Bariatric Surgeries, in 2015, over 195 000 bariatric surgeries were performed in the US in adults or adolescents. Over 50% of patients had the gastric sleeve procedure, and approximately 25% underwent the Roux-en-y-gastric bypass (RYGB). The adjustable gastric band is another surgical option for severe obesity in adults but has not been approved for use in adolescents under 18 years of age.

Surgical Procedures

RYGB, laparoscopic adjustable gastric band (LAGB), and laparoscopic sleeve gastrectomy (LSG) are the most commonly performed weight loss surgeries (Figures 3.1–3.3). Gastric band and sleeve gastrectomy are restrictive procedures (meaning that they cause limitation to food intake), while the RYGB has been described as a procedure whose effects are related to a combination of gastric restriction and intestinal malabsorption. Despite these

Emergency Management of the Hi-Tech Patient in Acute and Critical Care, First Edition. Edited by Ioannis Koutroulis, Nicholas Tsarouhas, Richard J. Lin, Jill C. Posner, Michael Seneff, and Robert Shesser.
© 2021 John Wiley & Sons Ltd. Published 2021 by John Wiley & Sons Ltd.

Roux-en-Y gastric bypass

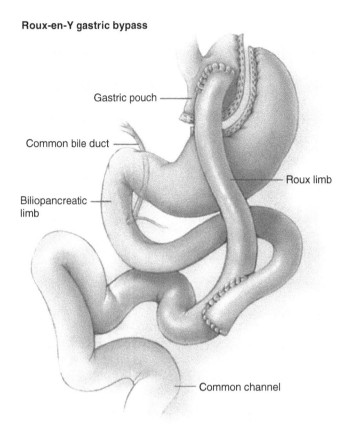

Gastric pouch

Common bile duct

Roux limb

Biliopancreatic limb

Common channel

Figure 3.1 Pencil drawing of RYGB. *Source:* Penn Medicine

classifications, it has become clear that all weight loss procedures have metabolic effects, which may contribute more significantly to postoperative weight loss than can be explained simply by gastric restriction and intestinal malabsorption alone.

In the RYGB, a small stomach pouch is created and the jejunum is divided. The distal limb of the jejunum is then connected directly to the small gastric pouch, bypassing the rest of the stomach and the proximal intestine. The small bowel is then placed in continuity with itself more distally, thereby providing a route for biliopancreatic secretions to mix with food. The small size of the stomach limits the capacity of food intake, while calorie and fat absorption is limited as the majority of the stomach and duodenum are bypassed.

The LAGB is a laparoscopic procedure where an inflatable silicone band is placed around the upper part of the stomach, creating a tiny new stomach pouch that limits the capacity to take in large amounts of food. The band position results in a small stomach outlet that leads to slowing of upper gastric emptying and increases the sensation of satiety. The band is able to be inflated and deflated by injecting a needle through the skin into a port connected to the band to adjust the size of the opening from the gastric pouch. Gastric banding

Laparoscopic adjustable gastric banding

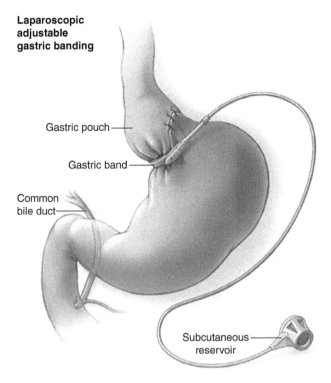

Gastric pouch

Gastric band

Common bile duct

Subcutaneous reservoir

Figure 3.2 Pencil drawing of LAGB. *Source:* Swedish Health Services

Vertical sleeve gastrectomy

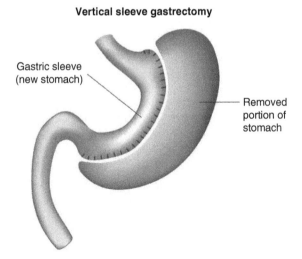

Gastric sleeve (new stomach)

Removed portion of stomach

Figure 3.3 Pencil drawing of LSG. *Source:* UNC Medical Center

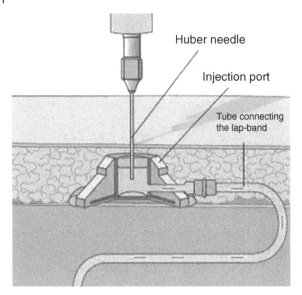

Huber needle

Injection port

Tube connecting
the lap-band

Figure 3.4 Pencil drawing of how to deflate port on LAGB. *Source:* Reproduced from Hamdan et al. (2011)

has the benefit of being relatively reversible and minimally invasive, as it requires no cutting or stapling of the stomach or bowel (Figure 3.4).

The LSG is performed by removing 75–80% of the stomach and leaving a long gastric tube or sleeve of the stomach, thereby restricting intake. This procedure was initially part of a staged approach to more complex weight -loss procedures but has been shown to offer significant weight loss and improvement of comorbid conditions such that it is currently offered as a stand-alone procedure.

Indications

Bariatric surgery is available to patients with severe obesity who have a low probability of successful weight loss with nonoperative measures, and who demonstrate motivation to continue medical treatment and lifestyle changes after surgery. In adults, criteria for bariatric surgery include those with a BMI > 40 or those with a BMI > 35 with comorbid diseases. As the risks of bariatric surgery in adolescents are not yet completely understood, adolescents are typically offered bariatric surgery primarily if they have comorbidities. Adolescents with severe comorbidities such as type 2 DM, moderate to severe sleep apnea, or pseudotumor may be considered surgical candidates with a BMI as low as 35. Adolescents with mild comorbidities and a BMI of 40 or greater are also potential candidates for weight loss surgery. While degree of obesity and weight-related medical problems are the most basic determinants of potential candidacy, adolescent patients should undergo a thorough workup to rule out medically reversible causes of obesity or contraindications to surgery. The workup typically involves evaluation by a multidisciplinary team, including a pediatric/adolescent medical weight loss specialist, a bariatric surgeon (or pediatric surgeon with expertise in performing bariatric procedures), a dietician, a mental health professional with experience in evaluating bariatric patients, an exercise specialist, and others. In addition, most patients undergo an intensive medical weight management program throughout the evaluation period prior to proceeding to weight loss surgery.

Complications

An estimated 5–25% of patients who undergo bariatric surgery will have complications. Most surgical complications will occur in the immediate postoperative period, perhaps while the patient is still in the hospital. These include anastamotic leak, pulmonary embolism, and bleeding. We will not discuss these complications in depth in this chapter.

Delayed complications occur in an estimated 10% of patients who undergo weight loss surgery. Patients may present to the emergency department (ED) with these delayed complications. Complications may be related to the device itself (if one is placed), to intermediate or late surgical complications (such as bowel obstruction), or they may relate to gastrointestinal (GI) symptoms that occur as a result of changing the GI tract anatomy (Table 3.1). Practitioners treating patients who have had bariatric surgery must be alert to the fact that these patients can have GI disorders that are not secondary to their weight loss

Table 3.1 GI symptoms and associated causes.

1) Diarrhea
    Malabsorption
    Bile salts
    Dumping syndrome
    Food intolerance
    Lactose intolerance
    Irritable bowel syndrome
    Bacterial overgrowth
    Infection
2) Vomiting
    Overeating
    Noncompliance with bariatric surgery diet
    Obstruction
    Marginal ulcers
    Stomal stenosis
    Gastric band slippage with gastric prolapse
    Roux stasis syndrome
    Excessively tight gastric band
    Gallstones
    Gastroesophageal reflux
3) Constipation
    Dehydration due to decreased fluid intake
    Iron supplementation
    Multivitamin supplementation

surgeries as well. Any patient with significant abdominal symptoms who has had bariatric surgery in the past should be evaluated by a surgeon experienced with such patients. Such consultation may be helpful in directing the most appropriate workup and management, and early consultation is essential in those cases where a prompt return to the operating room is indicated. The main bariatric surgery complications with timing, symptoms, diagnostics and treatment are summarized in Table 3.2.

All patients who present with abdominal pain, nausea, vomiting, or diarrhea after having weight loss surgery should have a full exam, with close attention to signs of dehydration and shock. Tachycardia is especially worrisome, as it may indicate dehydration, sepsis or infection (particularly in the setting of a postoperative leak), GI bleeding, pulmonary embolism, or even acute myocardial infarction. Intravenous access and full laboratory evaluation, including complete blood count, complete metabolic panel, and urinalysis, should be obtained. Blood gas, as well as stool hemoccult, may help acutely ill patient. The patient should be fluid resuscitated, antiemetics should be given for nausea and vomiting, and abdominal imaging should be considered. If there is concern for ileus or obstruction, abdominal radiographs should be performed. In a patient who is particularly toxic, or who has persistent abdominal tenderness, or nausea or vomiting after an antiemetic and fluids, abdominal CT or UGI study may need to be performed. This would help identify obstruction or staple line leak. Rapid weight loss can be a risk factor for development of gallstones. All bariatric surgery patients who have colicky abdominal pain and vomiting with no other identified cause should be evaluated for gallstones.

In the first month after surgery, patients who have undergone RYGB may present with nonspecific signs of infection: tachycardia, mental status changes, and dyspnea, with or without abdominal pain. This should immediately raise concern for anastomotic or staple line leak. Full labs, fluid resuscitation, and broad-spectrum antibiotics should all be initiated, along with abdominal imaging via UGI or abdominal CT. Anastomotic leak is the most serious complication patients may develop after RYGB or sleeve gastrectomy and requires urgent surgical consultation and operative exploration.

Patients who have had RYGB are also particularly at risk for the development of marginal ulcers. These occur in 5–10% of patients and present several months after surgery. Patients classically present with epigastric abdominal pain, nausea and vomiting, dyspepsia, or signs of an upper GI bleed. Perforation may also occur, with signs and symptoms of infection and sepsis. Stable patients may respond to IV fluids, sucralfate, and a proton pump inhibitor, while more acutely ill or hemodynamically unstable patients will require aggressive fluid resuscitation and packed red blood cell transfusion, along with emergent endoscopy. RYGB patients may also develop stomal stenosis in the first months after surgery. This presents as epigastric pain after eating and may also be accompanied by vomiting, initially only of solids, and ultimately of all food and liquids. Stomal stenosis is identified via UGI or endoscopy and can be corrected with endoscopic balloon dilation the majority of the time.

LSG and LAGB are technically more simple surgical procedures than RYGB and are, therefore, associated with fewer complications than RYGB. Patients do not experience dumping syndrome, stomal ulceration, nutritional deficiencies, or small bowel obstruction in the way that they may after RYGB. LSG does carry the risk of leaking at the staple line.

Table 3.2 Bariatric surgery complications.

Complication	Timing	Weight loss procedure	Signs and symptoms	Diagnostic testing	Management
Small bowel obstruction	Within 1 month	RYGB	nausea/vomiting and abdominal pain	Abdominal Xray	Nasogastric decompression and fluids
Staple line leak	Within 1 month	RYGB and LSG	Abdominal pain, tachycardia, and sepsis	UGI abdominal CT	Fluids, antibiotics, and surgery
Marginal ulcers	2–4 months	RYGB	Epigastric abdominal pain, upper GI bleeding, and dyspepsia	N/V endoscopy	PPI, sucralfate, fluid, or PRBC resuscitation
Upper GI bleeding	First 6 months	RYGB and LSG	Hematemesis, melena, anemia, and hypotension	Bleeding scan, and endoscopy	acid blocker, packed red blood cells, and fluid resuscitation, and endoscopy
Dumping syndrome	Variable, typically first 6 months	RYGB	Diarrhea, abdominal cramping, flushing and sweating, N/V, palpitations, and hypotension	None	Supportive, small frequent meals and fluids
Cholelithiasis/ cholecystitis	Anytime	RYGB, LSG, and LAGB	Colicky abdominal pain and N/V	Ultrasound	Supportive, cholecystectomy
GERD	Anytime	RYGB, LSG, and LAGB	Reflux, epigastric pain, and N/V	None	Acid blocker, small frequent meals
Gastric slippage	Anytime	LAGB	Epigastric pain, reflux, and food intolerance	AXR and UGI	Surgery
Gastric band erosion	Months to years	LAGB	Infected port site, weight gain, abdominal pain, and vomiting	UGI	Surgery for band removal
Gastric necrosis	Variable	LAGB	Acutely ill, abdominal pain, and N/V	UGI	Surgery

RYGB = Roux-en-y-gastric bypass
LSG = laparoscopic sleeve gastrectomy
LAGB = laparoscopic adjustable gastric band
UGI=Upper GI radiography
AXR = abdominal xray
N/V=nausea/vomiting
CT=computerized tomography scan
PPI = proton pump inhibitor
PRBC = packed red blood cells

This occurs in less than 5% of patients, typically in the first month after the weight loss surgery. Patients may present with infection or abdominal pain and will have the staple line leak identified on UGI or abdominal CT.

LAGB is the least complicated surgical procedure, but has not taken hold as a major bariatric surgery option because of the frequent band complications, and the significant segment of patients who do not achieve the weight loss results desired with this procedure. LAGB is considered reversible, though, after the band is removed, a significant amount of scar tissue will remain, complicating further surgical procedures. While the lap band is associated with fewer severe surgical complications such as leak and significant bleeding, the complication rate itself is higher. Complications include reflux symptoms, food intolerance, esophageal dilation, band slippage, gastric prolapse above the band, and erosion of the band, among others.

Gastric slippage, which occurs in 15–20% of LAGB patients, occurs when a part of the stomach becomes prolapsed above the gastric band and creates an unnecessarily large gastric pouch and potential obstruction. Patients will develop reflux symptoms and dysphagia and, in severe cases, can develop significant abdominal pain and vomiting. Abdominal upright radiographs or a UGI study will likely show the gastric slippage and dilation of the proximal gastric pouch. Even those patients who appear clinically well typically require surgery to correct the gastric slippage and should be aggressively fluid resuscitated and have electrolytes checked and corrected prior to surgery. Surgeons may attempt to deflate the gastric band by advancing a Huber needle into the port site at the skin until the needle hits the plate at the back of the port, and then withdrawing fluid to deflate the band completely. This should allow the stomach to return to its normal size and obviate the need for immediate surgery until a bariatric surgeon can evaluate the band. Nonsurgical practitioners are typically advised not to deflate the band themselves, though in EDs, where there is no timely access to a general or bariatric surgeon, ED physicians may do so.

Gastric band patients may also develop erosion of the band into the stomach. Band erosion may present subtly, with few abdominal complaints. Oftentimes, the presenting feature will be an infection at the band port site and can occur months or even years after the initial band placement. All patients with a port infection thus require evaluation for band erosion. Band erosion will require UGI or endoscopy to diagnose and will then require band removal. This is typically done surgically but endoscopic retrieval has been reported.

Finally, gastric band patients may also develop gastric necrosis. Gastric necrosis is typically a late complication of lap LAGB that occurs from a combination of pressure from the band and gastric prolapse. Patients will present acutely ill, with a surgical abdomen. UGI or abdominal CT studies demonstrate the gastric prolapse.

Though unlikely to cause someone to present to the ED, after LAGB, patients will sometimes present with weight gain, as the band is no longer functioning to restrict food intake or if patients themselves develop maladaptive eating strategies (ingesting high-calorie liquids such as ice cream or milkshakes or foods that can easily pass through the small stoma, e.g. potato chips).

Further Reading

1 Alqahtani, A., Alamri, H., Elahmedi, M., and Mohammed, R. (2012). Laparoscopic sleeve gastrectomy in adult and pediatric obese patients: a comparative study. *Surg. Endosc.* 26 (11): 3094–3100.

2 Alqahtani, A.R., Antonisamy, B., Alamri, H. et al. (2012). Laparoscopic sleeve gastrectomy in 108 obese children and adolescents aged 5 to 21 years. *Ann. Surg.* 256: 266–273.

3 American Society for Metabolic and Bariatric Surgeries [Internet]. Estimate of bariatric surgery numbers, 2011-2015. [cited Feb 14 2017]. Available from https://asmbs.org/resources/estimate-of-bariatric-surgery-numbers

4 Ellison, S.R. and Ellison, D.S. (2008). Bariatric surgery: a review of the available procedures and complications for the emergency physician. *J. Emerg. Med.* 34 (1): 21–32.

5 Hamdan, K., Somers, S., and Chand, M. (2011). Management of late postoperative complications of bariatric surgery. *Br. J. Surg.* 98: 1345–1355. doi:10.1002/bjs.7568.

6 Hsia, D.S., Fallon, S.C., and Brandt, M.L. (2012). Adolescent bariatric surgery. *Arch. Pediatr. Adolesc. Med.* 166 (8): 757–766.

7 Huang, C.S. and Farraye, F.A. (2006). Complications following bariatric surgery. *Tech. Gastrointest. Endosc.* 8: 54–65.

8 Inge, T.H., Zeller, M.H., Jenkins, T.M. et al. (2014). Perioperative outcomes of adolescents undergoing bariatric surgery. The Teen-Longitudinal Assessment of Bariatric Surgery (TEEN-LABS) study. *JAMA Pediatr.* 168 (1): 47–53.

9 Khwaja, H.A. and Bonanomi, G. (2010). Bariatric surgery: techniques, outcomes and complications. *Curr. Anaesth. Crit. Care* 21: 31–38.

10 Michalsky, M., Recihard, K., Inge, T. et al. (2012). ASMBS pediatric committee best practice guidelines. *Surg. Obes. Relat. Dis.* 8: 1–7.

11 https://www.pennmedicine.org/for-patients-and-visitors/find-a-program-or-service/bariatric-surgery/procedures/roux-en-y-gastric-bypass-rgb

12 https://www.swedish.org/services/adjustable-gastric-band

13 https://www.uncmedicalcenter.org/uncmc/care-treatment/bariatric-surgery/types-of-bariatric-surgery/gastric-sleeve-surgery/

4

Transjugular Intrahepatic Portosystemic Shunt

Heather House[1,2] and Anne Marie Cahill[1,3]

[1] *Perelman School of Medicine at the University of Pennsylvania, Philadelphia, PA, USA*
[2] *Division of Emergency Medicine, Department of Pediatrics, Children's Hospital of Philadelphia, Philadelphia, PA, USA*
[3] *Division of Interventional Radiology, Department of Radiology, Children's Hospital of Philadelphia, Philadelphia, PA, USA*

Introduction

The hepatic portal system is a group of vessels that supply nutrient-rich blood from the gastrointestinal tract to the liver. The hepatic portal vein drains the superior mesenteric vein and the splenic vein, as well as receives blood from the inferior mesenteric, gastric, and cystic veins. Within the liver, the portal vein branches to right and left, dividing further into portal venules. Portal venules and hepatic arterioles empty into hepatic sinusoids where hepatocytes receive nutrients, process toxins, and mix oxygenated blood. After processing, blood is returned to the systemic circulation via the hepatic vein.

Portal hypertension exists when the pressure in the portal venous system of the liver exceeds 10 mmHg. There are myriad causes of portal hypertension, which are broken down to three categories. Presinusoidal causes affect the portal vein and venous system. Portal vein thrombosis may be related to hypercoagulable states, or in neonates, a complication of umbilical central venous access. Direct mass effect or invasion of intrahepatic tumor may cause obstruction. Schistosomiasis causes fibrosis within the portal venules prior to the sinusoids. Other etiologies prior to sinusoids include hepatic fibrosis, congenital extrahepatic portal vein occlusion, arterioportovenous fistulae (Osler–Weber–Rendu syndrome), and hyperdynamic splenomegaly. Etiologies affecting the sinusoids (sinusoidal causes) include cirrhosis, congenital hepatic fibrosis, cystic liver disease, sclerosing cholangitis, and primary biliary cirrhosis. Cirrhosis is the most common cause of portal hypertension and may be related to viral hepatitis or alcoholic cirrhosis. Less commonly, Wilson's disease and hemochromatosis may lead to sinusoidal fibrosis and hypertension. Postsinusoidal obstruction is rare and caused by hepatic outflow obstructions, including Budd–Chiari syndrome, veno-occlusive disease after bone marrow transplantation, and mass effect.

Emergency Management of the Hi-Tech Patient in Acute and Critical Care, First Edition. Edited by Ioannis Koutroulis, Nicholas Tsarouhas, Richard J. Lin, Jill C. Posner, Michael Seneff, and Robert Shesser.
© 2021 John Wiley & Sons Ltd. Published 2021 by John Wiley & Sons Ltd.

In the event of portal hypertension, portal systemic collateral vessels form in order to bypass the obstruction. Increase in the blood flow through collateral vascularity can then lead to engorgement in gastroesophageal vessels to return to systemic circulation. Patients may develop esophageal varices that have an increased tendency to bleed when portal pressure rises. Other complications of portal hypertension include the development of ascites and progressive liver dysfunction.

The transjugular intrahepatic portosystemic shunt (TIPS) is an interventional radiology procedure where a stent is inserted to ameliorate the complications from portal hypertension.

Equipment/Device

The TIPS creates an artificial channel between the portal vein and the hepatic vein, thereby decreasing the resistance of blood flow returning to the systemic circulation. Placement of a TIPS is performed with interventional radiology.

Preferably, access occurs through the right internal jugular vein; however, the left internal jugular vein may be used as well. A vascular sheath is introduced and placed into the intrahepatic inferior vena cava. In most cases, the right hepatic vein is isolated and then the radiologist identifies the right portal vein. The shunt is introduced by cannulating the right portal vein from the right hepatic vein. Using the sheath introduced via the jugular access, a needle is passed into the right portal vein. Contrast is used to confirm placement of the needle tip. A wire is passed through the portal vein, and the fibrotic liver tissue is dilated with a small-caliber balloon. A stent is passed over the wire between the hepatic vein and the portal vein, and as the original vascular sheath is withdrawn, the stent opens. It is then balloon dilated to an appropriate width based on measurements of portal venous pressure.

Indications

The TIPS device is used to combat the downstream effects of portal hypertension. Patients who have experienced esophageal variceal bleeding that has not been controlled via medical or endoscopic management may benefit from the insertion of a TIPS. Patients who have recurrent worsening ascites that is not improved with traditional medication and diet management also may be candidates for insertion. TIPS may be similarly beneficial in extravascular shifts causing hepatic hydrothorax refractory to medical management.

Hepatorenal syndrome occurs when cirrhotic changes of the liver lead to poor perfusion. Response of vasoactive hormones causes vasodilation of the splanchnic circulation and compensatory vasoconstriction of renal arteries leading to increasing renal failure. Some effect of fluid shifts of increased ascites may also play a role in renal hypoperfusion, and there is some suggestion that TIPS may reduce these shifts leading to improvement in renal function.

Contraindications

Given the increase in systemic circulation through the hepatic vein, which then returns to the heart via the inferior vena cava, patients with severe elevation in right heart pressures or pulmonary hypertension are not ideal patients to receive a TIPS. Similarly, patients with congestive heart failure should not experience the increased systemic return. Patients with active infections either systemically or within the liver should not receive TIPS. Finally, patients with concurrent bleeding diatheses should be corrected prior to the procedure.

Management

Creation of a TIPS occurs with interventional radiology. Once the shunt device is in place, there is no further external equipment the patient requires.

Complications

Hepatic Encephalopathy

The liver processes toxins when blood is drained from the mesenteric system and filtered prior to returning to systemic circulation. Creation of a portosystemic shunt allows for the mixing of unfiltered intestinal blood into the hepatic vein. Hepatic encephalopathy occurs when unprocessed toxins are not removed effectively. Encephalopathy, if left untreated, may lead to patients progressing from mild confusion to altered levels of consciousness and even coma.

Most patients with portosystemic shunt related hepatic encephalopathy present two to three weeks after the TIPS procedure. Mild forms may be missed, as patients present initially with confusion and forgetfulness. Reversal in the sleep–wake pattern, with patients being awake at night and asleep during the day, is the first stage indicator of encephalopathy. Second stage may move to personality changes and worsening lethargy with altered consciousness. Severe encephalopathy can cause coma, seizures, and neurologic changes, including clonus and asterixis.

While encephalopathy may be noted after the initial TIPS procedure is performed, there are usually background causes that aggravate the symptoms. Episodes of esophageal bleeding, increased protein intake, worsening renal function, or constipation cause an increased gastrointestinal nitrogen load. Some medications or drugs of abuse (including alcohol) can be implicated. Patients who experience infection are at an increased risk of encephalopathy. Finally, many cases, up to 30%, have an unknown trigger.

Encephalopathy is a clinical diagnosis. While lab investigations may reveal elevation in liver enzymes and ammonia, there are no specific levels at which these tests are diagnostic. Most commonly, brain imaging does not show abnormalities. However, once the diagnosis of encephalopathy is suspected, investigation into the other attributing factors listed above may help with therapy.

Treatment of encephalopathy focuses on reversal of any of the secondary factors in combination with decreasing gut reabsorption of nitrogen waste products. Lactulose increases gut transit and may decrease production of nitrogen by intestinal bacteria. Addition of antibiotics, including rifaximin or metronidazole, also decreases intraluminal nitrogen production by decreasing intestinal bacterial load. Patients are encouraged to eat a nutritious diet with an appropriate amount of protein. Often, encephalopathy in patients with TIPS resolves spontaneously or with minimal change. In about 5% of patients with TIPS, if medical management of encephalopathy is not effective, the TIPS procedure may need to be reversed.

Infection

Clinicians need to consider stent infection in patients with a history of a TIPS procedure that present with intermittent or continuous fever. Most patients with vegetative infection present weeks to months after their TIPS, and infection may be related to clot formation or direct bacterial seeding (endotipsitis). Clinicians should assess with blood cultures from multiple sites and evaluation of the stent initially with Doppler ultrasound for the presence of stenosis or clot. In the absence of other etiologies for fever, patients should receive intravenous antibiotics targeted toward enteric organisms.

Bleeding

Worsening liver function due to the underlying liver disease can cause a decrease in hepatic production of clotting factors. Prior to TIPS insertion, assessment of coagulation panel should be performed and any bleeding diathesis corrected. Most patients who will experience bleeding as a complication to their TIPS insertion do so perioperatively, and it is not a common presentation to the emergency department.

Stent Obstruction

Creation of a TIPS introduces a stent across hepatic tissue from the hepatic vein to the portal vein. Hepatic tissue reacts to this placement and begins to create a pseudo-intima around and into the shunt. Increase in tissue into an uncoated stent begins to narrow the lumen of the stent and decrease the portosystemic blood flow, making the stent less effective. This then allows portal hypertension to recur, and patients have an increased risk in esophageal variceal bleeding and redevelopment of ascites.

Doppler ultrasonography is used as the initial screening method for shunt stenosis. Two main parameters are used for shunt patency. First, the velocity of flow within the TIPS is measured in multiple locations across the shunt. Single velocity measurement has a lower sensitivity and specificity than multiple measurements, with decrease in shunt velocity between 40 and 60 cm/s of significant elevated velocity over 200 cm/s identifying local stenosis. Main portal vein velocity is the second parameter. Stenotic shunts demonstrate lower main portal velocity and a change in the direction of flow toward the liver instead of normally away from the liver in a functioning stent. CT angiography can also be used in the evaluation of shunt stenosis; however, the gold standard of diagnosis of shunt stenosis is angiography. Stenotic shunts can be dilated during angiography and the placement of an additional stent ensures unobstructed flow of the TIPS.

Hemolytic Anemia

Patients presenting with an increase in jaundice after TIPS placement should be evaluated for hemolysis. TIPS-related hemolysis develops one to two weeks after TIPS creation and seems to be related to shearing of red blood cells or mechanical trauma of cells within the stent. Often, in patients, there is an evidence of increased unconjugated bilirubin and high reticulocytosis, which may mean the patient is only slightly anemic, if at all. If patients develop severe hemolytic anemia, the clinician can consider blood transfusion. Most TIPS patients will spontaneously improve as their stent endothelializes.

Consultation

Patients receive TIPSs as a stabilizing entity for portal hypertension, which has numerous causes. TIPS placement is not curative, and these patients will continue to be managed with gastroenterologists for their underlying disease. When considering consultation and management of these patients, the involvement of gastroenterology is often helpful.

Mechanical complications of TIPS stents, including occlusion or malplacement that leads to worsening liver disease, will need to be addressed with interventional radiology. While the patient needs to be stabilized medically for their presenting problem, clinicians need to consider either the involvement of interventional radiology (IR) or transfer to a center with IR capabilities for definitive management.

Further Reading

1 Chockalingam, A., Holly, B., and Hong, K. (2017). Transjugular intrahepatic portosystemic shunt. In: *Current Surgical Therapy* (eds. J. Cameron and A. Cameron), 402–411. Philadelphia: Elsevier.

2 Colambato, L. (2007). The role of transjugular intrahepatic portosystemic shunt (TIPS) in the management of portal hypertension. *J. Clin. Gastroenterol.* 41 (Suppl. 3): 344–351.

3 Conn, H. (1996). Hemolysis after transjugular intrahepatic portosystemic shunting: the naked stent syndrome. *Hepatology* 23 (1): 177–181.

4 Darcy, M. (2012). Evaluation and management of transjungular intrahepatic portosystemic shunts. *Am. J. Roentgenol.* 199: 730–736.

5 Jakhete, N. and Kim, A. (2017). The management of hepatic encephalopathy. In: *Current Surgical Therapy* (eds. J. Cameron and A. Cameron), 417–421. Philadelphia: Elsevier.

6 Li, J. and Henderson, J.M. (2001). Portal hypertension. In: *Surgical Treatment: Evidence Based and Problem Oriented* (eds. R.G. Holzheimer and J.A. Mannick), 306–319. Munich: Zuckschwerdt.

7 Somberg, K.A., Riegler, J.L., LaBerge, J.M. et al. (1995). Hepatic encephalopathy after transjugular intrahepatic portosystemic shunts: incidence and risk factors. *Am. J. Gastroenterol.* 90 (4): 549–555.

Section II

Central Catheters

5

Indwelling Central Venous Catheter Devices

Anna Weiss

Perelman School of Medicine at the University of Pennsylvania, Philadelphia, PA, USA
Division of Emergency Medicine, Department of Pediatrics, Children's Hospital of Philadelphia, Philadelphia, PA, USA

Introduction

The continual advancement of treatment for chronic diseases has brought with it an increased emphasis on allowing patients with long-term medical needs to receive much of their care in the outpatient setting. In this context, the use of indwelling central venous catheters (CVCs) has become a mainstay in the management of adults and children with chronic illness. CVCs provide patients with stable routes for life-saving infusions – including parenteral nutrition, blood transfusions, and chemotherapeutic agents – and allow for reliable venous access in patients who require frequent blood draws or whose peripheral vasculature no longer adequately supports recurrent venipuncture. Because of their placement in the large vessels of the central vasculature, CVCs can be used to infuse medications that are otherwise vesicants in peripheral vessels, and they are often the preferred means of administration for infusions containing high concentrations of electrolytes and/or dextrose.

As the number of patients receiving care in the community via CVCs increases, so too does the number of patients with CVCs presenting to the emergency department (ED). For this reason, ED practitioners must be familiar with both the routine care of these devices, as well as with the workup and management of their most common and most serious complications. When a patient with an indwelling CVC presents to the ED, the clinician must have a high index of suspicion for – and must be able to recognize – the symptoms of catheter-related complications, particularly as the patient's presenting complaint may not initially implicate the device.

Emergency Management of the Hi-Tech Patient in Acute and Critical Care, First Edition. Edited by Ioannis Koutroulis, Nicholas Tsarouhas, Richard J. Lin, Jill C. Posner, Michael Seneff, and Robert Shesser.
© 2021 John Wiley & Sons Ltd. Published 2021 by John Wiley & Sons Ltd.

Central Venous Catheter Types

The first tunneled CVC was introduced by Broviac in 1973, and since then, the variety of indwelling CVCs on the market has increased dramatically as their use has become more commonplace. As the list of available CVCs is extensive, practitioners should make a particular effort to become familiar with the devices most commonly encountered in their practice setting. In general, devices are referred to either by their trade name (e.g. Broviac©, Hickman©) or by their type (e.g. implanted port, peripherally inserted central catheter [PICC]). They can be externalized, as is the case with the Broviac, Hickman, and PICC devices, or they can be fully implanted – requiring needle access through intact skin – as is the case with implanted ports. Both externalized and implanted CVCs can have multiple lumens, and knowledge of a particular CVC's lumen count is often important when managing the device's complications.

Catheter Anatomy

The catheter tip of most CVCs terminates at the junction of the superior vena cava (SVC) and the right atrium (RA). The venous path each catheter takes to get to the central circulation depends on the type of device. Tunneled, externalized catheters are usually inserted in the subclavian, external jugular, or cephalic vein, while implanted devices are usually inserted in the subclavian or internal jugular vein (Figure 5.1. *CHOP Family Information Line Drawing w/anatomy*). Externalized catheters are tunneled from the point of venous access to an exit point in the patient's chest, where a Dacron cuff stimulates tissue adherence, thereby discouraging both catheter migration and microbial infiltration (Figure 5.2). Fully implanted catheters (ports) are tunneled from their point of venous access to a subcutaneous pocket in the chest wall, where they terminate in a reservoir that is sutured in place for stability. The reservoir of the port communicates with the catheter portion of the device and is topped by a silicone self-sealing septum that is accessed through the skin with a noncoring needle (Figure 5.3). PICC lines, which have no tunneled component, are generally inserted in the upper arm through the basilic, brachial, or cephalic vein from which they are advanced into the SVC.

Routine Management and Use

The overarching principles of routine management for CVCs in the ED is similar for all devices. As none of these indwelling catheters is initially placed in the ED, routine CVC use in the emergent setting consists primarily of accessing and de-accessing the device for blood drawing and/or medication infusion. In all cases, a sterile field and meticulous sterile technique should be maintained when accessing or caring for a CVC. Forceps with teeth should not be used to clamp externalized lines, as these increase the risk of catheter breakage; if only toothed forceps are available, the teeth should be wrapped in sterile gauze prior to using the forceps to clamp the line. While povidone-iodine may be used to sterilize both

(a) **Externalized indwelling CVC**
Tunneled catheter

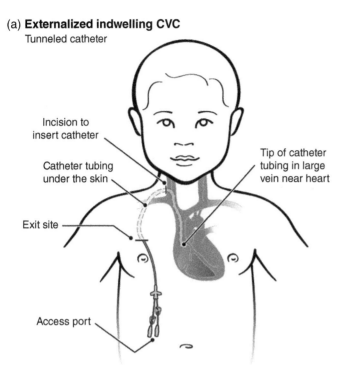

Incision to
insert catheter

Catheter tubing
under the skin

Tip of catheter
tubing in large
vein near heart

Exit site

Access port

(b) **Implanted port**
Implantable venous port

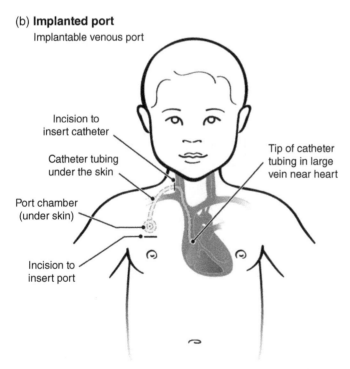

Incision to
insert catheter

Catheter tubing
under the skin

Tip of catheter
tubing in large
vein near heart

Port chamber
(under skin)

Incision to
insert port

Figure 5.1 Schematic of CVC anatomy. (a) Externalized indwelling CVC and (b) implanted port. (*Source:* ©2020 The Children's Hospital of Philadelphia, CHOP Family Information Line Drawing w/anatomy, (a): https://www.chop.edu/treatments/tunneled-catheter-placement; (b): https://www.chop.edu/treatments/implantable-venous-port.)

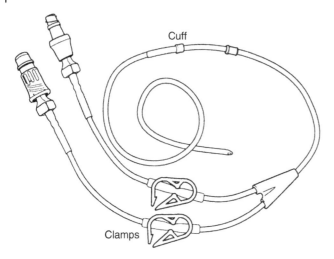

Figure 5.2 Schematic of externalized indwelling CVC.

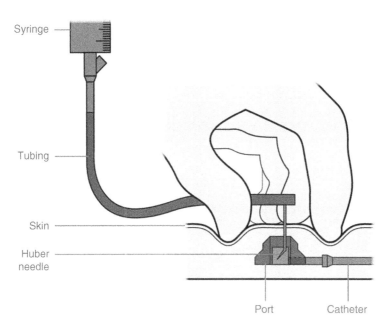

Figure 5.3 Schematic of fully implanted CVC. (*Source:* Image courtesy of Macmillan Cancer Support, UK.)

externalized catheter hubs and the skin overlying implanted CVCs, neither tincture of iodine nor acetone should be used to clean an externalized line, as it may dry the catheter and increase the risk of line breakage. When flushing fluids or drawing back blood from a CVC, a 10 cc syringe or larger should be used; smaller syringes may cause excessive pressure in the catheter, leading to rupture. Practitioners should have all specimen tubes for blood-drawing, all fluids to be infused, and all heparin and saline flushes ready prior to accessing the line. Fluids should never be infused into a line that does not draw back blood after flushing. To avoid instilling an air embolus, externalized catheters should always be clamped whenever a cap, syringe, or intravenous (IV) tubing is not attached to the distal end of the device. The specifics of accessing and de-accessing each device type are described below.

Accessing and Drawing Blood from an Externalized CVC (Broviac, Hickman, PICC)

As noted above, the procedure for accessing an externalized CVC must follow strict aseptic technique. ED personnel should have all necessary equipment open and ready prior to accessing the line. Table 5.1 describes the steps necessary to access an externalized CVC. If blood samples are to be drawn from the catheter, an attempt should be made to use the CVC's largest lumen of the for this purpose. If blood cultures are needed, a sample should be drawn from each lumen of the catheter and labeled carefully to indicate its lumen of origin. In general, blood samples withdrawn from a CVC should be labeled as such, so that

Table 5.1 Procedure for accessing an externalized central venous catheter.

1) Identify the patient and explain the procedure to the patient and family.
2) Position the patient safely. Supine positioning is preferred; women and adolescent girls should have their brassiere removed on the side of the catheter.
3) Perform hand hygiene and don sterile gloves. Some institutions will also require practitioners to wear a mask and/or sterile gown.
4) Prime all tubing and connectors to be used in the procedure to purge them of air.
5) Place a sterile towel or drape under the externalized portion of the catheter.
6) If the patient's CVC does not have its own clamp, clamp the line at least 3 in. proximal to the cap using forceps without teeth.
7) Remove the catheter cap and scrub the hub with alcohol, allowing it to dry fully (at least 5–10 seconds).
8) Attach a 10 cc syringe of normal saline; unclamp the catheter and slowly inject up to 5 cc of saline. If the line flushes easily, aspirate the instilled fluid and check for blood return.
9) If there is resistance to fluid infusion or no blood return with aspiration, the line is likely occluded (see the section on troubleshooting an occluded CVC). Recap the line and do not inject fluids or medications into the occluded line.
10) If there is successful blood return with aspiration, instill the remaining saline in the syringe. Clamp the line and remove the syringe.
11) If the line is needed for blood drawing, aspirate 3–5 cc from the line prior to clamping, as in Step 10. Discard this saline-and-blood mixture, and attach a new, empty syringe to the catheter cap. Unclamp the catheter and withdraw the needed volume of blood. Reclamp the catheter, attach a second 10 cc syringe of saline, unclamp the catheter, and flush the line to clear blood from the line. Clamp the catheter after flushing and remove the syringe.
12) If the line is needed for infusion of medications or fluids, connect primed IV tubing to the catheter hub, unclamp the catheter, and administer fluids or medications as care dictates.

any erroneous or unusual lab results may be interpreted in the context of the line's usual use (e.g. an extremely high blood glucose level drawn from a line ordinarily used to infuse parenteral nutrition).

Accessing and Drawing Blood from a Fully Implanted Catheter ("Port")

Accessing an implanted CVC requires puncturing the skin overlying the device; therefore, if line access is not required emergently, practitioners may wish to numb the skin over the port with a topical, lidocaine-containing anesthetic. Care must be taken to access the port with a noncoring (Huber©) needle, as standard hypodermic needles will damage the septum of the port and prevent it from resealing properly when the line is de-accessed. While the closed system of the implanted port boasts a decreased infection rate than that of externalized CVCs with routine use, it is critical to maintain proper aseptic technique when accessing these lines in the ED to avoid introducing infection at the access site. The skin overlying the implanted device should be cleansed with povidone-iodine or chlorhexidine (for patients older than two months) prior to attempting access. Table 5.2 details the steps necessary to access an implanted port. As noted above in the section on accessing externalized CVCs, all equipment should be prepared prior to attempting port access, and any blood samples drawn from a port should be labeled carefully to indicate their origin.

Complications

Both externalized and indwelling CVCs bring with them a host of common complications, including infection, catheter breakage and/or migration, catheter occlusion, and air embolism. Each of these complications will be discussed in detail below.

Infection

Catheter-related infections are among the most common reasons for ED visits among patients with indwelling venous-access devices. Because CVCs provide direct access to the central venous circulation, the risk of sepsis in patients with infected lines is a significant concern. This risk is exacerbated by the fact that the patients in whom these lines tend to be placed (e.g. immunocompromised oncology patients, gastrointestinal patients with diminished bowel-wall integrity) are by the nature of their underlying illness more likely to succumb to invasive infections. Therefore, any patient presenting to the ED with fever and an indwelling CVC should be considered septic until proven otherwise. Standard care for febrile patients with indwelling CVCs includes culturing each lumen of the catheter as well as a peripheral site, and initiation of broad-spectrum antibiotics (usually vancomycin and a third- or fourth-generation cephalosporin – though antimicrobial recommendations vary

Table 5.2 Procedure for accessing an implanted central venous catheter.

1) Identify the patient, and explain the procedure to the patient and family.
2) Position the patient safely. Supine positioning is preferred; women and adolescent girls should have their brassiere removed on the side of the catheter.
3) If anesthetic cream was applied to the skin overlying the port, wipe it away before cleansing with povidone-iodine or chlorhexidine (for patients over 2 months).
4) Perform hand hygiene and don sterile gloves. Most institutions will also require practitioners and patients to wear a mask.
5) Place a sterile towel or drape on the patient's chest below the port to create a sterile field.
6) Attach a 10 cc syringe of saline to extension tubing; attach the other end of the tubing to the noncoring needle. Flush the length of tubing and needle to remove air and lay it on the sterile field.
7) Triangulate the dome of port between the thumb and fingers of nondominant hand. Aiming for the center point of these fingers, use dominant hand to insert noncoring needle perpendicular to the skin and through the septum of the port.
8) Unclamp extension tubing and slowly infuse 2–5 cc of saline; if the line flushes easily, aspirate saline and check for blood return.
9) If there is resistance to fluid infusion or no blood return with aspiration, do not force fluid into the reservoir. Reclamp the tubing and see section on troubleshooting an occluded CVC.
10) If there is successful blood return with aspiration, instill the remaining saline in the syringe. Tape the needle in place at 90° to the dome of the port and apply a clear, sterile dressing. Clamp the tubing and remove the syringe.
11) If the line is needed for blood drawing, aspirate 3–5 cc from the line prior to clamping, as in Step 10. Discard this saline-and-blood mixture, and attach a new, empty syringe to the extension tubing. Unclamp the tubing and withdraw the needed volume of blood. Reclamp the tubing, attach a second 10 cc syringe of saline, unclamp the tubing, and flush to clear blood from the line. Clamp the tubing after flushing and remove the syringe.
12) If the line is needed for infusion of medications or fluids, connect primed IV tubing to the catheter hub, unclamp the catheter, and administer fluids or medications as care dictates.

widely by institution and according to local resistance patterns). CVC infections can range from systemic infections (bacteremia, fungemia, and sepsis) to local infections (exit-site or tunnel cellulitis, or "pocket infections" in the chest wall of patients with implanted ports). Practitioners should carefully examine the catheter exit site, the skin overlying an implanted port, and the entire palpable length of the subcutaneous tunnel for signs of redness, swelling, warmth, drainage, or tenderness. Streaking overlying the tunneled portion of an indwelling CVC is highly suggestive of a tunnel infection and is usually grounds for removal of the line in addition to administration of IV antibiotics. The most common organisms cultured from infected CVCs include *Staphylococcus aureus*, coagulase-negative staphylococci, gram-negative organisms such as *Klebsiella pneumoniae* and *Escherichia coli*, and fungi, especially *Candida* species. Catheter infections and catheter-associated soft tissue infections are most likely to occur in the first 100 days after device insertion, and in patients who were neutropenic at the time of placement, so practitioners should take care to inquire about these risk factors when working up a patient in whom they have a concern for CVC infection. When treating a patient for presumed CVC infection, the treatment team managing the patient's primary underlying condition should be contacted to assist with the selection of antimicrobial therapy.

Catheter Breakage and Dislodgement

Catheter breakage can occur for a variety of reasons, including inadvertent cutting during a dressing change, a patient pulling away during an attempt to access the line, snagging of the externalized portion of a CVC during daily activities or play, or blunt-force injury during contact sports or accident. Any fluid or blood reported by the patient or witnessed in the ED should be treated as a catheter break. Visualization of the catheter's Dacron cuff outside the chest wall should be treated similarly. To prevent infection, air embolus, or bleeding, broken externalized lines should be immediately clamped with nontoothed forceps proximal to the site of breakage and the damaged portion of the line should be cleaned with povidone-iodine and covered with sterile dressing. While repair kits specific to each type of CVC are available in many centers, they should be deployed only by those with expertise in their use – usually in consultation with an institutional IV team or interventional radiology. Less commonly, externalized CVCs can fracture proximal to their point of exit in the chest. In these cases, it is critical to apply pressure to the catheter's entrance to the vein and not to the chest wall exit site itself. A chest radiograph should be performed to determine the location of the proximal line fragment. Rarely, fractured catheter fragments are discovered in the pulmonary circulation, from which they must be removed by interventional radiology – usually via a femoral approach. Trauma or patient manipulation may dislodge an implanted port from its subcutaneous pocket in the chest wall. For this reason, practitioners should always check the stability of the port reservoir before attempting to access it with a needle. If port dislodgement is suspected, obtain a chest radiograph to interrogate the integrity of the implanted system. If dislodgement is confirmed by an X-ray, immediately discontinue any infusions running through the port and notify the interventional radiology or surgery department of the need for catheter replacement.

Catheter Occlusion

CVC occlusion is brought to the attention of ED providers either when patients complain of their catheter not working in the outpatient setting, or when ED's attempts to instill fluid or draw back blood from a CVC are unsuccessful. CVCs are considered to be partially occluded if fluid can be instilled in them, but blood cannot be drawn back. A CVC is fully occluded if neither fluid instillation nor blood aspiration can be completed successfully. If occlusion is suspected, the first step should be to obtain a chest radiograph to determine the position and integrity of the catheter tubing. Catheter occlusion occurs for a variety of reasons, from formation of medication precipitates within the lumen of the line to development of fibrin sheaths and/or thrombus either within or surrounding the catheter tubing. If a small clot is suspected within the lumen of the CVC, the ED practitioner can attempt to aspirate it from the line with a 10 cc syringe that is half-filled with saline. This technique is rarely successful in removing clots from implanted CVCs, as the small caliber of the noncoring needle used to access the catheter reservoir makes clot aspiration extremely difficult. If clot aspiration is unsuccessful, lysis of the occlusion can be attempted with a variety of lytic agents, depending on the nature of the blockage (e.g. clot vs. waxy precipitate vs. particulate matter). Practitioners should refer to their institution's guidelines for management of CVC occlusion for details on the use of each lytic agent. In centers where catheter fibrinolysis is not within the usual scope of practice of the ED nurses or providers, lytic maneuvers can also be attempted in consultation with an institutional IV team or with interventional radiology. Because it is possible for fibrin sheaths and large thrombi to embolize into the central venous circulation, it is critical that ED providers be able to recognize the signs and symptoms of pulmonary embolus – tachycardia, tachypnea, chest pain, and hypoxemia – and have a high index of suspicion for catheter-related thromboembolus if a patient exhibits these symptoms. Indwelling CVCs also bring with them an increased risk of catheter-associated deep- or central-vein thrombosis. Patients with PICC-associated thrombosis may demonstrate unilateral limb pain and swelling on the side of catheter insertion. Patients with central venous thrombosis associated with either an externalized CVC (Broviac, Hickman) or an implanted port may demonstrate signs and symptoms of SVC syndrome, including edema of the face, neck, or chest and neurologic changes. Both deep and central venous thrombosis are usually indications for removal of the catheter and initiation of anticoagulation.

Air Embolism and Other Rare Complications

While rare, air embolism is a potentially fatal complication of CVCs with which ED practitioners must be familiar. A patient with CVC-associated air embolism may demonstrate acute-onset chest pain, dyspnea, hypotension, tachycardia, dizziness, and anxiety. Because such patients may progress to loss of consciousness and cardiac arrest, ED providers suspecting air embolus must act quickly to prevent further air entry into the CVC circuit. Externalized catheters should be clamped immediately, and the patient should be placed in Trendelenburg in the left lateral decubitus position to trap any air bubbles in the right ventricle. Patients with suspected air embolus should be put on 100% supplemental oxygen, and alternate IV access should be obtained as quickly as possible. To prevent air emboli, patients, their care providers, and all ED personnel must keep the externalized portion of any indwelling CVC clamped whenever the line is not actively in use. Finally, because the proximal tip of most CVCs terminates at the SVC-RA junction, it is important to note that fracture or migration of an indwelling line can lead to other rare intrathoracic complications, including cardiac arrhythmia, cardiac tamponade, or – more commonly during catheter placement – pneumothorax or hemothorax. Patients presenting with these complications are unlikely to implicate the CVC in their chief complaint, so it is incumbent upon the ED provider to have a high index of suspicion in screening for them.

Further Reading

1 Campbell, P.M. (1996). Troubleshooting central venous catheters in the emergency department. *J. Emerg. Nurs.* 22 (5): 416–419; quiz 419-421.
2 Carde, P., Cosset-Delaigue, M.F., Laplanche, A., and Chareau, I. (1989). Classical external indwelling central venous catheter versus totally implanted venous access systems for chemotherapy administration: a randomized trial in 100 patients with solid tumors. *Eur. J. Cancer Clin. Oncol.* 25 (6): 939–944.

3 Castagnola, E., Molinari, A.C., Giacchino, M. et al. (2007). Incidence of catheter-related infections within 30 days from insertion of Hickman-Broviac catheters. *Pediatr. Blood Cancer* 48 (1): 35–38.

4 Cesaro, S., Corro, R., Pelosin, A. et al. (2004). A prospective survey on incidence and outcome of Broviac/Hickman catheter-related complications in pediatric patients affected by hematological and oncological diseases. *Ann. Hematol.* 83 (3): 183–188.

5 Chopra, V., Fallouh, N., McGuirk, H. et al. (2015). Patterns, risk factors and treatment associated with PICC-DVT in hospitalized adults: a nested case–control study. *Thromb. Res.* 135 (5): 829–834.

6 Chopra, V., Ratz, D., Kuhn, L. et al. (2014). PICC-associated bloodstream infections: prevalence, patterns, and predictors. *Am. J. Med.* 127 (4): 319–328.

7 Chow, L.M., Friedman, J.N., Macarthur, C. et al. (2003). Peripherally inserted central catheter (PICC) fracture and embolization in the pediatric population. *J. Pediatr.* 142 (2): 141–144.

8 Christianson, D. (1994). Caring for a patient who has an implanted venous port. *Am. J. Nurs.* 94 (11): 40–44.

9 Coles, C.E., Whitear, W.P., and Le Vay, J.H. (1998). Spontaneous fracture and embolization of a central venous catheter: prevention and early detection. *Clin. Oncol. (R. Coll. Radiol.)* 10 (6): 412–414.

10 Debets, J.M., Wils, J.A., and Schlangen, J.T. (1995). A rare complication of implanted central-venous access devices: catheter fracture and embolization. *Support. Care Cancer* 3 (6): 432–434.

11 Duggan, C. (1995). Central venous catheters in the emergency department: access, utilization, and problem solving. *Pediatr. Emerg. Care* 11 (5): 322.

12 Dyer, B.J., Weiman, M.G., and Ludwig, S. (1995). Central venous catheters in the emergency department: access, utilization, and problem solving. *Pediatr. Emerg. Care* 11 (2): 112–117.

13 Greene, M.T., Flanders, S.A., Woller, S.C. et al. (2015). The association between PICC use and venous thromboembolism in upper and lower extremities. *Am. J. Med.* 128 (9): 986–993.e1.

14 Hendrickson, M.L. (1993). How to access an implanted port. *Nursing* 23 (1): 50–53.

15 Hogan, M.J., Coley, B.D., Shiels, W.E. 2nd et al. (1998). Recurrent deep venous thrombosis complicating PICC line placement in two patients with cystic fibrosis and activated protein C-resistance. *Pediatr. Radiol.* 28 (7): 552–553.

16 Johansson, E., Hammarskjold, F., Lundberg, D., and Arnlind, M.H. (2013). Advantages and disadvantages of peripherally inserted central venous catheters (PICC) compared to other central venous lines: a systematic review of the literature. *Acta Oncol.* 52 (5): 886–892.

17 Kao, C.L. and Chang, J.P. (2002). Catheter fracture and embolization from an implanted venous access device. *J. Emerg. Med.* 22 (1): 95–96.

18 Larouere, E. (1999). Deaccessing an implanted port. *Nursing* 29 (6): 60–61.

19 Larouere, E. (1999). The art of accessing an implanted port. *Nursing* 29 (5): 56–58.

20 Wesley, J.R. (1992). Permanent central venous access devices. *Semin. Pediatr. Surg.* 1 (3): 188–201.

21 Yi, X.L., Chen, J., Li, J. et al. (2014). Risk factors associated with PICC-related upper extremity venous thrombosis in cancer patients. *J. Clin. Nurs.* 23 (5–6): 837–843.

22 Yukisawa, S., Fujiwara, Y., Yamamoto, Y. et al. (2010). Upper-extremity deep vein thrombosis related to central venous port systems implanted in cancer patients. *Br. J. Radiol.* 83 (994): 850–853.

23 Zochios, V., Umar, I., Simpson, N., and Jones, N. (2014). Peripherally inserted central catheter (PICC)-related thrombosis in critically ill patients. *J. Vasc. Access* 15 (5): 329–337.

6

Vascular Access for Hemodialysis

Sarah Fesnak[1,2], Xenia Morgan[3], and Kimberly Windt[3]

[1] *Perelman School of Medicine at the University of Pennsylvania, Philadelphia, PA, USA*
[2] *Division of Emergency Medicine, Department of Pediatrics, Children's Hospital of Philadelphia, Philadelphia, PA, USA*
[3] *Hemodialysis Unit, Division of Nephrology, Children's Hospital of Philadelphia, Philadelphia, PA, USA*

Introduction

Hemodialysis is a procedure to regulate fluid status and remove waste products and/or toxic substances from a patient's blood. Vascular access allows a patient's blood to be circulated extracorporeally through a dialysis machine, where it filters past a semipermeable membrane in contact with a washing solution (diasylate). Fluid and solutes are removed via diffusion, osmosis, and convection. Hemodialysis is one of three forms of renal replacement therapy (the others are peritoneal dialysis and renal transplant) available to patients with advanced renal failure. Patients may require hemodialysis on a long- or short-term basis, depending on their underlying disease process and potential for transplant, with many patients undergoing years of dialysis. Nearly 300 000 patients in the US have end-stage renal disease, and more than 60% of these undergo hemodialysis. The vast majority of these patients are adults, with fewer than 1% of hemodialysis patients under age 20 years. In both pediatric and adult patients, however, complications of vascular access remain a significant source of morbidity and mortality.

Equipment/Device

All forms of vascular access in hemodialysis allow blood to be pumped from the patient through the dialysis machine and back into the patient in a closed circuit. This circulation requires large-caliber access for rapid circulation of patient's blood volume. There are several options for short- and long-term vascular access in patients requiring hemodialysis.

Emergency Management of the Hi-Tech Patient in Acute and Critical Care, First Edition. Edited by
Ioannis Koutroulis, Nicholas Tsarouhas, Richard J. Lin, Jill C. Posner, Michael Seneff, and Robert Shesser.
© 2021 John Wiley & Sons Ltd. Published 2021 by John Wiley & Sons Ltd.

Hemodialysis Catheters

These are large-bore double lumen central venous catheters. Benefits of this type of access are that it can be placed rapidly and used immediately after placement and does not require any additional needle sticks for use. Drawbacks of this form of access include the risk of infection, potential for the catheter to become dislodged or removed inadvertently, and long-term risk of vascular stenosis.

Nontunneled hemodialysis catheter: This is a short-term form of access that can be placed emergently for acute use or to bridge to a longer-term access option. It is typically placed in the internal jugular (<3 weeks) or femoral veins (<5 days) and then stitched into place.

Tunneled hemodialysis catheter: This is a long-term tunneled and cuffed central venous catheter, typically placed in the right internal jugular vein, but may be placed femorally. It may be kept in place for years (Figure 6.1).

Arterio-Venous Access

These forms of access are surgically created anastomoses of the arterial and venous system used for hemodialysis. Venipuncture is used to access the anastomosis at each dialysis session. Benefits of these forms of access are decreased risk of infection as compared with

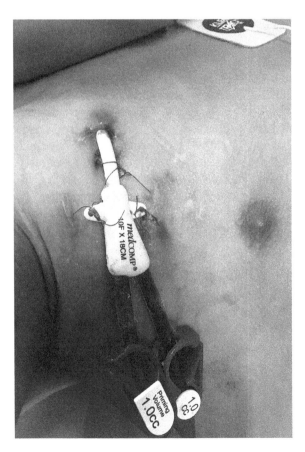

Figure 6.1 Photo of tunneled catheter in deidentified patient. (*Source:* Photo credit Xenia Morgan.)

Figure 6.2   Photo of graft in situ. (*Source:* Photo credit Kimberly Windt.)

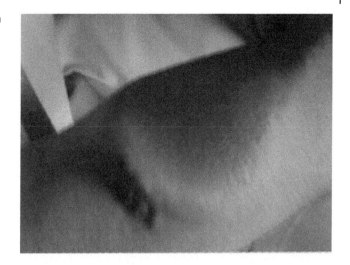

central venous catheters and long use life. Note that the risk of infection remains higher in graft. Drawbacks include potential for thrombosis at the anastomosis, delay between placement and maturation/use, need to use needle sticks to access at each use, and potential cosmetic issues.

- **Graft**: This is a synthetic material that is surgically placed between an artery and a vein in the nondominant arm. It may be placed in a straight, looped, or curved configuration and is palpable under the skin. Gentle palpation will reveal a thrill. Maturation takes at least two weeks before it may be used (Figure 6.2).
- **Fistula**: This is a surgical connection of patient's native artery to native vein in nondominant arm. It will be palpable under the skin. Gentle palpation will reveal a thrill. Maturation takes one to four months.

Indications

Hemodialysis may be used to replace renal function in acute and chronic renal failure. Some of the elements of renal function that may be controlled include the removal of naturally occurring metabolic waste products, regulation of acid–base status and electrolyte balance, regulation of intra- and extra-vascular volume, and removal of toxic materials (e.g. after toxic ingestion).

Management

Hemodialysis Catheters

- Contact with the institution's or patient's renal and/or dialysis team is appropriate early during the patient's evaluation.
- Like all forms of central access, these devices should be handled by individuals trained in appropriate infection control and following the existing protocols of the home institution.

- Dressings vary by institution but may include a transparent dressing or one with a dry gauze component. Antiseptic and topical antibiotic use at exit site should conform to institutional policies.
- Note that catheters are locked with anticoagulant (e.g. high-dose heparin, altepase, and citrate), and this must be removed prior to blood draws or instillation of medications (e.g. antibiotics) through the catheter. If not otherwise instructed by dialysis team, typically the volume removed should be three times the volume of the lumen (listed on the clamp of the device).

Arterio-venous Access

- Contact with the institution's or patient's renal and/or dialysis team is appropriate prior to access. In general, access should be avoided aside from dialysis procedure This site should not be used for blood draws, administration of medications, etc.
- Avoid any other intravenous access or needle sticks in the extremity; avoid taking blood pressures or constricting clothing on the extremity.
- Note that only gentle palpation of the site is appropriate; firm pressure may occlude blood flow.

Complications/Emergencies

Hemodialysis Catheters

- Inability to draw blood from catheter: If the patient requires blood draw from the central access (e.g. in the setting of workup for fever) and clinician cannot draw from the lumen, contact the dialysis or renal team prior to attempting to flush. Recall that there is anticoagulant in the lumen which should not be flushed into patient without careful consideration. Conversation with renal or dialysis team will assist in planning appropriate approach.
- Hole or break in catheter: This should be treated, as with all compromise of central access, as a potential bloodstream infection. Cultures should be drawn, and the access should not be used pending repair or replacement by interventional radiology. Note that lab draws may be inaccurate for up to four hours after a dialysis session.
- Fever or evidence of exit site infection: Cultures should be drawn and antibiotics administered through both lumens of the catheter. Contact with renal and/or dialysis team will help direct therapy; in general, broad-spectrum empiric antibiotic coverage is appropriate but review of prior culture data may further determine care. Note that lab draws may be inaccurate for up to four hours after a dialysis session.
- Displacement or migration of catheter: Displaced or migrated (for example, cuff is now visible outside of skin (as in Figure 6.3) catheters require replacement by interventional radiology. X-ray may help determine the positioning of the catheter. Conversation with renal and/or dialysis team can determine urgency and protocol. Recall that this is a form of central access, and care should be used to apply appropriate pressure to stop bleeding.

Figure 6.3 **Figure 6.3** Photo of fistula in situ.
(*Source:* Photo credit Xenia Morgan.)

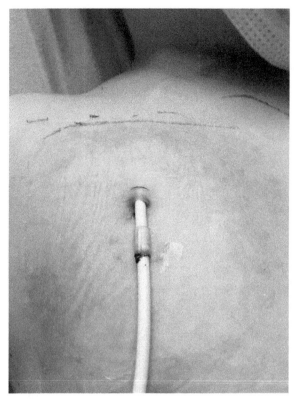

Arterio-venous Access

- Decreased or absent thrill: Patients will typically be familiar with the location and quality of the thrill at their access site. They will have been instructed on assessing it daily. If a patient presents with concern for a decreased or absent thrill at their site, assessment by Doppler ultrasound and rapid communication with the renal and/or dialysis team is appropriate. Delay in treatment may lead to worse outcomes for the access site.
- Swelling or discoloration surrounding access: This may indicate thrombosis or infection. Any evidence of discoloration, induration, swelling, pain, or warmth should be discussed with the renal and/or dialysis team. Peripheral cultures and Doppler ultrasound are often appropriate. Recall that lab draws may be inaccurate for up to four hours after a dialysis session.

Consultation

All forms of hemodialysis access are best managed by, or in consultation with, a patient or institution's own renal or dialysis experts. Early communication with these teams will reduce complications and morbidity for these patients.

Further Reading

1 National Kidney Foundation (2001a). K/DOQI clinical practice guidelines for hemodialysis adequacy, 2000. *Am. J. Kidney Dis.* 37 (Suppl. 1): S7–S64.
2 National Kidney Foundation (2001b). NKF-K/DOQI clinical practice guidelines for vascular access: update 2000. *Am. J. Kidney Dis.* 37 (Suppl. 1): S139–S140.

7

Peritoneal Dialysis Catheters

Jamie Lovell

Division of Emergency Medicine, Department of Pediatrics, Cincinnati Children's Hospital Medical Center, Cincinnati, OH, USA
University of Cincinnati College of Medicine, Cincinnati, OH, USA

Introduction

Peritoneal dialysis catheters are placed for patients in end-stage renal failure requiring dialysis. Although most patients requiring dialysis undergo hemodialysis, around 10% of patients in the US receive peritoneal dialysis. Within the pediatric population, about 90% of infants and 50% of adolescents requiring dialysis undergo peritoneal dialysis. Indications for peritoneal dialysis over hemodialysis include poor vascular access or peripheral vascular disease, younger children, and long distance to hemodialysis center as well as other practitioner and patient preference factors.

Equipment Device

A peritoneal dialysis catheter is a flexible, silicone tube with three portions: an external segment, a tunneled segment, and an intraperitoneal segment. The intraperitoneal portion has several small holes to optimize dialysis. The tunneled segment is from the subcutaneous tissue to the rectus muscles and contains the Dacron cuffs (see Figure 7.1). Most peritoneal dialysis catheters have two cuffs: the first sitting in the subcutaneous tissue to maintain positioning of the catheter and a second cuff sitting within the abdominal wall to act as a barrier for infection.

Catheters vary in terms of length, number of cuffs, and shapes. The typical shapes include straight, swan-neck, and pigtail-curled. Most include a radio-opaque line along the intraperitoneal portion of the catheter that identifies its positioning on x-ray. They are placed most often by laparoscopic or open surgical technique, but can be placed by percutaneous method as well. The tunneled portion of the tube runs medially and should be palpable in thinner patients.

The dialysate is typically in a clear bag, containing up to 5 liters of fluid. It is often buffered with lactate, and dextrose is used as the osmotic agent. The dialysate may contain varying concentrations of sodium, calcium, magnesium, and chloride.

Emergency Management of the Hi-Tech Patient in Acute and Critical Care, First Edition. Edited by Ioannis Koutroulis, Nicholas Tsarouhas, Richard J. Lin, Jill C. Posner, Michael Seneff, and Robert Shesser.
© 2021 John Wiley & Sons Ltd. Published 2021 by John Wiley & Sons Ltd.

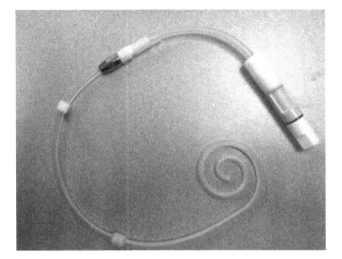

Figure 7.1 Example of pigtail-curled peritoneal catheter.

A dressing is placed over the catheter site after initial insertion. This dressing should remain in place for at least one week to maintain immobilization and minimize risk of infection.

Indications

Peritoneal dialysis catheters are used for patients in end-stage renal failure requiring dialysis. Peritoneal dialysis utilizes the catheter both to infuse the dialysate solution and to remove the effluent. The peritoneal membrane acts as the blood-dialysate interface so that fluid and solutes can flow by both chemical and pressure gradients. This allows clearance of solutes as well as excess fluid from the body.

Management

With the exception of emergency placement of peritoneal dialysis catheters, most catheters are placed by laparoscopic or open surgical technique. An advantage to this placement choice includes precision of catheter placement within the peritoneum and the ability to perform omentectomy and lyse adhesions, if necessary. The patient or family members can perform peritoneal dialysis at home. Accessing a catheter for laboratory studies should be done after discussion and coordination with Nephrology.

Complications

Complications of peritoneal dialysis catheters can by classified as early or late as well as mechanical versus infectious. Early complications occur within the first month of placement and are related to the insertion, anatomic abnormalities, and the change in intra-abdominal pressure due to dialysate.

On presentation to the emergency department, it is important to inquire about the patient's cause of end-stage renal disease, recent complications of their peritoneal dialysis, the patient's baseline weight and laboratory values, and symptoms of uremia. Physical exam should focus on assessing for peritoneal signs, inspection of hernias, auscultation of bowel sounds, and inspecting the catheter exit site and its surrounding skin.

Infusion Pain

Patients may complain of pain during infusion of the dialysate. This is typically due to the positioning of the catheter, an increased sensitivity to the low pH of the dialysate solution, or poor connection with infusion of air during dialysis. Constipation may also worsen infusion pain.

Once peritonitis is excluded, treatment of infusion pain depends on the cause. Confirming the location of the catheter may be useful for patients complaining of localized pain as the catheter tip may be resting against the pelvic wall or intra-abdominal organs. An abdominal x-ray will be able to identify the location of the catheter with the tip of the catheter expected to be in the pelvis. If the tip of the catheter has migrated into the abdomen, it will need to be replaced. Treating constipation with stool softeners may alleviate some symptoms. Otherwise, discussion with Nephrology may lead to adjustments in the length of the catheter or the contents of the dialysate solution.

Bleeding

Patients with hemoperitoneum may present with blood tinged to grossly bloody dialysate effluent. There are many causes, which include peritonitis, menstruation or ovulation, neoplasm, splenic infarct or vessel damage, pancreatitis, and polycystic diseases. Menstruation can be a common cause in premenopausal women. Occasional, transient bleeding can occur when tension is placed on the catheter causing damage to the abdominal wall vessels.

Bloody effluent can be seen after the placement of a new catheter and clears over time. In patients with chronic peritoneal dialysis, the finding of blood within the effluent should prompt evaluation for infection. The dialysate effluent should be sent for culture, white blood cell count, and hematocrit, if possible. Consider sending amylase as well if there are concerns for pancreatitis. Baseline electrolytes and complete blood count (CBC) should be obtained. An effluent hematocrit level >2% can suggest severe bleeding, and further imaging should be obtained.

Leakage

Pericatheter leakage is typically an early complication. Patients are at higher risk with larger dwell volumes, history of multiple abdominal surgeries or pregnancies, diabetes, or malnourishment. Leaks are typically suspected with soiling of the dressing and visible fluid from the catheter site. The location of the leak can also be determined by infusing contrast material through the catheter, followed by computerized tomography (CT) imaging in adults. It is recommended that the catheter be allowed to heal for two weeks before use to prevent leaks. If the catheter requires use before two weeks, low dialysate volumes are recommended.

The optimal treatment is to hold dialysis to facilitate healing. Fibrin glue may be used to seal the site as well. If dialysis cannot be held, decreasing the dwell volume, minimizing physical activity, or performing dialysis with the patient in a supine position can minimize leakage.

Pleuroperitoneal Leakage

A pleural effusion, especially located on the right side in the absence of heart failure or peripheral edema, is likely secondary to a pleuroperitoneal leak. This is typically an early complication, with half of cases occurring within the first month of initiating peritoneal dialysis. Acute thoracentesis is rarely indicated for pleuroperitoneal leaks, and temporarily discontinuing dialysis is the first step in management. Further down the line, chemical or thoracoscopic pleurodesis may be indicated, though most patients with a pleuroperitoneal leak require transition to hemodialysis.

Obstruction/Outflow Failure

The inability to remove the instilled dialysate is a common complication of peritoneal dialysis. It is most commonly related to catheter malposition, constipation, and intra- or extra-luminal catheter obstruction. Plain films should be obtained to determine the positioning of the catheter. This can identify malposition, kinking of the distal catheter, and diagnose constipation.

Catheter malposition causes obstruction due to the distal portion of the catheter abutting omentum or intestine. It can also be associated with infusion pain and typically occurs as an early complication. It may also occur as a later complication if there is migration of the catheter, though this is uncommon due to the use of Dacron cuffs. Newer catheters contain titanium tips to ensure positioning of the catheter. The catheter may also migrate under the liver, which also requires replacement.

Intra- or extra-luminal catheter obstruction occurs most frequently due to fibrin clots or catheter kinking. Catheter kinking can interfere with both inflow and outflow of dialysate. It may improve with patient positioning, but often requires removal of the superficial cuff or catheter replacement. If fibrin clots are visualized within the catheter, first, attempt to "milk" the tubing toward the drain bag. If this is unsuccessful, infusion of heparin or alteplase in discussion with Nephrology can be used to relieve an obstruction secondary to a fibrin clot. Heparin or alteplase should not be used in patients with bleeding disorders or active bleeding, recent abdominal surgery, or presenting with abdominal trauma. If the obstruction is not relieved, patients may need to undergo surgical exploration to determine the cause and visualize the function of the catheter.

Infection

Patients with peritoneal dialysis catheters are at risk for exit site infections, tunnel infections, and peritonitis. Exit site infections can present as surrounding erythema and induration, pain at the catheter site, or purulent drainage. Grading systems are typically used to evaluate the exit site and the risk of infection. The scoring tool includes an assessment of swelling, crust, redness, pain with pressure, and drainage at the exit site. A higher combination of these findings indicates an exit site infection. In pediatrics, purulent drainage alone can indicate an infection. Wound cultures should be sent and antibiotics initiated. Antibiotics are typically given for at least two weeks. For mild to moderate infections, oral therapy is just as effective as intraperitoneal antibiotics. Antibiotic therapy should include coverage of previous positive cultures and skin flora, especially methicillin-resistant *Staphylococcus aureus* (MRSA). *Pseudomonas aeruginosa* is also a commonly cultured bacterium for exit site infections and should be considered if the patient is not improving on their antibiotic regimen.

The skin overlying the tunneled portion of the catheter should also be evaluated. Infections of the tunneled portion may be less obvious than exit site infections and can occur independently. Tunneled infections can present as pain along the skin overlying the tunneled catheter. They may also have erythema and drainage from the exit site. Ultrasound of the tunneled portion may be beneficial to evaluate for infection in the case that pain is the only presenting symptom. Failure to treat exit site and tunneled catheter infections can lead to peritonitis.

Peritonitis is a common and major complication of peritoneal dialysis, occurring at a rate of 1 episode per 18 dialysis months. The mortality rate for primary infections ranges from 2 to 5%. Patients may present with a recent history of exit site or tunnel infections, though many do not have preceding symptoms. The most common presenting symptoms are abdominal pain and cloudy peritoneal effluent. Patients may also have fever, nausea, vomiting, or diarrhea and show signs of rebound tenderness, tachycardia, or hypotension on physical exam.

Peritoneal fluid should be sent for cell count, gram stain, and culture. Also, consider sending amylase and lipase from peritoneal fluid if a secondary cause of peritonitis is being considered. Accessing the peritoneal catheter for labs should be done in coordination with Nephrology and only by trained individuals. Blood work should include CBC and culture. A white blood cell count of >100 cells/mm^3 from the peritoneal fluid with $>50\%$ polymorphonuclear leukocytes (PMNs) is consistent with bacterial peritonitis. However, patients with rapid exchanges and short dwell times presenting with bacterial peritonitis may not exhibit a leukocytosis within the peritoneal effluent, so a clinical suspicion should still prompt treatment.

Patients with elevated amylase levels or feculent material from the peritoneal effluent should prompt immediate surgical consult. If secondary causes of peritonitis are suspected, further imaging such as abdominal CT should be pursued.

Intraperitoneal antibiotics are the preferred treatment for peritonitis. The choice of antibiotics should be based on center-specific susceptibility patterns to cover both gram-positive and gram-negative organisms. Cefepime monotherapy and a combination of vancomycin and a third-generation cephalosporin are used as empiric therapy. Typically, no further imaging or lab work is necessary. In mild cases, patients may be treated as outpatient with close Nephrology follow-up.

Hernia

Patients who are on peritoneal dialysis are at increased risk of developing an abdominal hernia, including incisional, inguinal, ventral, or umbilical. The occurrence rate is about 5%, and the risk increases with dwell volume, length of time on peritoneal dialysis, previous hernias, previous abdominal surgeries, malnutrition, and other causes of increased abdominal pressure such as weightlifting or constipation.

Patients can present with painless swelling, general discomfort, or complications arising from the abdominal hernia. Presenting features may include abdominal wall or genital edema in the setting of an inguinal hernia, intestinal obstruction or strangulation, or symptoms of peritonitis. If not clinically apparent, the location of the hernia can be determined by instilling contrast into the catheter and obtaining imaging. This should be done after discussion with Nephrology. Patients with an abdominal hernia require surgical consult to repair the hernia and should take measures to not increase intra-abdominal pressure, such as treating constipation, temporarily stopping peritoneal dialysis, and avoiding strenuous activity.

Catheter Cuff Extrusion

The superficial cuff may become visible through the skin and can be secondary to exit site infection or catheter migration. If an exit site infection is likely, the patient should be treated as described above. Typically, conservative management is attempted in the absence of infection. For more severe cases with eroding exit site, the cuff or entire catheter may need to be removed.

Further Reading

1 Burkart JM, Bleyer AB. "Tunnel and peritoneal catheter exit site infections in continuous peritoneal dialysis." UpToDate. 2016.

2 Cadnapaphornchai, M.A. and Lum, G.M. (2020). Kidney and urinary tract. In: *Current Diagnosis and Management: Pediatrics* (eds. W.W. Hay Jr., M.J. Levin, R.R. Deterding and M.J. Abzug), 726–751. McGraw-Hill Education.

3 Foley, M., Mehta, N., and Sinert, R. (2016). End-stage renal disease. In: *Tintinalli's Emergency Medicine: A Comprehensive Study Guide* (eds. J.E. Tintinalli, J. Stapczynski, O. Ma, et al.), 584–588. New York, NY: McGraw-Hill.

4 García Ramón, R. and Carrasco, A.M. (1998). Hydrothorax in peritoneal dialysis. *Perit. Dial. Int.* 18: 5.

5 Greenberg, A., Bernardini, J., Piraino, B.M. et al. (1992). Hemoperitoneum complicating chronic peritoneal dialysis: single-center experience and literature review. *Am. J. Kidney Dis.* 19 (3): 252–256.

6 Guest, S. (2014). Catheter dysfunction. In: *Handbook of Peritoneal Dialysis*, 83–92. CreateSpace Independent Publishing Platform.

7 Hoffman, B.B. (2018). Chapter 51. Peritoneal dialysis. In: *Current Diagnosis and Treatment: Nephrology and Hypertension* (eds. E.V. Lerma, J.S. Berns and A.R. Nissenson), 606–618. New York, NY: McGraw-Hill.

8 Leblanc, M., Ouimet, D., and Pichette, V. (2001). Dialysate leaks in peritoneal dialysis. *Semin. Dial.* 14: 50–54. https://doi.org/10.1046/j.1525-139x.2001.00014.x.

9 Lew, S.Q. (2007). Hemoperitoneum: bloody peritoneal dialysate in ESRD patients receiving peritoneal dialysis. *Perit. Dial. Int.* 27 (3): 226–233.

10 Li, P.K.-T., Szeto, C.C., Piraino, B. et al. (2016). ISPD peritonitis recommendations: 2016 update on prevention and treatment. *Perit. Dial. Int.* 36 (5): 481–508.

11 Oliveira, L.G., Luengo, J., Caramori, J.C. et al. (2012). Peritonitis in recent years: clinical findings and predictors of treatment response of 170 episodes at a single Brazilian center. *Int. Urol. Nephrol.* 44: 1529.

12 Piraino, B., Bernardini, J., Brown, E. et al. (2011). ISPD position statement on reducing the risks of peritoneal dialysis-related infections. *Perit. Dial. Int.* 31 (6): 614–630.

13 Rocco M, Burkart JM. Abdominal hernias in continuous peritoneal dialysis. UpToDate. 2016.

14 Schmidt, RJ., and Holley JL. "Noninfectious Complications of Peritoneal Dialysis Catheters." UpToDate. 2017

15 Warady BA, Scafer F et al. International Society of Peritoneal Dialysis (ISPD) Guidelines/Recommendations Peritoneal Dialysis-Related Infections Recommendations: 2010.

16 Warady, B.A. (2012). Peritoneal dialysis and the pediatric patient. *Perit. Dial. Int.* 32: 393–394.

Section III

ENT and OMFS Devices

8

Orthopedic Devices

Carmelle Wallace[1], Andrew Tyler[2], and Keith D. Baldwin[3,4]

[1] Division of Emergency Medicine, Department of Pediatrics, University of Alabama at Birmingham, Birmingham, AL, USA
[2] Department of Orthopedic Surgery, Vanderbilt University Medical Center, Nashville, TN, USA
[3] Department of Orthopedic Surgery, Perelman School of Medicine at the University of Pennsylvania, Philadelphia, PA, USA
[4] Department of Orthopedic Surgery, Children's Hospital of Philadelphia, Philadelphia, PA, USA

Introduction

Orthopedic injuries comprise nearly one-third of general emergency department visits and up to one-half of pediatric emergency department visits. As such, the emergency department physician should be prepared to manage not only acute orthopedic complaints but also any complications that may arise from orthopedic devices. Some orthopedic devices, such as splints and casts, are often placed by nonorthopedists, while others, such as external fixators or prosthetic joints, are exclusively placed by orthopedic surgeons in the operating room. Regardless, the emergency department physician is responsible for the initial evaluation and management of these devices when complications occur. This chapter aims to describe the key complications, emergencies, and initial management related to the most common devices.

Splints and Casts

Indications

In the emergency department, splints and casts are the most common orthopedic devices encountered, as they are the mainstay of treatment for the stabilization of fractures. Typically, splints are applied in the acute scenario shortly after an injury and are used for shorter periods of time (up to two weeks). They are most often a temporizing measure to provide stability to an injured bone or joint prior to more definitive fixation. Casts, on the other hand, are meant to provide more definitive stabilization and are designed to maintain alignment for a longer time period (up to a few months if necessary) (Figure 8.1).

Emergency Management of the Hi-Tech Patient in Acute and Critical Care, First Edition. Edited by
Ioannis Koutroulis, Nicholas Tsarouhas, Richard J. Lin, Jill C. Posner, Michael Seneff, and Robert Shesser.
© 2021 John Wiley & Sons Ltd. Published 2021 by John Wiley & Sons Ltd.

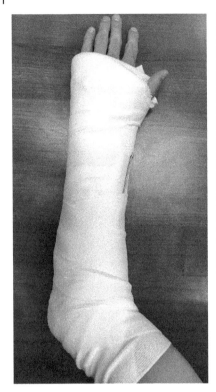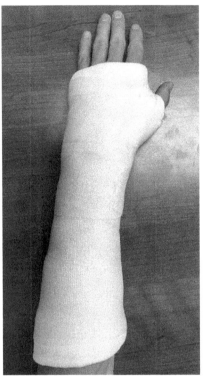

Figure 8.1 Example of a splint (left) and cast (right).

Equipment/Devices

While there are many types of splints for various fracture patterns and injured areas, the basic structure and function of the splint are universal. A splint consists of a stiff or rigid component that provides external stabilization, soft padding between this component and the skin to prevent irritation, and an elastic overwrap to maintain correct positioning. The rigid component is usually made of plaster, although prefabricated fiberglass splints are becoming more popular in many emergency departments. The rigid component is usually noncircumferential, allowing for anticipated swelling of the affected limb, more accessible monitoring of the skin, and easier removal if further intervention is required. For many orthopedic injuries, a splint will be the initial and, sometimes, the only intervention required on the part of the emergency physician.

Conversely, casts are meant to provide long-term immobilization and are, therefore, constructed out of more durable material. Although historically plaster was used to make casts, fiberglass has supplanted plaster as the material of choice due to enhanced strength and lighter weight (Figure 8.2). Unlike splints, casts are applied circumferentially to provide rigid support in all directions. Casts usually consist of a cotton stockinet liner overwrapped with cotton padding, then surrounded by fiberglass that is molded to provide maximal stability to the broken bone or joint. "Waterproof" cast materials are also becoming more popular in the community. These cast materials provide water resistance and thus

Figure 8.2 Plaster (top) and fiberglass (bottom) casting material.

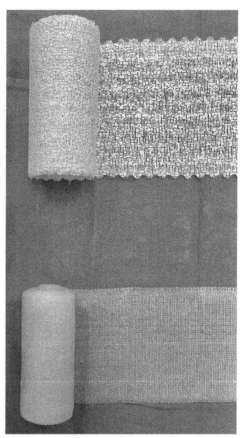

allow the patient to get the cast wet (via swimming, bathing, etc.) without damaging the materials. They also may be less likely to develop odors over time. Though these waterproof materials allow for the benefit of participating in water activities, particularly during the summer, they are more expensive, often not covered by insurance, and may take several hours to dry.

Complications, Emergencies, and Their Management

Compartment Syndrome

The most serious clinical emergency that may occur in a patient with a splint or cast is compartment syndrome. Compartment syndrome is the sequelae of increased pressure in a closed fascial space, often due to edema following traumatic injury, burns, prolonged limb compression, or gunshot wounds. Elevated pressures within the compartment compromise perfusion and the resultant ischemia may lead to necrosis and muscle/nerve death within hours. Patients with compartment syndrome may present with pain out of proportion to injury, persistent deep ache or burning pain, paresthesias, tense compartments on

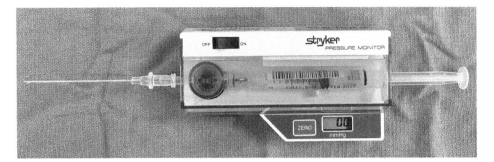

Figure 8.3 Intracompartmental monitoring device.

palpation, pallor of the extremity, diminished sensation, or muscular weakness. Paralysis and pulselessness are late clinical findings. Normal pulses on examination do not rule out compartment syndrome. Casts, circumferential splints, and even elastic wraps can produce symptoms similar to compartment syndrome.

If compartment syndrome is suspected, immediately remove as much external compression of the limb as possible. In a splint, this involves unwrapping or splitting the bandage and cotton padding; in a cast, this involves splitting the cast along the long axis of the limb using an oscillating cast saw, and releasing the underlying padding. If this completely relieves all of the aforementioned symptoms, and the underlying limb is soft and nontender, the likelihood for compartment syndrome is low.

If there is any concern for compartment syndrome, orthopedic consultation is indicated, as the definitive treatment for compartment syndrome is surgical fasciotomy to completely release the skin and underlying fascia of the affected compartment. The "Stryker" test is used by some clinicians to "rule out" compartment syndrome. This involves the use of a hand-held intracompartmental pressure monitor to measure compartment pressure at the bedside. While some nonorthopedic clinicians are comfortable using this device, this is most commonly employed by orthopedic surgeons (Figure 8.3).

If compartment syndrome is highly suspected, emergent fasciotomy, as above, is indicated. This may be performed by orthopedic, general surgery, and/or trauma specialists. If fasciotomy cannot be accomplished at the initial clinical site, emergent transfer to a facility capable of fasciotomy is mandatory. Delay in treatment is limb-threatening, so all efforts should be made to accomplish fasciotomy at the presenting clinical site.

Deep Vein Thrombosis

Deep vein thrombosis (DVT) is a known complication most commonly seen in adult patients, particularly those with lower extremity immobilization. Physical examination may reveal calf or thigh pain, a palpable cord of a thrombosed vein, unilateral edema, difference in calf diameters, warmth, tenderness, erythema, or superficial venous dilation. However, physical signs and symptoms are often nonspecific for diagnosis of DVT.

If DVT is suspected, an ultrasound is usually indicated. In adult patients, clinicians may apply the Wells' criteria or modified Wells' criteria (Table 8.1) to assess the clinical pretest probability of DVT. This scoring system helps guide the need for ultrasound. The d-dimer

Table 8.1 Modified Wells' criteria for risk stratification for DVT.

Clinical feature	Score
Active cancer (treatment or palliation within 6 months)	1
Bedridden recently >3 days or major surgery within 4 weeks	1
Calf swelling >3 cm compared to other leg (10 cm below tibial tuberosity)	1
Collateral (nonvaricose) superficial veins present	1
Entire leg swollen	1
Localized tenderness along the deep venous system	1
Pitting edema, confined to symptomatic leg	1
Paralysis, paresis, or recent plaster immobilization of the lower extremity	1
Previously documented DVT	1
Alternative diagnosis to DVT as likely or more likely	−2

Score of 0 is considered low risk. Consider proceeding to d-dimer testing. A negative d-dimer warrants no further imaging. A positive result warrants ultrasound imaging.
Score of 1–2 is considered moderate risk. Consider proceeding to high-sensitivity d-dimer testing (moderate sensitivity d-dimer testing is not sufficient). A negative high-sensitivity d-dimer warrants no further imaging, but a positive result warrants ultrasound imaging.
Score of 3 is considered high risk with a high likelihood of DVT. Proceed with ultrasound.

test further helps risk stratification. Importantly, other conditions may also be associated with an elevated d-dimer. The Wells' criteria system is not validated for pediatric patients, so the test of choice is ultrasound. Of course, high suspicion for DVT should warrant imaging regardless of the Wells score.

As long as compartment syndrome is not a concern and the indicated imaging may be completed without removing the device, it is best to leave the splint or cast on. However, if this is not possible, removing the device to obtain the ultrasound imaging is imperative. Obtain a radiograph, as well, to assess fracture alignment.

If a thrombus is found, anticoagulation is indicated, typically for three months. If the fracture is stable, the patient may not necessarily require transfer to a tertiary care center, but consultation with an orthopedic surgeon for follow-up within a week after discharge is appropriate. If the fracture appears to be maligned on imaging, more urgent consultation with an orthopedic surgeon is indicated.

Nerve Palsy

Nerve palsy can be caused by local edema from an injury compromising the nerve, but more often results from the compression of the cast or splint itself. It presents with decreased, altered, or painful sensation and is generally limited to the dermatome of the affected nerve. If a sensory deficit is noted on exam, compartment syndrome must be paramount on the differential. Once compartment syndrome is excluded, the diagnosis of isolated nerve palsy should be considered.

The median nerve at the wrist, ulnar nerve at the elbow, and common peroneal nerve at the fibular head are particularly susceptible to pressure injuries from casting and splinting.

Iatrogenic nerve palsy from splinting/casting typically resolves within hours or days once the device has been removed and the pressure is relieved. After the cast or splint has been removed, and a careful physical examination had ruled out compartment syndrome, a radiograph should be obtained to assess for fracture alignment. If both the x-ray and physical exams are reassuring, the patient may be carefully re-splinted, with follow-up with an orthopedic surgeon within a week for repeat evaluation and potential recasting.

The development of an acute nerve palsy immediately following orthopedic reduction is an orthopedic emergency. Additionally, an acute foot drop should be assessed by an orthopedic surgeon to determine if urgent decompression is an option.

Skin Breakdown, Irritation, and Infection

Skin complications are far more common complications of casts and splints and include skin breakdown and wound infection. Skin damage following casting can be benign or more serious. These complications commonly result from inappropriate cast care by the patient or caregiver. Skin irritation and breakdown may be caused by a wet or soiled cast. In some cases, patients experiencing pruritus use a foreign object inserted between the skin and cast to scratch the itch.

While some casts include waterproof padding, the majority of casts should not be exposed to moisture, as this may lead to both skin breakdown or infection. If the cast or splint is foul smelling, or any or drainage (including blood) is present, the physician should be concerned for wound infection. Additionally, patients with sensory loss, including those with diabetic neuropathy, spina bifida, or spinal cord injury, are at great risk for pressure ulcers, especially over bony prominences.

All wet casts should be removed, and the skin/tissues carefully inspected underneath. A splint or new cast may be placed if there is no evidence of skin breakdown, infection, pressure ulcer, or foreign body. Of course, any of these complications should be appropriately treated if found. Radiographs should be considered to confirm maintenance of the fracture reduction. Orthopedic consultation should be arranged urgently to closely monitor the limb, as well as repeat casting, if not already accomplished.

Finally, casts that only have light external moisture exposure may be dried with a hair dryer on cool or low heat. This should only be considered when there is absolutely no concern for internal moisture, skin irritation, or infection.

Muscle and Joint Complaints

Joint stiffness, muscle atrophy, weakness, and contracture are also potential complications in patients who have been splinted or casted, particularly when the period of immobilization has been prolonged. The management of these complications involves physical therapy, stretching, serial casting, or manipulation and strengthening exercises once the cast or splint is removed.

Screws, Pins, Plates, and Wires

Open reduction and internal fixation (ORIF) of fractures is indicated for fractures that are otherwise unstable or cannot be reduced in a closed (i.e. nonoperative) manner. When

ORIF is performed, orthopedic surgeons place metallic hardware in the form of screws, pins, plates, and wires as necessary to provide precise apposition of bone surfaces and stability to fracture fragments. These same devices are used in other orthopedic procedures as well, including osteotomies for limb length discrepancies or boney deformities, bone fusions, and bone tumor resections.

Equipment/Devices

Screws have a variety of uses, including compressing (lagging) two pieces of bone together, holding plates in correct position by compressing or locking into the plate, serving as anchors for wires or sutures, or serving as fulcrums to redirect other orthopedic hardware such as intramedullary nails. They are typically made of titanium but can also be made of stainless steel or cobalt chrome. They are composed of a head, shaft, and point, with a thread wrapped around the shaft. Figure 8.4 demonstrates screws and screw and plate combinations used to stabilize fractures.

Pins often serve a similar function to screws, in that they maintain the position of fracture fragments relative to each other. There are two key differences, however: (i) While pins are sometimes threaded at the distal tip, they cannot provide compression and (ii) pins

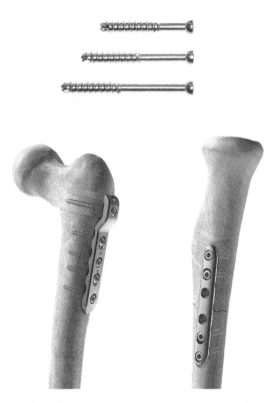

Figure 8.4 Orthopedic screws (top) and examples of screw and plate combinations used to stabilize fractures (bottom).

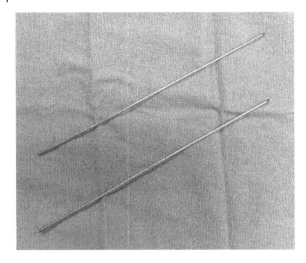

Figure 8.5 Orthopedic pins.

often have an extracutaneous portion so that they can be removed in clinic, while screws are always used as internal hardware. Like screws, they can be made of a variety of metals. They are rod-shaped, but longer and of smaller diameter than screws (Figure 8.5).

Plates have several functions, including compression, bridging, neutralization, and buttressing. They sometimes interlock with screws to provide a fixed angle construct between the screw and the plate. Their primary function is to provide stability between two or more fragments of bone. They are typically flat and rectangular-shaped but can be curved in many different ways depending on their application. They too can be made of several different types of metal (Figure 8.4).

Wires are less commonly used than screws, pins, and plates. They are utilized for tension band constructs, in situations when a strong distracting force may pull apart the fractured pieces of bone that have been aligned. Examples of fractures that may require wire placement include olecranon or patella fractures. Wires are typically thin, pliable, and are made out of stainless steel.

Complications, Emergencies, and their Management

Infection

As with any foreign body, infection is a potential complication of orthopedic hardware. This includes osteomyelitis, soft tissue infection, or joint infection. Due to the presence of hardware, a biofilm may develop which makes organism eradication more difficult. Clinically, a patient with suspected hardware-associated infection may present with point tenderness over the affected bone or joint, or pain with motion of the joint. Some patients complain of subacute symptoms such as diffuse pain or instability. A classic presentation is a patient whose symptoms had initially been improving, who then abruptly worsens over one to three days. If local soft tissue infection is present, there may be erythema, swelling, and warmth. A draining sinus with or without purulence may also be present. The patient may or may not exhibit systemic symptoms such as fever or hemodynamic instability. Infection should also be suspected if the device has failed or imaging indicates any loosening of hardware ("halos" around the screws). The skin around pin heads is also susceptible to superficial infections, given their extracutaneous exposure.

Management includes obtaining radiographs to assess stability, and to look for signs of loosening or failure. Radiographs may reveal periosteal reaction or osteolysis; however, osteomyelitis and cellulitis typically have no radiographic findings. Consequently, a negative radiograph does not rule out infection. If radiographs are normal, bone scintigraphy or a magnetic resonance imaging may be helpful for diagnosis of infection. However, metal hardware will often degrade the quality of the image. Ultrasound may demonstrate a fluid collection around the hardware, which can, in some cases, be aspirated.

If infection is suspected, the patient requires orthopedic consultation. The orthopedic surgeon may opt for debridement, revision of the hardware, bone biopsy, culture collection, etc. If joint involvement is suspected, the emergency department physician may initiate a workup to include complete blood count (CBC) with differential (looking specifically at the white blood cell count), C-reactive protein (CRP), and erythrocyte sedimentation rate (ESR). If any or all of these indicators are elevated, needle aspiration may be indicated to rule out septic arthritis. The most important joint fluid studies include synovial fluid Gram stain with culture and fluid cell count with differential.

If the patient is not systemically ill, antibiotics should be deferred until the surgical cultures and biopsies have been obtained. However, if patient is ill-appearing or unstable in any way, broad-spectrum antibiotics with *Staphylococcus aureus* coverage, such as intravenous cefazolin and vancomycin, should be started immediately. When possible, a blood culture should be drawn prior to the administration of antibiotics.

Loosening, Migration, or Catastrophic Failure

Loosening or migration of the device may occur over time and may be present in a patient who has had a history of internal fixation or other orthopedic hardware. If the fracture has not yet healed, the patient may report a new instability to the affected joint or limb. Physical exam may reveal instability, pain, catching, or locking of the joint. However, if the fracture has healed, the clinical exam may be nonspecific or have minor local soft tissue irritation.

Catastrophic failure occurs when the device breaks or becomes dislodged from the bone (Figure 8.6). Clinically, the presentation may be similar to loosening or migration of the device, with the patient reporting new instability of the affected area. Carefully inspect and palpate the subcutaneous tissue for broken components, as well signs of infection, as infection may increase the device's susceptibility to failure.

While all orthopedic hardware is at risk of failing over time due to repetitive stress, catastrophic failure is relatively rare. Literature reports, however, do reveal a few clinical circumstances that may be at higher risk for device failure.

One circumstance for which failure is possible occurs with fixation of hip fractures. They may be fixed by either a sliding hip screw (SHS) or a cephalomedullary rod and screw. The SHS repair consists of a compression screw inserted into the femoral head; this is attached to a plate that is fixed to the lateral proximal femur by several screws.

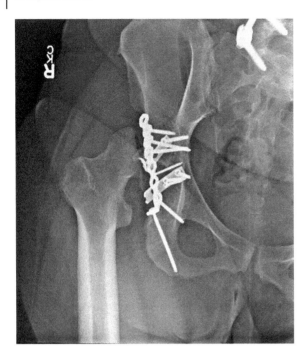

Figure 8.6 Acetabular fixation failure.

Alternatively, the cephalomedullary rod and screw repair consists of a screw inserted into the femoral head; this is attached to an intramedullary rod, which is inserted into the proximal femur. While SHSs have been widely used for decades, they can be prone to failure in specific types of intertrochanteric hip fracture patterns (Figure 8.7). In addition, unintended extrusion of the femoral head screw is a complication encountered for both types of devices. The screw is extruded out of the bone superiorly and into the joint. This complication, referred to in the orthopedic literature as "cut-out," may occur even several months postoperatively.

Another notable orthopedic procedure with high potential for screw-related complication is the screw fixation of the tibiofibular syndesmosis. The tibiofibular syndesmosis is the bony articulation between the distal tibia and fibula. In unstable ankle fractures requiring fixation, the orthopedic surgeon may place any number of screws, typically at least two, just proximal to the syndesmosis, through the fibula and into the tibia. The syndesmosis experiences significant rotational forces with even normal ankle movement. Thus, the screws experience torque and are at high risk of breakage, especially if the patient is weight bearing. This may require further surgical intervention; orthopedic consultation is warranted.

If loosening, migration, or catastrophic failure is suspected, radiographs should be obtained. Prior radiographs, if available, are very useful for comparison. Radiographs may reveal a new lucency around a loosened device, or dislodged or displaced components, if the device has had a catastrophic failure.

In general, if a patient is found to have broken hardware but an otherwise stable joint, healed bone, and no concern for infection, the patient may be referred for close orthopedic

Figure 8.7 Sliding hip screw failure with intertrochanteric fracture.

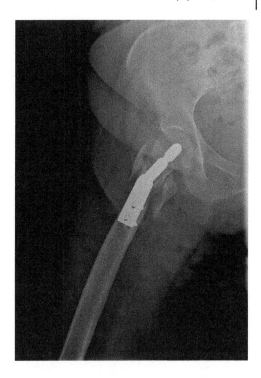

follow-up within the next week. Alternatively, if the joint is unstable, urgent orthopedic consultation is mandatory. The emergency department physician may splint the joint to provide temporary stability while awaiting orthopedic consultation. A revision surgery to remove or replace the hardware may be required, but this is usually not an emergent procedure. Patients in whom there is concern for bone or joint infection associated with internal hardware warrant the initial infectious workup described above (CBC, CRP, ESR, blood culture). Again, urgent orthopedic consultation is indicated.

Intramedullary Rods or Nails

Intramedullary rods or nails (rods and nails are interchangeable names for the same device and will be referred to as rods in this chapter) are placed by an orthopedic surgeon for the stabilization of diaphyseal long bone fractures, most commonly the femur and tibia. Similar to the previously discussed orthopedic hardware, intramedullary rods are usually made from titanium and, less commonly, from cobalt chrome.

Equipment/Devices

Intramedullary rods are long and cylindrical, with a diameter of 1 cm. They fill the narrowest part of the bone marrow cavity and are tapped into place in an anterograde or retrograde fashion. The rod may be held in place proximally and/or distally with screws. In children, narrower and sometimes flexible rods are placed (Figure 8.8).

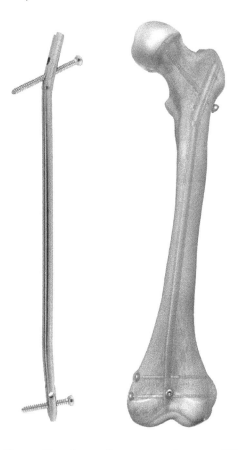

Figure 8.8 Example of an intramedullary rod (left) and intramedullary rod placed in a femur (right).

Complications, Emergencies, and Their Management

Pain

Patients with recent placement of intramedullary rods may present with pain, most commonly at the point of insertion, or at the site of fracture. It is important to note that the patient who has had an intramedullary rod inserted may be allowed to bear weight as tolerated in the immediate postoperative period. Therefore, the development of new pain or difficulty weight bearing that was not present immediately postoperatively is concerning. Radiographs should be obtained to assess for nonunion or malalignment. Orthopedic consultation may be warranted depending on the clinical severity and/or x-ray findings.

Nonunion and Malalignment

Nonunion and malalignment are other known complications of intramedullary rods. These complications are more common with more highly comminuted fractures or fractures where bone loss has occurred. Consider these complications persistent postoperative pain or swelling, joint instability, or leg length discrepancy.

If there is a nonunion, infection must be considered. Fortunately, infections are rare, as most intramedullary nail placements are performed in a closed fashion. This results in minimal soft tissue dissection and exposure, as compared with the placement of plates and screws. If infection is suspected (fever, local warmth, swelling, drainage, etc), the orthopedic consultation is indicated. Initial workup again includes CBC, CRP, ESR, and blood culture. If the patient is stable and well appearing, antibiotics should be deferred until orthopedic consultation is accomplished.

Patients with nonunion or malalignment, with no concern for infection, should have orthopedic follow-up within a week. Nonunion usually will require orthopedic surgical intervention; this is not always the case with malalignment. Fractures of the proximal third of the femur are more likely to be associated with malalignment.

Late Fracture

Late fracture is also a potential complication of intramedullary devices. Patients may present with pain, swelling, or new joint instability. Known risk factors include old age, female gender, or osteopenia. In the immediate postoperative period, increasing pain should be evaluated for a new fracture or malalignment. As always, radiographs should be obtained (Figure 8.9). A new fracture warrants orthopedic consultation.

Hardware Prominence

While this complication is certainly possible with any orthopedic implant, the distal interlocks of femoral and tibial nails, as well as the tips of flexible pediatric nails, are notorious for prominence. Typical complaints include pain directly over the implant and mechanical

Figure 8.9   Periprosthetic tibial fracture with an intramedullary device.

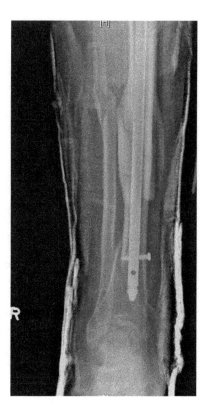

pain. Other complications, including infection and hardware failure, should be ruled out. Outpatient follow-up is appropriate, as the orthopedic surgeon may eventually choose to electively remove the irritating hardware when the fracture is fully healed.

Anchors

Anchors are utilized by orthopedic surgeons to attach soft tissue to bone when there is not adequate soft tissue to suture. As an example, this is common during rotator cuff surgery.

Equipment/Devices

Anchors consist of a suture attached to a metal or bioabsorbable screw. The screw firmly implants the end of the suture to the bone, and the suture is sewn into the soft tissue (Figure 8.10).

Complications, Emergencies, and Their Management

Failure of the Anchor or Suture

Common complications of anchors include loosening of the anchor, or suture failure. Either complication may present as decreased strength in the extremity or decreased function of the affected joint. Local edema or swelling may be present if tearing of the attached tissue

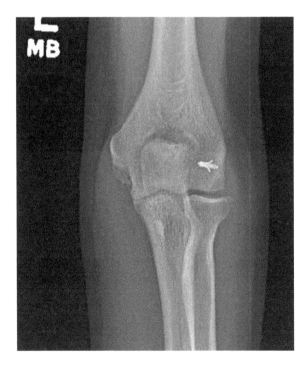

Figure 8.10   Anchor attached to distal humerus.

has occurred. Radiographs may demonstrate dislodgement of the screw, or, with bioabsorbable anchors, lucencies around the anchors due to excessive bone resorption after placement of the device. Occasionally, periprosthetic fractures may occur around larger anchors.

Suture failure may be more difficult to diagnose, as it may have no abnormal radiograph findings. Suspected suture failure requires close orthopedic follow-up within a few days. If the joint is unstable, it should be splinted prior to discharge.

External Fixators

External fixators are orthopedic devices that have both internal and external components. They are commonly used for temporary or primary stabilization of a limb. Typically, they are replaced by more definitive internal fixation later.

Equipment/Devices

External fixators typically consist of one or more external bars that connect to two or more pin-gripping clamps (Figure 8.11). The pins are inserted into the bone. External fixators come in unilateral, bilateral, or multiplanar configurations.

Complications, Emergencies, and Their Management

Vascular Injury

Vascular injury due to external fixator hardware is most likely to be seen in the immediate postoperative period and may present as excessive bleeding through a pinhole. Vascular bleeding may be due to a pin resting on a vessel eroding over time, or, less commonly, associated with a puncture from the initial procedure. While collateral circulation may in the acute phase prevent vascular compromise of the limb, in severe cases, even the collateral circulation may be disrupted and serious bleeding may occur. The lateral distal tibia is at an increased risk of undetected neurovascular injury due to the anatomical positioning of the anterior tibial artery and deep peroneal nerve directly on the bone periosteum. Patients with severe vascular compromise will show signs of hypovolemia, but milder cases, with slower bleeding, may not. Consequently, the clinician should still suspect vascular injury if there are any signs of postoperative bleeding at the surgical sites.

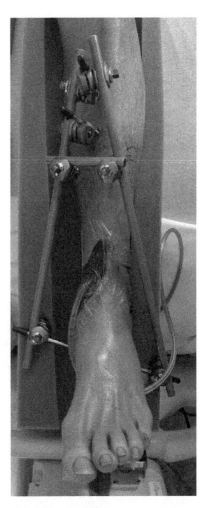

Figure 8.11 Example of an external fixator device.

If vascular injury is suspected, initial management should include resuscitation and transfusion as appropriate. Transfer the patient to a tertiary center with orthopedic consultants available as soon as the patient is stable.

Pressure Necrosis

Pressure necrosis is another known complication of external fixators and is caused by continuous contact of the metal frame on surrounding tissues causing local pain and ischemic necrosis. The affected tissues are at risk for infection. Gauze can be placed between the metal component and the tissue to relieve some of the pressure. Orthopedic follow-up within the next few days should be ensured to allow for any necessary adjustments to the device.

Pin Tract Infection

External fixators are susceptible to pin tract infections, including cellulitis, osteitis, or abscess formation. Clinical exam may reveal local swelling, erythema, and drainage from or around the pin site (Figure 8.12). Radiographs should be performed to ensure there is no loosening or disruption of the hardware.

The majority of pin site infections are mild and will resolve with local hygiene care and oral antibiotics. Typical causal organisms include *S. aureus* and *Pseudomonas* species. Various cleaning solutions are effective, but chlorhexidine has been associated with fewer positive cultures and fewer days of antibiotic use. Twice-daily use of chlorhexidine, along

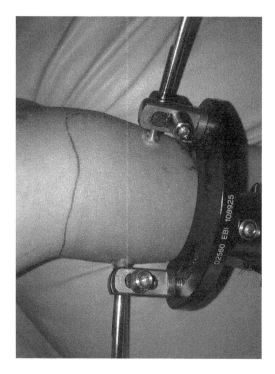

Figure 8.12 Pin site infection and surrounding cellulitis.

with a seven-day course of oral antibiotics with good skin flora coverage, such as cefadroxil or cephalexin, is a reasonable initial course of management. If methicillin-resistant *S. aureus* is suspected, sulfamethoxazole/trimethoprim or clindamycin may be prescribed. If the patient has skin irritation due to chlorhexidine, mild soap and water may be substituted.

If the hardware is intact, and the infection appears to be localized to the soft tissue around the pin, the patient may be discharged with orthopedic follow-up within a few days. Signs of systemic illness warrant inpatient orthopedic and medical management, including intravenous antibiotics. Toxic shock syndrome and necrotizing fasciitis are serious complications of pin tract infections.

Broken Components

Broken components may occur due to falls or trauma to a patient with an external fixator applied. If any external components appear to be broken, radiographs should be obtained to ensure the internal components have not been dislodged or broken. Infection should be ruled out, as broken components should alert the physician to the potential for associated infection. If the external rods are broken or bent, a splint should be applied to stabilize the joint, and orthopedic consultation sought.

Pain

Pain is a common complaint in patients with external fixators. Pain may be radicular due to nerve stretching or compression, or postoperative pain from the procedure itself. Nerve transection is relatively rare in orthopedic procedures, but nerve compression or stretching may develop over time. Postoperative pain typically improves after a week, so postoperative pain persisting beyond a week should raise suspicion for infection. Pain persisting beyond a few days after removal of an external fixator should also raise concern for infection. Radiographs are indicated to assess positioning of the hardware.

If there are no signs of infection, the patient should follow up with an orthopedic surgeon in a few days. More urgent follow-up is required in patients whose radiographs reveal dislodgement or breakage of the hardware. If there is suspicion for infection, a CBC, CRP, ESR, and blood culture should be obtained and orthopedic consultation sought. Antibiotics should be deferred in the stable patient until orthopedic evaluation has been completed.

Compartment Syndrome

Compartment syndrome is uncommon with external fixators, but should be considered in the appropriate clinical setting. This complication is described in detail in the "Splints and Casts" section above.

Joint Replacements

The most common joint replacements are for the hip, knee, and shoulder. They are seen in adult patients who have painful or disabling osteoarthritis or inflammatory arthropathies. In pediatric patients, joint replacements may be performed for patients with avascular necrosis of the hip (e.g. sickle cell patients), bone malignancy with joint involvement, or severe disabling juvenile arthritis.

Equipment/Devices

Hip arthroplasty consists of an acetabular shell, acetabular liner, femoral head, and femoral stem. The acetabular shell and femoral stem are typically made out of titanium, although other metals have been used in the past. The acetabular liner and femoral head can be made of plastic (polyethylene), metal, or ceramic. The most popular combination currently is a polyethylene liner with a ceramic head. Bone cement is typically not used in the modern total hip replacement (THR), but is commonly used in the elderly following a hip fracture if a hemiarthroplasty (femoral component only) is placed. A screw may be used to stabilize the acetabular shell.

The knee arthroplasty consists of a femoral implant, tibial implant, patellar implant, and joint liner. The femoral and tibial implants, much like the hip components, are usually composed of titanium, whereas the liner and patellar components are made of polyethylene. Cement is always used for total knee replacement (TKR) to stabilize the metal components in the bone.

The classic shoulder arthroplasty consists of a humeral component and a glenoid liner. A more recent variation on the shoulder replacement is the "reverse" total shoulder arthroplasty, which incorporates a "glenosphere" on the glenoid with a concavity on the humeral component.

Complications, Emergencies, and Their Management

Infection

As with all orthopedic devices in the body, joint replacements are at risk for infection. An infected joint may present with joint pain with range of motion, joint instability, erythema, edema, or effusion. The patient may appear well or be systemically ill. The most common organisms implicated are *Staphylococcus epidermidis* and *S. aureus*. If infection is suspected, as above, CBC, CRP, ESR, and blood cultures should be obtained. An effort should be made to contact the surgeon who placed the implant for decisions regarding joint aspiration. If the patient is ill-appearing, broad-spectrum antibiotics with good *S. aureus* coverage should be administered. Options include intravenous cefazolin, clindamycin, and/or vancomycin. If the patient is not ill, antibiotics should be withheld pending orthopedic decision-making about surgical intervention, as intraoperative cultures are best obtained without antibiotic pretreatment.

Deep Vein Thrombosis

TKR and THR have proven to be associated with an increased risk of DVT. Though uncommon in children, patients who are older and have significant comorbidities such as congestive heart failure, peripheral artery disease, and end-stage renal disease are at higher risk for DVT. Therefore, any patient presenting with worsened postoperative pain or swelling should be worked up for DVT. Additional signs and symptoms are discussed previously.

If a DVT is diagnosed, the physician should discuss anticoagulation for DVT with the patient's orthopedic surgeon. The decision to anticoagulate and the strategy are both challenging and somewhat controversial. Anticoagulation is a known risk factor for developing an infection in the perioperative period after total joint replacement. There is evidence that the risk of pulmonary embolism is not increased in patients with confirmed DVT distal to the popliteal vein.

Periprosthetic Fracture

Periprosthetic fractures of any joint replacement in the postoperative period may occur. They may be due to the positioning of the components during surgery, the removal of bone during surgery, osteolysis, or simply the result of trauma. Female gender and small size are known risk factors for periprosthetic fracture in patients who have undergone THR. The most common clinical presentation is new pain and swelling of the affected joint. There may be point tenderness on the bone or joint instability. Periprosthetic fractures identified by x-ray require urgent orthopedic evaluation (Figure 8.13).

Figure 8.13 Periprosthetic fracture associated with a total hip arthroplasty.

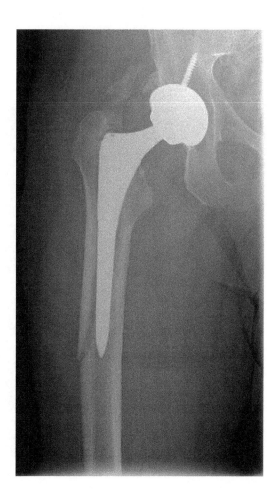

Joint Instability

Joint instability may occur after any joint replacement. If there are no signs of infection and radiographs confirm that there is no periprosthetic fracture or dislocation, the patient may follow up with an orthopedic surgeon in the next week.

Joint Dislocation

Prosthetic joint dislocation occurs more commonly in total hip arthroplasty but can also occur in other types of prosthetic joints. While the implications are less serious than those for a native hip, prosthetic dislocation should be treated in an urgent manner with expedient orthopedic evaluation and intervention with closed reduction typically accomplished in the emergency department setting.

Hardware Failure

A relatively rare but documented complication of joint replacements is catastrophic failure (Figure 8.14). The risk is higher in patients who have had a revision. These patients will demonstrate joint instability, usually with a visible deformity on exam. This complication requires urgent orthopedic evaluation.

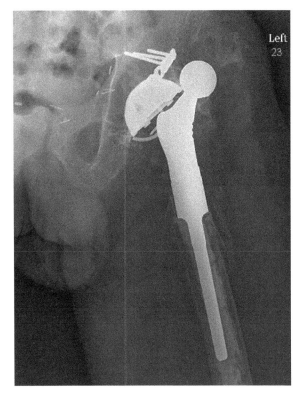

Figure 8.14 Catastrophic failure of a total hip arthroplasty with hip dislocation.

Prosthetic Limbs

A comprehensive discussion about prosthetic limbs is beyond the scope of this text. However, the clinician should be aware that complications include local pressure wounds or ulcers, iatrogenic nerve palsy due to positioning of the device, and limb malfunction. After the limb is removed, minor complications may be treated. The prosthetic limb itself will need to be evaluated by an orthopedic surgeon. The patient may be discharged with outpatient orthopedic follow-up arranged promptly.

Further Reading

1 Rui P, Kang K, Albert M. National Hospital Ambulatory Medical Care Survey: 2013 Emergency Department Summary Tables; c2016 [cited 2017 Jan 30]. Available from: http://www.cdc.gov/nchs/data/ahcd/nhamcs_emergency/2013_ed_web_tables.pdf

2 Thornton, M.D., Della-Giustina, K., and Aronson, P.L. (2015 May). Emergency department evaluation and treatment of pediatric orthopedic injuries. *Emerg. Med. Clin. North Am.* 33 (2): 423–449.

3 Vanderhave, K. (2015). Orthopedic surgery. In: *Current Diagnosis and Treatment Surgery*, 14e (ed. G.M. Doherty), 1061–1147. New York: McGraw-Hill.

4 Elliott, K.G. and Johnstone, A.J. (2003 Jul). Diagnosing acute compartment syndrome. *J. Bone Joint Surg. Br.* 85 (5): 625–632.

5 Goodacre, S., Sutton, A.J., and Sampson, F.C. (2005 Jul 19). Meta-analysis: the value of clinical assessment in the diagnosis of deep venous thrombosis. *Ann. Intern. Med.* 143 (2): 129–139.

6 Bates, S.M., Jaeschke, R., Stevens, S.M. et al. (2012 Feb). Antithrombotic therapy and prevention of thrombosis, 9th ed: American College of Chest Physicians Evidence-Based Clinical Practice Guidelines. *Chest* 141 (2 Suppl): e351S–e418S.

7 Modi, S., Deisler, R., Gozel, K. et al. (2016 Jun 8). Wells criteria for DVT is a reliable clinical tool to assess the risk of deep venous thrombosis in trauma patients. *World J. Emerg. Surg.* 11: 24.

8 Antoniadis, G., Krestschmer, T., Pedro, M.T. et al. (2014 Apr 18). Iatrogenic nerve injuries: prevalence, diagnosis and treatment. *Dtsch. Arztebl. Int.* 111 (16): 273–279.

9 Parvisi, J. and Della Valle, C.J. (2010 Dec). AAOS Clinical Practice Guideline: diagnosis and treatment of periprosthetic joint infections of the hip and knee. *J. Am. Acad. Orthop. Surg.* 18 (12): 771–772.

10 Lobo-Escolar, A., Joven, E., Iglesias, D., and Herrera, A. (2010 Dec). Predictive factors for cutting-out in femoral intramedullary nailing. *Injury* 41 (12): 1312–1316.

11 Davis, T.R., Sher, J.L., Horsman, A. et al. (1990 Jan). Intertrochanteric femoral fractures. Mechanical failure after internal fixation. *J. Bone Joint Surg. Br.* 72 (1): 26–31.

12 Bava, E., Charlton, T., and Thordarson, D. (2010 May). Ankle fracture syndesmosis fixation and management: the current practice of orthopedic surgeons. *Am. J. Orthop.* 39 (5): 242–246.

13 Xenos, J.S., Hopinson, W.J., Mulligan, M.E. et al. (1995 Jun). The tibiofibular syndesmosis. Evaluation of the ligamentous structures, methods of fixation, and radiographic assessment. *J. Bone Joint Surg. Am.* 77 (6): 847–856.

14 Smith, W.R., Stahel, P.F., Susuzki, T., and Peacher, G. (2006). Musculoskeletal trauma surgery. In: *Current Diagnosis and Treatment in Orthopedics*, 5e (eds. H.B. Skinner and P.J. McMahon), 18–87. New York: McGraw-Hill.

15 Chapman, J.R., Bradford, H.M., Agel, J., and Benca, P.J. (2000 Mar-Apr). Randomized prospective study of humeral shaft fracture fixation: intramedullary nails versus plates. *J. Orthop. Trauma* 14 (3): 162–166.

16 Patton, J.G., Cook, R.E., Adams, C.I., and Robinson, C.M. (2000 Sep). Late fracture of the hip after reamed intramedullary nailing of the femur. *J. Bone Joint Surg. Br.* 82 (7): 967–971.

17 Ricci, W.M., Bellabarba, C., Lewis, R. et al. (2001 Feb). Angular malalignment after intramedullary nailing of femoral shaft fractures. *J. Orthop. Trauma* 15 (2): 90–95.

18 Berber, F.A. and Herbert, M.A. (2013 May). Cyclic loading biomechanical analysis of the pullout strengths of rotator cuff and glenoid anchors: 2013 update. *Arthroscopy* 29 (5): 832–844.

19 Green, S.A. (2015). Principles and complications of external skeletal fixation. In: *Skeletal Trauma: Basic Science, Management, and Reconstruction*, 5e (eds. B.D. Browner, J.B. Jupitor, C. Krettek and P.A. Andersa), 177–220. Philadelphia: Elsevier Saunders.

20 Ferreira, N. and Marais, L.C. (2012 Aug). Prevention and management of external fixator pin track sepsis. *Strategies Trauma Limb Reconstr.* 7 (2): 67–72.

21 Jareugui, J.J., Bor, N., Thakral, R. et al. (2015 Sep). Life- and limb-threatening infections following the use of an external fixator. *Bone Joint J.* 97-B (9): 1296–1300.

22 Davis, K.W. (2015). Principles and complications of orthopedic hardware. In: *Musculoskeletal Imaging*, 2e (eds. T. Pope, H. Bloem, J. Beltran, et al.), 1107–1122. Philadelphia: Elsevier Saunders.

23 Fehring, T.K., Odum, S., Griffin, W.L. et al. (2001 Nov). Early failures in total knee arthroplasty. *Clin. Orthop. Relat. Res.* (392): 315–318.

24 Dua, A., Desai, S.S., Lee, C.J., and Heller, J.A. (2017 Jan). *Ann. Vasc. Surg.* 38: 310–314.

25 Jacobs, J.J., Mont, M.A., Bozic, K.J. et al. (2012 Apr 18). American Academy of Orthopaedic Surgeons clinical practice guideline on: preventing venous thromboembolic disease in patients undergoing elective hip and knee arthroplasty. *J. Bone Joing Surg. Am.* 94 (8): 746–747.

26 Oishi, C.S., Grady-Benson, J.C., Otis, S.M. et al. (1994 Nov). The clinical course of distal deep venous thrombosis after total hip and total knee arthroplasty, as determined with duplex ultrasonography. *J. Bone Joint Surg. Am.* 76 (11): 1658–1663.

27 Bonnin, M.P., Neto, C.C., Aitsiselmi, T. et al. (2015 Jun). Increased incidence of femoral fractures in small femurs and women undergoing uncemented total hip arthroplasty – why? *Bone Joint J.* 97-B (6): 741–748.

28 Alberton, G.M., High, W.A., and Morrey, B.F. (2002 Oct). Dislocation after revision total hip arthroplasty: an analysis of risk factors and treatment options. *J. Bone Joint Surg. Am.* 84-A (10): 1788–1792.

9

Spine Devices

Susan E. Nelson[1] and Keith D. Baldwin[2,3]

[1] Department of Orthopedic Surgery, University of Rochester Medical Center, Rochester, NY, USA
[2] Department of Orthopedic Surgery, Children's Hospital of Philadelphia, Philadelphia, PA, USA
[3] Department of Orthopedic Surgery, Perelman School of Medicine at the University of Pennsylvania, Philadelphia, PA, USA

Introduction

Spine instrumentation is used from the very young to the elderly, for stabilization during fusion, deformity correction, and fracture fixation. In children, through the use of growth-friendly implants, spine instrumentation can also be used to manage deformity, while maintaining growth. Lack of familiarity with spine instrumentation and devices may cause unnecessary anxiety when patients with implants or devices present to the emergency department. Investigation of common complications in these patients can often begin similarly for many devices, simplifying and streamlining medical management.

Devices

Most spine instrumentation consists of a rod spanning several vertebral segments that is anchored to the spinal column. Different types of anchors exist for spinal instrumentation. The key component of modern spine surgery is the pedicle screw (Figure 9.1). This screw is placed through the boney pedicle and into the vertebral body. Other anchors that may be seen include pedicle and transverse process hooks (Figure 9.2), rib hooks, wiring or cable constructs, sublaminar bands, and pelvis anchors. Constructs can consist of multiple different types of fixation, termed hybrid fixation (Figure 9.3). In terms of metallurgy, screws may be made of stainless steel or titanium alloy. Rods can be composed of stainless steel, titanium, titanium alloy, and cobalt chromium alloy. The pedicle screw and rod construct is the most commonly used in modern spine surgery (Figures 9.4 and 9.5). The following discussion will focus on devices other than the pedicle screw constructs.

Emergency Management of the Hi-Tech Patient in Acute and Critical Care, First Edition. Edited by Ioannis Koutroulis, Nicholas Tsarouhas, Richard J. Lin, Jill C. Posner, Michael Seneff, and Robert Shesser.
© 2021 John Wiley & Sons Ltd. Published 2021 by John Wiley & Sons Ltd.

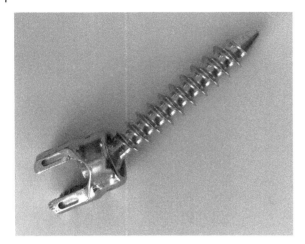

Figure 9.1 Clinical photograph of a polyaxial pedicle screw.

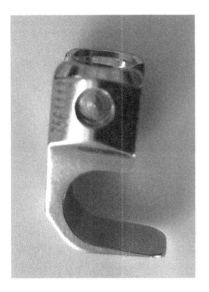

Figure 9.2 Clinical photograph of a transverse process hook.

Growing Constructs

Unique to the pediatric population are devices that allow for continued growth of the immature spine, either through distraction or guided growth. Examples of these growing constructs include traditional growing constructs (Figure 9.6), the vertical expandable prosthetic titanium prosthetic rib (VEPTR, Depuy/*Synthes*), the magnetically controlled growing rod (MAGEC, *NuVasive*), and the Shilla construct (*Medtronic*). Two devices that are unique in design are the VEPTR and MAGEC rods. The VEPTR is semimodular and can be constructed in a rib-to-rib, rib-to-spine, or rib-to-pelvis construct (Figures 9.7 and 9.8). The MAGEC rod system consists of an adjustable growing rod with magnet technology that allows for noninvasive distraction of the implant with an external remote

Figure 9.3 Hybrid construct in a child with cerebral palsy; wires can be seen transfixing the lamina proximally with a cross-link at the top of the construct. Cables can be seen between pedicle screws lower in the construct, and pelvic fixation is achieved with pedicle screws.

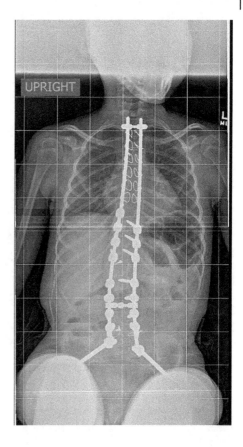

controller. The magnetic actuator can be easily identified on x-ray (Figure 9.9). While traditional growing rods, VEPTR devices, and MAGEC rods require distraction, the Shilla technique fuses the apex of the deformity to allow for guided growth without distraction.

It is important to note that in patients with MAGEC rods, magnetic resonance imaging (MRI) is currently contraindicated due to the presence of the magnetic actuator inside the device. The safety of obtaining an MRI on a MAGEC patient has not yet been verified, so it is not recommended by the manufacturer. Recent research on the use of MRI on *in vitro* phantom and *in vivo* animal models has not shown any dislodgement, heating, movement, or other adverse effects. However, there is significant scattering effect of the MRI, which degrades visualization of the area around the implant.

Interbody Cages

Interbody cages may be placed between vertebrae when a discectomy or vertebrectomy has been performed. These devices are placed in the anterior column and consist of a cage filled with bone graft. These cages can be made of titanium, carbon fiber, or polyetherether-ketone (PEEK). Polymer varieties have metal markers that appear on imaging to assess positioning (Figure 9.10).

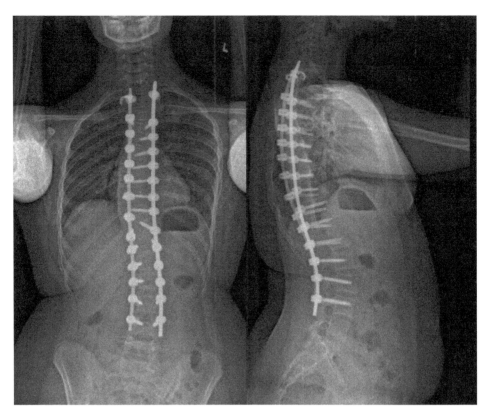

Figure 9.4 Anteroposterior and lateral view of a patient with adolescent idiopathic scoliosis after posterior spinal fusion.

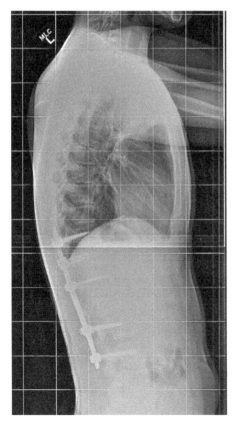

Figure 9.5 Lateral view of a patient with a congenital wedge deformity after posterior spinal fusion.

Figure 9.6 Growing rod construct; the site of expansion is circled.

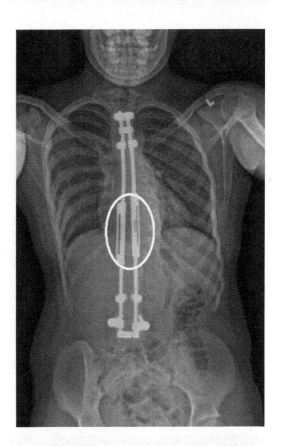

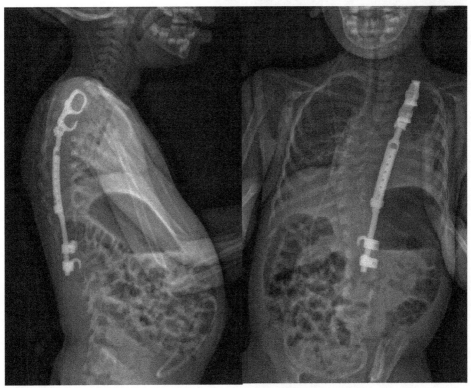

Figure 9.7 Anteroposterior and lateral view of a rib-to-spine vertical expandable prosthetic titanium prosthetic rib construct.

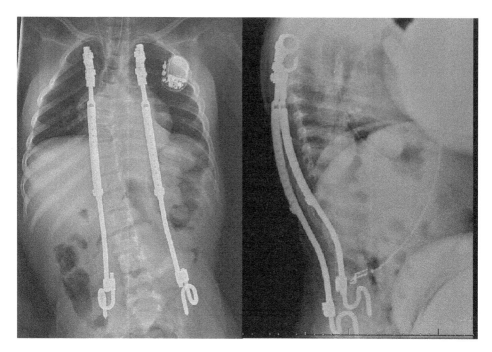

Figure 9.8 Anteroposterior and lateral view of a rib-to-pelvis vertical expandable prosthetic titanium prosthetic rib construct.

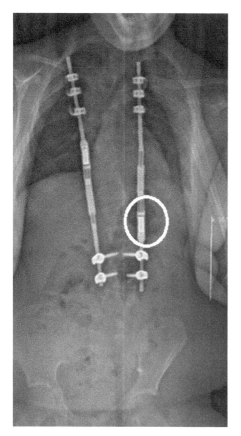

Figure 9.9 Anteroposterior view of a magnetically controlled growing rod with the magnetic actuator circled.

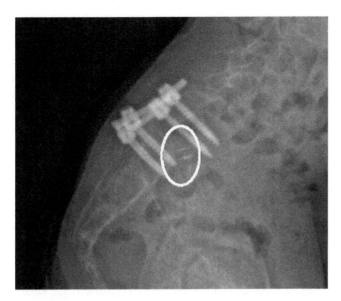

Figure 9.10 Lateral radiograph of a patient after fusion for spondylolisthesis; an anterior cage is circled.

Halo Orthosis

External bracing of the spine may also be seen in children and adults. The halo vest consists of a halo ring with bars connected to a halo vest for immobilization of the cervical spine. The halo may be a pinned or pinless construct. For pinned constructs in adolescents and adults, four pins are used to secure the halo ring, tightened to 8 in. lbs of torque; in children, six to eight pins with 2–4 in. lbs of torque are used. A less invasive "pinless" halo may be used in the pediatric population. This cervical orthosis consists of a padded forehead, occiput, and chin pieces connected to the halo vest with bars.

Indications

Spinal devices encountered in the emergency patient are placed for a heterogeneous group of indications. Pedicle screws and rod constructs are used in a variety of patients to stabilize the spine and allow fusion. In adults, this construct is used often in combination with interbody cages for addressing degenerative spine conditions. In younger patients, this construct is used during the correction of scoliosis and other spine deformities. In either population, pedicle screws and rod constructs may be required for deformity correction or stabilization after trauma or tumor resection.

Growing Constructs

The umbrella of growth-friendly constructs used to control pediatric spine deformity includes traditional growing rods, VEPTR, MAGEC, and Shilla, as described previously. The indication for any of these devices includes progressive early-onset scoliosis in patients who are too young to undergo a definitive spinal fusion. A surgeon may choose any of these options based on preference, patient characteristics, and deformity characteristics. Additionally, unique to the VEPTR device is its indication for treatment of thoracic insufficiency syndrome. The original VEPTR device is a rib-to-rib device used to expand the chest wall for children with thoracic insufficiency.

Interbody Cages

Interbody cages may be used for deformity correction and anterior column fusion in a variety of settings. Cages may be used in degenerative conditions after discectomy is performed, in the setting of spondylolisthesis, and after vertebrectomy for structural anterior column support in the spine.

Halo Orthosis

Halo application may be done as a primary or adjunct treatment for cervical spine pathology. It may be indicated as a primary immobilization method for certain cervical spine fractures, or postoperatively to immobilize and protect the cervical spine instrumentation.

Management

Of the devices presented, only the halo orthosis is external. This device may require management and manipulation in the emergency department for several reasons. In emergency situations, the halo may need to be removed for emergency cardiac or respiratory assessment or chest compressions if cardiopulmonary resuscitation is to be administered. Alternatively, patients may present with loosening or infection of the pins fixing the halo ring to the skull. This will be discussed under complications.

A wrench for the halo bolts should be attached to the halo vest at all times. In case of emergency, the patient should be placed supine, with c-spine precautions maintained, while the anterior bolts are loosened and the side straps of the halo vest are undone. The anterior vest can then be lifted up out of the way of the chest.

Patients with halo vest immobilization may require diagnostic imaging as part of their evaluation in the emergency department. Modern halo vests most often will be MRI compatible. MRI compatible halo vests are composed of graphite composites, titanium, aluminum, and plastic components; these have been tested for ferromagnetism, heating, and artifact. If any doubt exists as to MRI compatibility, the manufacturer's guide should be consulted.

Complications

The most common emergency department presentations of patient with spine devices will be related to pain. Underlying etiologies of pain include infection, hardware prominence or failure, adjacent segment degeneration, junctional kyphosis, fracture, pseudoarthrosis, or nerve compression. Patients presenting with pain should undergo initial imaging with orthogonal x-rays of the entire spine. These are important for assessing any change in implant position, overall alignment of the spine, and presence of boney or implant fractures. Lucency around the screws can indicate an infectious process or motion resulting from nonunion. If previous imaging is available for comparison, this can aid in assessment. Additional x-rays, coned down to the area of symptoms, as well as flexion/extension x-rays, may also be helpful. MRI advances have reduced metal artifact, making MRI a more valuable imaging modality to assess various complications. This is particularly true in the evaluation of infection, as well as the visualization of the central canal and neuroforamina.

Infection

Recent studies have demonstrated that neuromuscular patients are at higher risk of infection. Infection rates for posterior spinal fusions for adolescent idiopathic scoliosis (AIS) are reported to be <1–8.5%, while rates of 5.3–14% are noted in neuromuscular patients. Patients with growing constructs who require repeat operations for lengthening are at increased risk of infection, as well as wound and skin complications.

Delayed infections of spinal instrumentation can occur, so a high index of suspicion should be maintained when evaluating patients even beyond a year from surgery. Organisms typically with low virulence, such as *Propionibacterium acnes,* are associated with delayed infection; these patients may not present with typical infectious symptoms. Delayed infections have been reported in 2.77–6.7% of AIS patients. Moreover, wound appearance may appear benign in delayed infections.

Infection should also be considered when broken rods are discovered, as this may affect the fusion of the spine post instrumentation and the subsequent development of a pseudoarthrosis. Lucency around the screws can be a hint to an infectious etiology (Figure 9.11), although motion due to pseudoarthrosis is also possible.

If infection is suspected, laboratory evaluation is required, including a complete blood count, C-reactive protein (CRP), erythrocyte sedimentation rate (ESR), and blood cultures. Leukocytosis may be absent even in the presence of deep infection. Inflammatory markers (CRP and ESR) are sensitive for identifying and monitoring infection, but elevation must be interpreted with caution when a patient has recently had surgery. The CRP will normalize within two weeks of surgery, while the ESR may take six weeks.

Pseudoarthrosis

Pseudoarthrosis, or nonunion, refers to an area of an arthrodesis where the bone does not heal together, resulting in persistence of a mobile segment. Pseudoarthrosis is possible for any patient undergoing spinal fusion. Pseudoarthrosis is reported to occur <1–8.9% after posterior spinal fusion for AIS, but is less common with modern implants. However, it may become clinically symptomatic years after the initial fusion, with an insidious onset of pain. Broken hardware can also be a presenting sign on x-ray (Figure 9.12). Flexion and extension x-ray imaging may often be helpful in diagnosing a pseudoarthrosis. Advanced imaging in the form of computerized tomography (CT) or MRI may be appropriate based on clinical findings and initial radiographs. Although some artifact is expected, CT can be

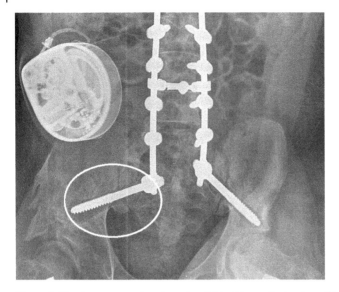

Figure 9.11 Anteroposterior view of a child with cerebral palsy with pelvic fixation with a lucency around the pelvic screw (circled).

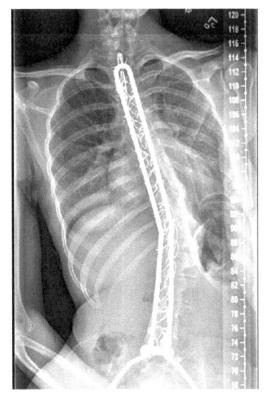

Figure 9.12 Anteroposterior view of a child with cerebral palsy with a unit rod (Depuy/Synthes) with a broken rod due to pseudoarthrosis.

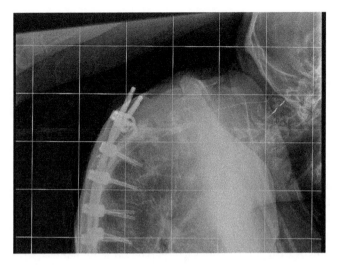

Figure 9.13   Lateral view of a child with cerebral palsy with proximal junctional kyphosis.

helpful to examine implant position, especially of pedicle screws, as well as to evaluate the presence of pseudoarthrosis. Ultimately, however, the definitive diagnosis is made by surgical exploration.

Junctional Complications

Junctional deformity or degeneration may occur adjacent to previously fused spinal levels (Figure 9.13). Junctional deformity is possible with growing constructs as well, particularly junction kyphosis. Junctional kyphosis is where the sagittal contour of the spine becomes acutely kyphotic above or below the level of a construct. Patients may be asymptomatic. Proximal junctional kyphosis has been reported in 17–39% of cases after spinal deformity surgery, though this may have no effect on quality of life. However, progression of deformity and/or degenerative changes at adjacent segments may cause pain and/or neurologic symptoms consistent with stenosis or radiculopathy, which may precipitate a visit to the emergency department.

Implant-related Complications

Specific to the use of interbody cages, migration, or retropulsion (ejection of the device into the canal) may occur. Although rare, patients may present with back and/or leg pain consistent with radiculopathy. Postoperative radicular pain is one of the most common symptoms of neurologic injury prompting evaluation in the emergency department. Patients who have growing instrumentation, such as growing rods or VEPTR implants, are at higher risk for implant complications. In cases where the caudal anchors are rib cradles, migration through the rib and subsequent implant prominence may be seen. The urgency of surgical revision will depend on the extent to which the soft tissue is under pressure from the prominent device, the degree of exposure, and/or the presence of any concomitant infection.

Drift of spinal laminar hooks and pelvic hook fixation is also common, and may or may not be symptomatic. Rod fracture may also occur.

Implant-related complications have been reported to be 0.64–1.37% of all surgeon-reported complications in spinal fusion surgery for AIS. Rod fracture or screw loosening after posterior spinal fusion may indicate pseudoarthrosis.

Halo-specific Complications

Minor complications are common after halo vest application (11–92%), with the most common complications being pin loosening and pin tract infection. If no signs of infection are present, and a torque wrench or torque caps are available, the pins can be retightened to the appropriate torque. Alopecia is a common complication of pinless halo application. If the patient presents with recurrent loosening, once infection is ruled out, an appointment with their treating spine surgeon for possible pin exchange should be recommended. Superficial pin site infection requires treatment with oral antibiotics; pin exchange is sometimes considered. Other complications of halo application that may require revision include dysphagia from relative neck extension, supraorbital or supratrochlear nerve injury, skull or dural penetration of pins, and neurologic deficit from loss of reduction.

Consultation

Migration or prominence of implants that are not causing symptoms may be managed non-urgently by the treating surgeon. In the case of a growing construct, revision often occurs at the time of a scheduled lengthening. However, up to 10% of pediatric patients will require revision of spinal instrumentation, so orthopedic surgical consultation is mandatory. Consultation should be prompt for any prominent implant that has nearly or fully eroded through the skin. Any change in spine alignment, hardware position, or hardware fracture should also be brought to the attention of treating surgeon. This is even more emergent if there are associated neurologic symptoms. In cases of infection, the instrumentation may be salvaged if the infection is diagnosed early and managed promptly with surgical debridement and intravenous antibiotics. Delayed presentations of infection are more likely to require removal of instrumentation. For infection of spinal instrumentation, a multidisciplinary team is usually necessary, including the spine surgeon, an infectious disease specialist, a nutrition consultant, and likely a pediatrician or general internal medicine specialist. Any neurological change or increasing pain associated with halo immobilization should raise suspicion for loss of reduction. Consultation with a spine surgeon is appropriate for any complication that may require adjustment of halo position or replacement of halo pins.

Summary

Although patients with spine devices are a heterogeneous population, this chapter has introduced common spine devices to help familiarize the emergency physician with potential complications and presentations. A high index of suspicion for the complications discussed in this chapter will help the emergency physician initiate an appropriate diagnostic workup with prudent consultation.

Further Reading

1 Gomez, J.A., Lee, J.K., Kim, P.D. et al. (2011). *"Growth friendly" spine surgery: management options for the young child with scoliosis. J. Am. Acad. Orthop. Surg.* 19 (12): 722–727.

2 Cheung, K.M., Cheung, J.P., Samartzis, D. et al. (2012). *Magnetically controlled growing rods for severe spinal curvature in young children: a prospective case series. Lancet* 379 (9830): 1967–1974.

3 Budd, H.R., Stokes, O.M., Meakin, J. et al. (2016). *Safety and compatibility of magnetic-controlled growing rods and magnetic resonance imaging. Eur. Spine J.* 25 (2): 578–582.

4 Eroglu, M., Demirkiran, G., Kocyigit, I.A. et al. (2017). *Magnetic resonance imaging safety of magnetically controlled growing rods in an in vivo animal model. Spine (Phila Pa 1976)* 42 (9): E504–E508.

5 Xiao, Y.X., Chen, Q.X., and Li, F.C. (2009). *Unilateral transforaminal lumbar interbody fusion: a review of the technique, indications and graft materials. J. Int. Med. Res.* 37 (3): 908–917.

6 Bono, C.M. (2007). *The halo fixator. J. Am. Acad. Orthop. Surg.* 15 (12): 728–737.

7 Campbell, R.M. Jr., Smith, M.D., and Hell-Vocke, A.K. (2004). *Expansion thoracoplasty: the surgical technique of opening-wedge thoracostomy. Surgical technique. J. Bone Joint Surg. Am.* 86-A (Suppl 1): 51–64.

8 Chrastil, J. and Patel, A.A. (2012). *Complications associated with posterior and transforaminal lumbar interbody fusion. J. Am. Acad. Orthop. Surg.* 20 (5): 283–291.

9 Diaz, F.L., Tweardy, L., and Shellock, F.G. (2010). *Cervical external immobilization devices: evaluation of magnetic resonance imaging issues at 3.0 Tesla. Spine (Phila Pa 1976)* 35 (4): 411–415.

10 Shellock, F.G. (1996). *MR imaging and cervical fixation devices: evaluation of ferromagnetism, heating, and artifacts at 1.5 Tesla. Magn. Reson. Imaging* 14 (9): 1093–1098.

11 Berquist, T.H. (2006). *Imaging of the postoperative spine. Radiol. Clin. N. Am.* 44 (3): 407–418.

12 Kim, H.J., Cunningham, M.E., and Boachie-Adjei, O. (2010). *Revision spine surgery to manage pediatric deformity. J. Am. Acad. Orthop. Surg.* 18 (12): 739–748.

13 Cornett, C.A., Vincent, S.A., Crow, J., and Hewlett, A. (2016). *Bacterial spine infections in adults: evaluation and management. J. Am. Acad. Orthop. Surg.* 24 (1): 11–18.

14 Sasso, R.C. and Garrido, B.J. (2008). *Postoperative spinal wound infections. J. Am. Acad. Orthop. Surg.* 16 (6): 330–337.

15 de Mendonca, R.G., Sawyer, J.R., and Kelly, D.M. (2016). *Complications after surgical treatment of adolescent idiopathic scoliosis. Orthop. Clin. North Am.* 47 (2): 395–403.

16 Murphy, R.F. and Mooney, J.F. 3rd (2016). *Complications following spine fusion for adolescent idiopathic scoliosis. Curr. Rev. Musculoskelet. Med.* 9 (4): 462–469.

17 Floccari, L.V. and Milbrandt, T.A. (2016). *Surgical site infections after pediatric spine surgery. Orthop. Clin. North Am.* 47 (2): 387–394.

18 Akbarnia, B.A. and Emans, J.B. (2010). *Complications of growth-sparing surgery in early onset scoliosis. Spine (Phila Pa 1976)* 35 (25): 2193–2204.

19 Lall, R.R., Wong, A.P., Lall, R.R. et al. (2015). *Evidence-based management of deep wound infection after spinal instrumentation. J. Clin. Neurosci.* 22 (2): 238–242.

20 Lykissas, M.G., Crawford, A.H., and Jain, V.V. (2013). *Complications of surgical treatment of pediatric spinal deformities. Orthop. Clin. North Am.* 44 (3): 357–370, ix.

21 Lee, D., Adeoye, A.L., and Dahdaleh, N.S. (2017). *Indications and complications of crown halo vest placement: a review. J. Clin. Neurosci.* 40: 27–33.

10

Facial Distractors

Cranial Vault, Midface, and Mandibular

Francesca Drake and Phuong D. Nguyen

Division of Plastic and Reconstructive Surgery, Children's Hospital of Philadelphia, Philadelphia, PA, USA

Introduction

Distraction osteogenesis, or the process of creating new bone by distraction along an oste-otomy, has a long history of use beginning with lengthening long bones. Distraction osteo-genesis in the craniofacial skeleton was first investigated by McCarthy in 1990 on the mandibles of dogs and subsequently used it successfully clinically in humans in 1992. As a result, facial distractors are now used as a standard of care in a variety of patient popula-tions and clinical scenarios. These include cranial vault expansion in craniosynostosis, midface advancement in syndromic and nonsyndromic midface retrusion, and mandibular advancement for obstructive sleep apnea and orthognathic applications. Distraction osteo-genesis relies on three phases of bony regeneration: latency, activation, and consolidation. The devices discussed here include cranial distractors, cranial springs, midface halo dis-tractors, and mandible distractors.

Equipment/Device

Midface Distraction (Halo)

Midface distraction is indicated in midface retrusion, which may cause obstructive sleep apnea and exorbitism. A midface distractor is most commonly used as an external device that consists of a halo (head frame) with attached wires that allows multivector distraction. There are two distraction pins that are placed bilaterally at the pyriform aperture. If addi-tional control is needed, other pins can be placed at the intersection of the frontal and nasal bones (nasion). These pins act as bone anchors for the distraction device. The frame of the distractor is a U-shaped device secured to the patient with external lateral screws. Steel wires are passed through the pins affixed in the patient and are attached to the halo. Distraction is performed by turning the screws on the device (Figure 10.1).

Emergency Management of the Hi-Tech Patient in Acute and Critical Care, First Edition. Edited by Ioannis Koutroulis, Nicholas Tsarouhas, Richard J. Lin, Jill C. Posner, Michael Seneff, and Robert Shesser.
© 2021 John Wiley & Sons Ltd. Published 2021 by John Wiley & Sons Ltd.

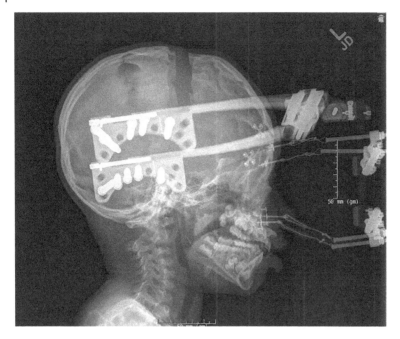

Figure 10.1 Lateral radiograph of halo device for frontal and midface advancement in an adolescent following monobloc procedure.

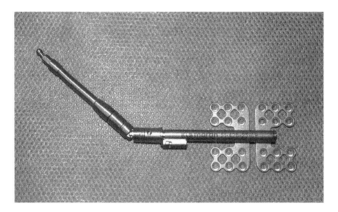

Figure 10.2 Mandibular distractor with spindle arm connected.

Mandibular Distraction

A mandibular distraction device consists of a fixed two-plate system along a spindle arm (Figure 10.2). An osteotomy is made, usually along the ramus, on the mandible. The plates of each device are fixated to the mandibular bone bilaterally on either side of the osteotomy. An extension device is attached to the distractor and passed through a channel in the skin. Most often, a latency period of 24 hours is given prior to activation. The extension arm is then turned 1–2 mm a day, based on the bony advancement ultimately required, using a custom screwdriver. The consolidation period then follows for two months before the patient is brought back to the operating room for device removal.

Mandible distractors come in several different variations including straight and curved shapes, as well as rigid and rotational plates. Device selection is determined by the vector of movement desired.

Cranial Vault Distraction

Cranial vault distraction can be performed for either posterior vault or anterior vault expansion. A cranial vault distraction device is a fixed two-plate system along a spindle arm (Figure 10.3). The scalp is elevated subperiosteally, and a craniotomy is performed. The plates of two distractors are fixated to the skull with screws on either side of the osteotomy. An extension device is attached to the distractor and passed through a channel in the skin. This extension arm is then turned 1–2 mm a day with a custom screwdriver until the desired bone length is achieved, usually 25–35 mm. The consolidation period then follows for two months before the patient is brought back to the operating room for device removal.

Cranial vault distractors come in several varieties including fixed and rotational plates. Cranial vault distraction is mostly used in the pediatric population, due to the closure of the cranial suture lines in adults, and inherent limitations of the distractors to produce necessary pressure.

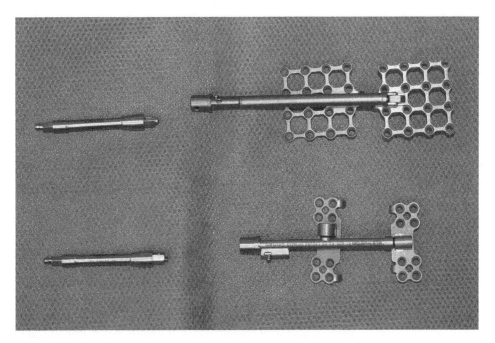

Figure 10.3 Cranial distractor with spindle arms.

Cranial Springs

Cranial springs are metal rods that are coiled into U-shaped segments to produce the desired pressure to create cranial expansion. Most often, these are used for patients with sagittal craniosynostosis. The springs are often custom-made at a hospital-affiliated laboratory by the surgical team. Two to three springs are placed through minimally invasive incisions in the scalp. The scalp is elevated above the periosteum, and the springs are placed over an osteotomy made in the cranium to allow for gradual expansion.

Indications

Midface Distraction (Halo)

A midface distraction device is utilized to treat patients with craniofacial syndromes including Apert, Crouzon, or Pfeiffer syndromes, who present with midface recession, shallow orbits, malocclusion, obstructive sleep apnea, exorbitism, and facial imbalance. Midface distraction allows larger advancements (>10 mm) without the need for interpositional bone grafting or creation of large gaps and dead space. Le Fort-type osteotomies are performed. These can be done in children as young as five years of age. A relatively slow distraction contributes to both a low infection rate and a decreased likelihood of relapse.

Additionally, gradual distraction provides expansion of the soft tissue envelope, which may aesthetically improve repositioning of the lips, cheeks, and eyelids. Furthermore, soft tissue expansion often allows patients with tracheostomies to be decannulated due to a now well-supported airway.

Mandible Distraction

The goal of mandibular distraction is to expand the lower jaw. Patients who receive this treatment in both the pediatric and adult patient populations suffer from mandibular retrognathia. Mandible anomalies are caused by more than 100 genetic syndromes such as Pierre Robin sequence and hemifacial macrosomia, as well as chromosomal anomalies. In the pediatric population, mandibular distractors are often placed in neonates to relieve severe airway obstruction and remedy feeding problems.

Cranial Vault Distraction

Cranial vault distraction is used in patients with craniosynostosis, or the premature fusion of one or more cranial sutures. The two major objectives of surgery for craniosynostosis are to expand the cranial vault volume to reduce or prevent increased intracranial pressure and to create an aesthetically pleasing skull shape. Distraction may be aimed at increasing the posterior vault (posterior vault distraction osteogenesis), or the anterior skull (fronto-orbital advancement). If raised intracranial pressure is left untreated, it may lead to blindness from optic nerve atrophy, or developmental delay.

Cranial Springs

Similar to cranial vault distraction, cranial springs are used to expand the cranial vault volume to reduce intracranial pressure and to create an aesthetically pleasing skull shape. Cranial springs are a minimally invasive option for patients with sagittal craniosynostosis who are less than six months old.

Management

Midface Distraction (Halo)

Distraction of the Halo device is achieved by placing a custom screwdriver into the cross frame over the patient's midface where the wires from the distraction pins attach to the distractor. The screws are turned gradually to produce the desired midface advancement.

Cranial springs are placed in the operating room, and no additional management is needed.

Cranial vault and mandibular distraction: Distraction of the device is achieved by placing the screwdriver on the end of the distractor activator arm; then, using the flat side of the screwdriver handle and the arrow as a guide, the screwdriver is turned in the direction of the arrow (Figure 10.4).

Complications/Emergencies

Midface Distraction (Halo)

The most common device complications are mechanical failures, such as distractor pin loosing, broken wires or pins, frame migration, and dislodgement of transcranial fixation pins.

During presentation to the hospital or outpatient clinic, patients should undergo physical examination with special attention directed to mechanical device failure and signs of infection at pin sites. Plain film radiographs (posteroanterior [PA] and lateral) should be performed. Radiographs are evaluated for device positioning and interpositional bone growth. If the patient is in an outside hospital, studies should be sent to the surgical team where the distractor was placed. The primary surgical team will then decide if immediate transfer to the primary hospital is necessary for management. If there is concern for migration of intracranial pins, the patient will need a computerized tomography (CT) scan to evaluate for dural perforation causing a cerebrospinal fluid (CSF) leak. This will require neurosurgical consultation. For other mechanical failures, determination will be made by the operating surgeon to replace or remove the broken distractor components.

Patients with midface distractors may have airway compromise. Once a patent airway is established, the surgical team may be consulted for ensuing steps. Patients should always have a wire cutter and screwdriver for the device with them to allow for quick removal of the head frame to establish airway support. Figure 10.5 outlines the management strategy of these patients.

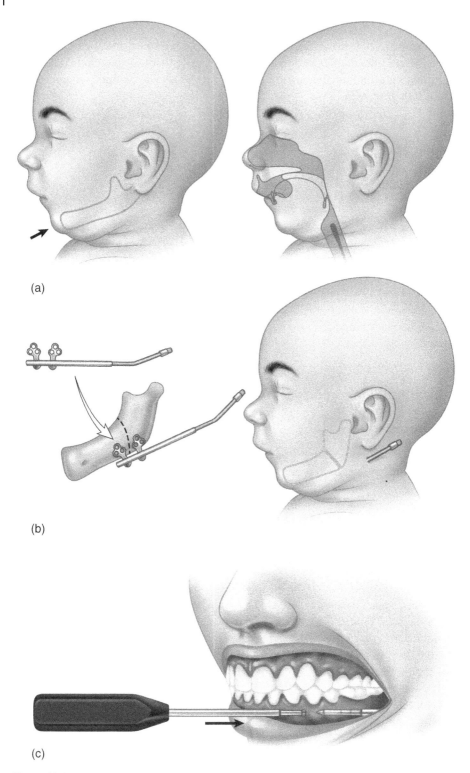

(a)

(b)

(c)

Figure 10.4 Illustration of retrognathic patient (a), mandibular distraction device placement and osteotomy (b), and screwdriver and turning of spindle arm (c).

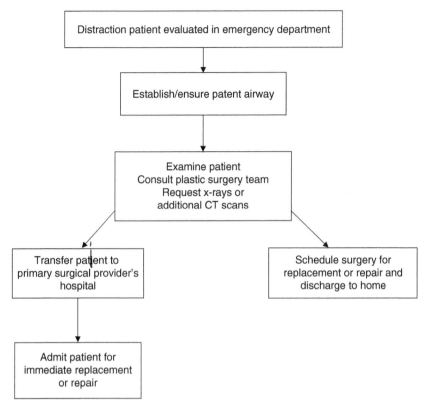

Figure 10.5 Algorithm for the management strategy of a distraction patient in the emergency department.

Cranial Springs

Complications of cranial springs include CSF leak from dural perforation during placement and dislodgement. A CT scan may be obtained to ascertain placement of the spring and assess for dural penetration. Plain film radiograph (PA/lateral) may be obtained initially to check for device placement. Bone formation within the craniotomy gap should be evaluated. If the springs are dislodged, consultation with the primary surgeon will determine replacement versus removal.

Cranial Vault and Mandible Distraction

The most common device complications are mechanical failure, such as a broken spindle, or dislodgement. Patients and their families often note that the distractor is no longer turning properly.

During admission to the hospital or outpatient clinic, the patient should be examined and have radiographs taken of the device to evaluate its integrity. Similar to midface distractors, determination will be made regarding replacement versus removal by the primary surgeon. Imaging should be forwarded to the surgical team responsible for the device.

Additional CT scan imaging may be required if there is concern for dural penetration. If there is evidence for CSF leak, neurosurgical consultation is paramount. There may also be higher risk of spindle malfunction in older patients due to increased scar burden placing undue stress on the distractor.

Mandibular distractor patients may have airway-related complications. Priority is given to establishing a patent airway, while the surgical team may be consulted for device management secondarily, as noted in Figure 10.5.

Consultation

Midface Distraction (Halo), Cranial Springs, and Distractors:

Ensuring airway patency is the priority, particularly for patients with midface and mandibular distractors. The primary plastic surgery team should be consulted, and the patient transferred as needed. Often, distraction devices necessitate secondary surgical procedures for repair, replacement, or removal. Neurosurgical consultation is required when there is concern for CSF leak.

Further Reading

1 Karp, N.S., Thorne, C.H., McCarthy, J.G., and Sissons, H.A. (1990). Bone lengthening in the craniofacial skeleton. *Ann. Plast. Surg.* 24: 231–237.

2 McCarthy, J.G., Schreiber, J., Karp, N. et al. (1992). Lengthening the human mandible by gradual distraction. *Plast. Reconstr. Surg.* 89: 1–8; discussion 9-10.

3 Hong, P. and Bezuhly, M. (2013). Mandibular distraction osteogenesis in the micrognathic neonate: a review for neonatologists and pediatricians. *Pediatr. Neonatol.* 54: 153–160.

4 Arko, L.t., Swanson, J.W., Fierst, T.M. et al. (2015). Spring-mediated sagittal craniosynostosis treatment at the Children's Hospital of Philadelphia: technical notes and literature review. *Neurosurg. Focus.* 38: E7.

5 Tahiri, Y. and Taylor, J. (2014). An update on Midface advancement using Le fort II and III distraction Osteogenesis. *Semin. Plast. Surg.* 28: 184–192.

6 Derderian, C.A., Wink, J.D., McGrath, J.L. et al. (2015). Volumetric changes in cranial vault expansion: comparison of fronto-orbital advancement and posterior cranial vault distraction osteogenesis. *Plast. Reconstr. Surg.* 135: 1665–1672.

11

Management of Facial Fractures in Adults and Children

Sameer Shakir[1] and Phuong D. Nguyen[2]

[1] *Division of Plastic Surgery, Children's Hospital of Philadelphia, Philadelphia, PA, USA*
[2] *Division of Plastic and Reconstructive Surgery, Children's Hospital of Philadelphia, Philadelphia, PA, USA*

Introduction

Traumatic injury accounts for 25% of all emergency department (ED) visits and one in eight hospital admissions nationally, with a substantial portion attributable to the cranio-maxillofacial (CMF) skeleton. Adult injuries may result from both low- and high-energy impacts and have resultant differences in fracture distribution. Low-energy impacts include falls from standing or sports injuries, while high-energy impacts include motor vehicle collisions, gunshot, and ballistic wounds. These facial trauma patients are four times more likely to be male than female, with a median age of 35 years.

In contrast, injuries to the growing pediatric CMF skeleton significantly diverge from their adult counterparts. The pediatric facial skeleton is more elastic, given its less ossified and pneumatized properties, allowing for a significant amount of energy to be absorbed without fracture when compared to adults. This elasticity often results in minimally displaced "green-stick" fractures, in contrast to comminuted eggshell or blow-out fractures seen in adults. The incidence of these facial fractures correlates with age, as there is a greater risk with contact activities and sports. Pediatric facial fractures present unique treatment dilemmas given the concern for ongoing growth and development. The cranial-to-facial ratio goes from 8 : 1 at birth, to 2 : 1 by adulthood, leading to a greater number of fractures of the skull vault and orbital roof in the young, while adolescents and adults exhibit a higher incidence of mandible fractures.

As a general rule, fractures of the growing CMF skeleton are often managed conservatively unless there is a complicating factor necessitating earlier operative intervention. The goal of management is to restore preinjury structure and function while minimizing the potential for future growth disturbance. Evaluation and treatment of pediatric CMF trauma has significantly improved with readily available computerized tomography (CT) imaging.

Emergency Management of the Hi-Tech Patient in Acute and Critical Care, First Edition. Edited by
Ioannis Koutroulis, Nicholas Tsarouhas, Richard J. Lin, Jill C. Posner, Michael Seneff, and Robert Shesser.
© 2021 John Wiley & Sons Ltd. Published 2021 by John Wiley & Sons Ltd.

Fine-cut CT scans through the CMF skeleton are now considered the standard of care. Significantly displaced CMF fractures may require closed or open reduction, internal or external fixation, or, for isolated indications, external splinting.

Anatomy

The CMF skeleton can be classified into facial thirds.

Mandible
Midface
Orbital roof, cranial base, and vault

Evaluation

Primary Survey

The assessment of a trauma patient remains universal. Advanced Trauma Life Support protocols should be followed by the treating emergency department and/or trauma surgery team. The CMF assessment should be initiated only after the primary survey has been completed with thorough evaluation of the airway, breathing, circulation, and central nervous system. Verschueren et al. found that greater than 95% of all patients with airways compromised due to laryngotracheal injuries had concomitant CMF injuries. These are often clinically identified by aspirated teeth, excessive upper airway bleeding, and/or bony fragments. Emergent airway management should be dictated by patient stability, with stable patients undergoing nasotracheal intubation with fiberoptic assistance, and unstable patients undergoing awake tracheostomy. Massive bleeding and hemorrhage should be initially managed with direct pressure, packing, or a compressive dressing. Vascular clamping, vessel ligation, and/or electrocauterization in the ED is to be avoided to prevent inadvertent injury to essential structures. All patients with facial fractures should be evaluated for underlying cervical spine injury with both clinical examination and CT imaging. Data suggest that 2–10% of patients presenting with CMF fractures are found to have concomitant cervical spine injuries, while 15–20% of patients with cervical spine injuries have concomitant CMF fractures. When orbital fractures are present, formal ophthalmologic evaluation and consultation should be performed to document visual acuity, extra-ocular movements, pupil size, and reactivity. Blindness resulting from CMF trauma is relatively rare, with a reported incidence of 2–5%. Blindness can be classified as immediate, delayed, or postoperative. Accepted treatments for traumatic optic nerve injury may include observation, corticosteroids, osmotic diuretics, and/or surgical decompression; a universally applicable algorithm does not exist. If there is suspicion for postoperative optic nerve injury, it is imperative to obtain CT imaging and urgently surgically decompress the orbit to prevent lasting visual deficits.

Secondary Survey

A secondary CMF survey is helpful in isolating specific fracture patterns prior to confirmation with CT imaging. Table 11.1 depicts classic history and physical examination findings associated with specific CMF fractures.

Indications and Equipment/Devices

Mandible Fractures

Approximately 40% of pediatric CMF fractures relate to the mandible, with an even greater proportion in the adult population. As children age, there is a caudal shift in fracture patterns from the condyle to the angle and body of the mandible. Evaluation of the injured mandible begins with inspection and palpation from condyle to condyle. Areas of swelling, tenderness, and misaligned teeth correlate to sites of fracture. Often, fractures result in paresthesia along the trigeminal nerve V3 distribution, related to neuropraxic injury or, rarely, transection of the infra-alveolar nerve. Both subjective and objective occlusal relationships are evaluated in addition to documentation of cross-bites and open-bites. Temporomandibular joint (TMJ) function can be assessed by roughly calculating protrusion, lateralization, and maximal incisor opening.

The goal of mandibular fracture treatment is to restore preinjury occlusion while minimizing stiffness and delay of function. Pediatric mandible fractures are treated more conservatively, as one aims to minimize growth disturbances. Mandible rest can be achieved with the use of a circumferentially wrapped ACE bandage known as a "jaw bra," or with a cervical collar.

Open reduction and internal fixation can affect future growth and injure underlying dental follicles and should be reserved for specific cases in pediatric mandibular trauma. After mandibular skeletal maturity (16–18 years in females, and 18–20 years in males), one treats fracture patterns similarly. Displaced mandibular body or angle fractures resulting in malocclusion may require surgical treatment, while (sub)condylar fractures are often managed conservatively due to concerns for growth impairment, TMJ ankylosis, and injury to the facial nerve. Condylar head fractures, for this reason, are treated with early joint physical therapy and range of motion exercises within three to five days postinjury to reduce the potential for TMJ ankylosis. Indications for operative management of condylar fractures include (i) malocclusion without successful closed reduction, (ii) condyle displacement into the middle cranial fossa, (iii) foreign body within joint, and (iv) bilateral neck fracture. Minimally displaced fractures with or without minor malocclusion are otherwise best managed conservatively.

Mandible fractures may be treated with maxillomandibular fixation (MMF) and/or rigid fixation. There are several methods of MMF, including Erich arch bars, intermaxillary fixation (IMF) screws, hybrid arch bar systems, and occasionally, less common methods such as drop wires and ivy loops (Figure 11.1). MMF is used in situations that require splinting, such as closed reduction, or when easy passive occlusion is unable to be obtained. Erich arch bars consist of a malleable steel bar with lugs to accommodate elastics or wires to immobilize the

Table 11.1 Commonly encountered craniomaxillofacial (CMF) fractures with associated history and physical examination findings.

CMF fracture type	Complaints	Findings
Mandible	• Malocclusion • Temporomandibular joint pain • Trismus	• Occlusal deviation • Floor of mouth ecchymosis • Paresthesia (mental)
Maxillary	• Malocclusion	• Midface edema • Periorbital ecchymosis • Epistaxis • Palpable step-offs • Crepitus • Maxillary mobility • Tenderness along pterygomaxillary buttresses
Zygomaticomaxillary complex	• Cheek/maxillary teeth numbness • Trismus	• Malar flattening • Enophthalmos • Dystopia • Downsloping palpebral fissure • Intraorbital paresthesia • Orbital rim, zygomatic arch, zygomaticomaxillary buttress step-offs
Nasal	• Epistaxis	• Visible deformity • Compressibility of the dorsum • Nasal edema • Nasal laceration • Epistaxis • Crepitus • Tenderness • Septal deviation • Septal hematoma
Orbital	• Diplopia • Visual change	• Periorbital edema • Periorbital ecchymosis • Orbital rim step-off • Subconjunctival hematoma • Limited eye excursions • Enophthalmos/exophthalmos • Diplopia • Infraorbital nerve hypoesthesia
Naso-orbital-ethmoid	• Epistaxis	• Telecanthus • Loss of dorsal nose projection • Periorbital edema/ecchymosis • Nasal lacerations • Orbital rim step-offs • Subconjunctival hemorrhage

Table 11.1 (Continued)

CMF fracture type	Complaints	Findings
Frontal sinus/ cribiform plate	• Rhinorrhea • Headache	• Upper face edema, ecchymosis • Palpable frontal bone step-off • Paresthesia (supraorbital, supratrochlear) • Rhinorrhea (CSF) • Globe displacement
Temporal bone	• Hearing loss • Otorrhea	• Hemotympanum • Mastoid ecchymosis (Battle's sign) • Facial paralysis • Otorrhea

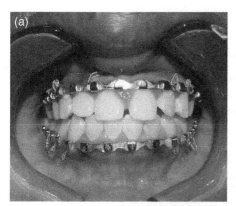
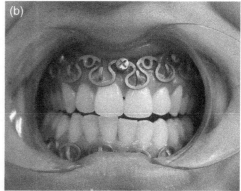
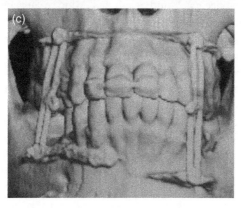

Figure 11.1 Examples of methods of maxillomandibular fixation (MMF). (a) Erich arch bars, (b) hybrid MMF, (c) intermaxillary fixation (IMF) screws.

maxillary and mandibular arches together. These are affixed to the dental arches using circumdental steel wires. The advantages of arch bars include multiple points of fixation for stability, as well as relative inexpensiveness. Disadvantages include prolonged time required for placement and potential injury from the sharp ends of the wires. IMF screws are self-drilling screws that contain a groove under the screw-head to secure wires or elastics and two cross-holes aligned with the cruciform head to accommodate wire passage. These are placed above or between the dental roots, most commonly lateral to the canines. Advantages of IMF screws include ease and reduced application time, as well as reduced potential for self-injury with wire sticks. Disadvantages include being applicable only in situations with simple fracture patterns and reduced number of points of fixation. More recently, there has been the advent of hybrid arch bar systems that combine the advantages of both IMF screws and traditional arch bars. These are essentially arch bars that have screw holes attached to them such that they do not require interdental wire fixation and are thus relatively quick to apply. The disadvantages include increased cost and their relatively large size, reducing the amount of space available for rigid fixation. Severely comminuted fractures may not be amenable for internal fixation, so an external fixator may be required.

Midface (Maxillary, Nasal, Tripod, Orbital, and NOE) Fractures

The midface patterns consist of maxillary, zygomatic, nasal, and orbital fractures. CT imaging is critical in identifying midface injuries, as physical examination is often limited. Examination findings may consist of bony step-offs, malocclusion, and mobile segments. There may be overlying soft tissue lacerations, hematoma, or ecchymoses. The infraorbital nerve distribution may also be affected, resulting in numbness of the cheek, upper lip, and nasal side wall. Any rhinorrhea observed in the setting of CMF trauma should be promptly tested for cerebrospinal fluid with a low threshold to obtain neurosurgical consultation. In the pediatric population, similar to mandible fractures, midface fractures are often treated conservatively, with adherence to a liquid or soft diet. Minor malocclusion is well tolerated and can be addressed with orthodontic treatment at a later age.

Nasal fractures are quite common and have been reported as the most common facial fracture. These may often result from low- or high-energy impacts and present with swelling, tenderness, and ecchymosis. Due to acute swelling, it is often difficult to confirm fracture and displacement on physical examination. X-rays may be helpful. When confirmation is necessary, CT imaging may be obtained. Confirmed nasal fractures should usually be referred to a surgeon specializing in facial fractures in one week. This allows for a reduction in swelling, and, thus, a better assessment of cosmetic implications. Nasal fractures are amenable to closed reduction within a two-week window from the time of injury.

Secondary deformities are best treated at the time of skeletal maturity with elective septorhinoplasty. The nasal septum is the growth center for nose, so aggressive premature manipulation is to be avoided. Suggestion of clear nasal discharge or rhinorrhea should be evaluated for CSF with prompt neurosurgical evaluation. An intranasal examination should be performed to evaluate for septal hematoma. Suggestion of evolving hematoma requires emergent drainage to prevent abscess formation, septal thickening, septal perforation, or saddle-nose deformity due to septal cartilage resorption. Nasal packing or splints are often placed postdrainage to provide compression at the site.

The classic pattern of malar flattening, enophthalmos, and lateral canthal displacement define zygomaticomaxillary complex (ZMC) fractures. Previously, these were misnamed as "tripod" fractures, as there are actually *four* sites of articulation: zygomaticofrontal (ZF), zygomaticomaxillary (ZM), zygomaticotemporal (ZT), and zygomaticosphenoid (ZS). Minimally displaced fractures with no obvious deformity are managed conservatively. When ZMC fractures require surgical treatment, reduction and rigid fixation occur at three anatomic sites: (i) ZF suture, (ii) inferior orbital rim/floor, and (iii) ZM suture, with care to avoid rigid fixation within developing maxillary tooth buds. Fixation is performed using titanium plates and screws, or, less commonly, steel wire.

Orbital fracture repair aims to release entrapped extra-ocular muscles, correct vertical orbital dystopia (VOD), and prevent enophthalmos. Pediatric orbital trauma is associated with an increased risk for blindness, as much as 3% according to one source. Providers must, therefore, have a low threshold for ophthalmologic consultation. Orbital trauma can be thought of as affecting the floor or roof. Upon direct impact to the orbit, the orbital floor is the weakest component of the bony orbit and is susceptible to blow-out fractures. In children, these may present as incomplete or "green-stick" fractures, as a result of less ossified bones, minimally pneumatized maxillary sinuses, and developing tooth buds that can absorb a significant amount of energy. During green-stick fracture of the orbital floor, the inferior rectus muscle may become entrapped when the inferior orbit snaps back into alignment, causing muscle edema and eventual ischemia. Consequently, the evaluation of orbital floor fractures should include testing of the extraocular movements, with emergent ophthalmologic consultation if there is concern for inferior rectus entrapment. Forced duction testing should be performed under local anesthesia and sedation if there is any concern for entrapment. True entrapment requires urgent decompression to prevent muscle ischemia and long-term complication. Large (>50%) orbital floor blow-out fractures should undergo open reduction and reconstruction with either split cranial bone graft or an implant, such as titanium or porous polyethylene (Figure 11.2).

A comprehensive evaluation of periorbital trauma should also include measurement of the interorbital distance (IOD), which can be affected in naso-orbital-ethmoid (NOE)

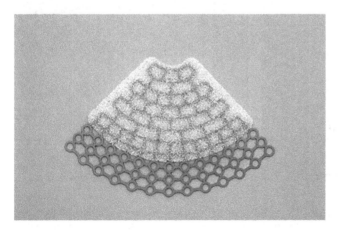

Figure 11.2 Titanium and porous polyethylene implant used for orbital floor reconstruction.

fractures. Radiographically, the IOD represents the distance from dacryon to dacryon. It may be clinically assessed by measuring the medial intercanthal distance and subtracting 4–6 mm to obtain the IOD. A bowstring test may be performed to evaluate for stability of the medial canthus in suspected NOE fracture. Other ophthalmologic emergencies associated with orbital trauma include superior orbital fissure (SOF) syndrome and orbital apex syndrome. SOF syndrome represents findings of proptosis, abducens nerve paresthesia, and internal or external opthalmoplegia. Orbital apex syndrome represents this constellation of findings with blindness. Concern for these findings warrants emergent ophthalmologic and surgical evaluation.

Orbital Roof, Cranial Base, and Vault Fractures

The orbital roof remains in continuity with the anterior cranial base, posing unique considerations when evaluating traumatic injuries. Moore et al. previously described obliquely oriented cranial base fractures extending into the facial skeleton, which are often observed in the pediatric patient with suspected skull fracture. Growing skull fractures result from underlying dural disruption at time of initial injury. Leptomeningeal cyst formation occurs with disruption of the leptomeninges and resulting brain pulsation. This pulsation causes a growing diastasis in the overlying bone, which can be clinically observed as orbital expansion, VOD, or pulsatile exophthalmos. Suspected injuries require long-term surveillance with CT imaging to ensure appropriate healing. When identified, surgical treatment of growing skull fractures involves resecting the cyst, patching the interrupted dura, and bone grafting the cranium. Our institution's experience with reconstruction of the anterior cranial base involves the utilization of pedicled pericranial flaps and/or galeal-frontalis flaps, with split thickness calvarial bone to separate intracranial and nasal contents (Figure 11.3).

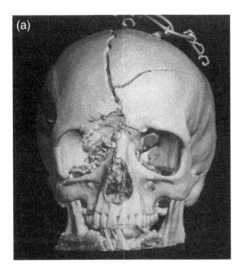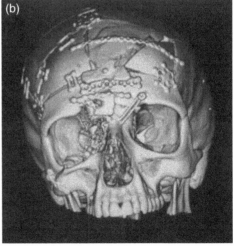

Figure 11.3 (a) Preoperative CT of severe craniofacial trauma from a gunshot wound involving the orbit, anterior cranial base, and frontal bone. (b) Postoperative CT demonstrating open reduction internal fixation, and reconstruction of the right orbit with titanium mesh, transnasal wiring medial canthopexy, reconstruction of anterior cranial base with split thickness cranial bone, and frontal bone reconstruction.

Initial evaluation of skull and/or forehead trauma should include careful sterile examination of the injuries to gauge the depth of involvement. Skull fractures underneath brow lacerations may be missed, given their inconspicuous location. Otorhinolaryngology consultation should be made when CT imaging is suggestive of basilar or temporal skull fracture, given the concern for CSF leak or facial nerve involvement. External auditory canal lacerations are often associated with underlying condylar fractures.

Complications

The goal of treatment in facial fractures is to restore anatomic alignment and function and to prevent long-term sequelae. Complications related to hardware may include malreduction and malposition, hardware extrusion, hardware failure, and infection. Reasons for hardware removal include pain, infection, loose plates/screws, prominence, sensitivity, and dehiscence. The concern for growth restriction in children has led to the development of biodegradable materials composed of various polymers that are resorbable, less prominent, and associated with fewer infections. However, these materials may still lead to osteolysis, soft tissue swelling, and foreign body reaction.

Upon symptomatic presentation following facial fracture repair, the duration of elapsed time from the surgical procedure and the specific surgical details are paramount aspects of the history. Physical examination suggestive of hardware malfunction or infection, such as fever, swelling, or tenderness, often requires CT imaging for assessment. Panorex radiographic imaging may be useful for isolated dental or mandibular assessment; however, access to this modality is often limited. For best CT resolution, thin-slice (1 mm) axial CT imaging should be obtained with 3D postprocessing reconstruction. Surgical intervention may be required for either infection or hardware malposition. In some cases, drainable collections or abscesses may be amenable to percutaneous aspiration.

Mandible

Fracture complications include malunion, nonunion, infection, ankyloses, and nerve injury. Malunion may present as occlusal changes, which may or may not be clinically significant. Minor malocclusion can be addressed with prolonged MMF or elastic bands, while significant postoperative malocclusion may require orthodontic treatment or future orthognathic correction.

For patients who have MMF, a wire cutter should be present at bedside at all times. These are to be used in emergent situations that may compromise the airway, such as emesis or bleeding. The wires should be cut at the midpoint; care should be taken to ensure that loose wires are completely removed to prevent foreign body aspiration or ingestion. If the wires are cut, the surgeon should be consulted for further management and follow-up.

Arch bars and IMF screws may often be removed in the office setting under local anesthesia. Most pediatric patients, however, and select adult patients, may require general anesthesia. In the event of acute infection in the setting of early bony healing, it is preferable to treat with antibiotics and aspiration/washout, rather than complete hardware removal. Long-term hardware failure, severe pain, or significant prominence may warrant secondary hardware removal. Screws penetrating dental roots, causing severe pain, may require removal as well. External fixator complications include pin site infection and migration of hardware. Routine pin site care includes antibacterial ointment application and wrapping of the pin with xeroform at the skin insertion site. Severe infections may require the removal of the external fixator.

Midface

Serious complications of maxillary fractures may include a compromised airway from soft tissue edema, hemorrhage due to bleeding from major branches of the external carotid artery, dacryocystitis from lacrimal duct injury, and CSF leak from fracture of the cribiform plate. Late complications of malunion or nonunion can be managed with reexposure, osteotomy of partially healed fractures, reduction, bone grafting, and IMF. Postoperative infections may be treated with antibiotics, and, possibly, hardware removal. Orbital injuries are associated with a myriad of complications ranging from visual changes, to ectropion, to persistent diplopia. As previously discussed, any visual change or loss necessitates prompt ophthalmologic evaluation. Approximately 5% of orbital trauma may be associated with ectropion or malposition of the lower lid, which may be prophylactically managed at the time of intervention with a temporary suture tarsorrhaphy (Frost stitch), which can be easily removed at bedside postoperatively. To determine the necessity for this maneuver, a lower lid "snap-back test" is performed to evaluate for excessive lower lid laxity. If an implant is utilized to reconstruct the orbit, resulting complications may include malposition, infection, and extrusion. Postoperative CT imaging is strongly encouraged for confirmation of accurate positioning and reduction. If suboptimal reduction and fixation are identified, the patient may require return to the operating room for correction.

Superior Orbit, Cranial Base, and Vault

Frontal sinus complications are classified as early or late, based on postinjury timing. Early complications include pain, sensory changes to the forehead, CSF leak, and, rarely, meningitis. CSF leaks may resolve spontaneously or require lumbar drain placement and antibiotic administration. Large leaks failing to respond to conservative measures may require operative exploration and direct dural repair. Signs suggestive of meningitis such as mental status change, high fevers, or severe neck pain should be promptly identified and treated. Intracranial abscesses may require exploration and drainage. Late complications include mucocele, osteomyelitis, and bony erosion exerting mass effect.

Conclusions

Facial fracture management may require closed or open reduction, and internal or external fixation. As such, successful outcomes depend on accurate reduction of bony fragments and rigid fixation. In cases treated conservatively with close reduction or observation, close follow-up is required to ensure adequate healing. Hardware complications may require reoperation or the need for antibiotics.

Further Reading

1 Prekker, M.E., Miner, J.R., Rockswold, E.G., and Biros, M.H. (2009). *The prevalence of injury of any type in an urban emergency department population. J. Trauma* 66 (6): 1688–1695.

2 Mithani, S.K., St-Hilaire, H., Brooke, B.S. et al. (2009). *Predictable patterns of intracranial and cervical spine injury in craniomaxillofacial trauma: analysis of 4786 patients. Plast. Reconstr. Surg.* 123 (4): 1293–1301.

3 Singh, D.J. and Bartlett, S.P. (2004). *Pediatric craniofacial fractures: long-term consequences. Clin. Plast. Surg.* 31 (3): 499–518, vii.

4 Eggensperger Wymann, N.M., Hölzle, A., Zachariou, Z., and Iizuka, T. (2008). *Pediatric craniofacial trauma. J. Oral Maxillofac. Surg.* 66 (1): 58–64.

5 Verschueren, D.S., Bell, R.B., Bagheri, S.C. et al. (2006). *Management of laryngo-tracheal injuries associated with craniomaxillofacial trauma. J. Oral Maxillofac. Surg.* 64 (2): 203–214.

6 Hackl, W., Fink, C., Hausberger, K. et al. (2001). *The incidence of combined facial and cervical spine injuries. J. Trauma* 50 (1): 41–45.

7 Jamal, B.T., Diecidue, R., Qutob, A., and Cohen, M. (2009). *The pattern of combined maxillofacial and cervical spine fractures. J. Oral Maxillofac. Surg.* 67 (3): 559–562.

8 Marcus, J.R., Erdmann, D., and Rodriguez, E.D. (2012). *Essentials of Craniomaxillofacial Trauma*, 333. St. Louis, MO: Quality Medical Pub. xvi.

9 Rowe, N.L. (1969). *Fractures of the jaws in children. J. Oral Surg.* 27 (7): 497–507.

10 Bartlett, S.P. and DeLozier, J.B. 3rd (1992). *Controversies in the management of pediatric facial fractures. Clin. Plast. Surg.* 19 (1): 245–258.

11 Erdmann, D., Follmar, K.E., Debruijn, M. et al. (2008). *A retrospective analysis of facial fracture etiologies. Ann. Plast. Surg.* 60 (4): 398–403.

12 Holt, G.R. and Holt, J.E. (1983). *Incidence of eye injuries in facial fractures: an analysis of 727 cases. Otolaryngol. Head Neck Surg.* 91 (3): 276–279.

13 Moore, M.H., David, D.J., and Cooter, R.D. (1990). *Oblique craniofacial fractures in children. J. Craniofac. Surg.* 1 (1): 4–7.

12

Cranial Orthotics and Ear Molding

Meg Ann Maguire and Phuong D. Nguyen

Division of Plastic and Reconstructive Surgery, Children's Hospital of Philadelphia, Philadelphia, PA, USA

Introduction

Cranial molding helmets (CMH) or bands are most commonly used for remodeling an infant's head shape secondary to asymmetry from positional plagiocephaly. In recent years, there has been an increased use of cranial molding devices as an adjunctive therapy following surgical correction of craniosynostosis.

Indications

Positional Plagiocephaly

Positional plagiocephaly refers to asymmetric flattening of the skull as a result of chronic positioning and restricted growth patterns of the skull, which is unrelated to premature closure of one or more of the major cranial sutures (craniosynostosis). The classic appearance of positional plagiocephaly is a parallelogram-shaped skull with flattening of the occiput on the affected side. Growth of the skull is dependent on patency of cranial sutures and the anterior and posterior fontanelles, driven by the growth of the brain. The posterior fontanelle will typically close between one and three months of life, while the anterior fontanelle will typically close between one and three years of life. The major cranial sutures are the metopic, coronal, sagittal, and lambdoid sutures (Figure 12.1).

Peak prevalence of positional plagiocephaly is within the first six months of life. While direct causation cannot be proven, there is suggestion of associated risk factors for positional plagiocephaly that include fetal deliveries requiring adjunctive maneuvers or devices, first-born children, male infants, cumulative time on the back, and torticollis. The cited incidence of positional plagiocephaly varies in the medical literature; however, it is widely accepted that there has been a marked increase in the incidence after the American Academy of Pediatrics instituted the "Back to Sleep Campaign" in 1992. This guideline

Emergency Management of the Hi-Tech Patient in Acute and Critical Care, First Edition. Edited by Ioannis Koutroulis, Nicholas Tsarouhas, Richard J. Lin, Jill C. Posner, Michael Seneff, and Robert Shesser.

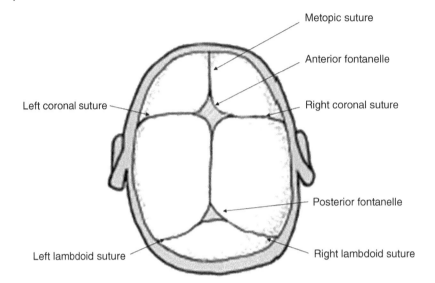

Figure 12.1 Major growth centers of the skull.

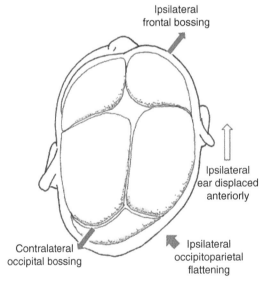

Figure 12.2 Diagrammatic demonstration of right unilateral plagiocephaly involving the right posterior occiput.

recommended that an infant, when not in direct supervision, should not be left in a prone position until they are able to roll and position themselves.

Plagiocephaly does not have an impact on intellectual development or the ability of the brain to develop. There is a deformation of the shape of the skull which can be classified as mild to severe, and patients may also present with significant facial asymmetry. With plagiocephaly, a flatness is seen in one side of the occiput, with a corresponding flatness in the contralateral anterior or temporal skull. This may result in an anterior displacement of the ear on the side of the flattened occiput, as well as asymmetry of the facial features. There is no difference in orbital height in plagiocephaly (Figure 12.2).

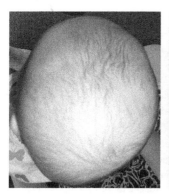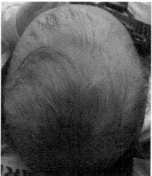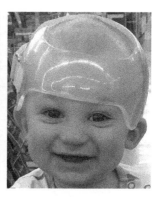

Figure 12.3 Bird's-eye view of patient with right positional plagiocephaly before (left) and after (middle) CMH. Note the right posterior occiput flatness in the premolded head shape that is improved after CMH. The photo on the right is an example of an infant with a CMH in place.

Torticollis can cause preferential head positioning and tilt, which may exacerbate positional plagiocephaly and reduce the infant's tolerance of tummy time. Torticollis may delay milestones of rolling, sitting, and crawling, which offset the pressure on the occiput. Physical therapy evaluation including home stretching by parents is recommended for the management of torticollis.

Treatment options for plagiocephaly include altering head position, or CMHs, with evidence that CMHs yield a better head shape than repositioning alone (Figure 12.3). Treatment is predicated on patient age. Physical repositioning should be consistent with the American Academy of Pediatric's "Back to Sleep" guideline. While there is some benefit of helmet therapy after a year of age, it has been shown that there is decreased amount of helmeting needed and improved cranial dimensions when helmet therapy is initiated prior to seven months of age.

Craniosynostosis

More recently, CMHs have been used to assist in molding of the skull after surgical correction of craniosynostosis. Craniosynostosis occurs when one or more of the major cranial sutures fuse prematurely and restrict the ability of the cranial bones to accommodate brain growth. Craniosynostosis typically results in predictable growth patterns of the cranial vault (Table 12.1) and is not correctable solely with cranial molding. The goal of a cranial orthotic is to adjunctively mold the skull after surgical osteotomies are performed to encourage growth in the previously restricted dimensions.

In some scenarios, craniosynostosis may cause increased intracranial pressure and affect brain development. CMH may be used as an augmentative device to surgical intervention in either the preoperative and/or postoperative period.

Protective Helmets

While somewhat similar in appearance, helmets used for protection of the head due to cranial defects from various etiologies, such as trauma, infection, or tumor, serve a different purpose and should not be confused with a cranial molding helmet. In this instance, the

Table 12.1 Common clinical findings of single suture synostosis.

Suture	Common clinical findings associated with suture synostosis
Metopic	• Trigonocephaly (triangulating shape of the forehead) • Bilateral temporal retrusion • Hypoterlorism (decreased distance between the inner canthus of the eyes)
Coronal (can be unilateral or bilateral)	• Turricpehaly (tall/towering head shape) • Brachycephaly (short head shape) • Facial asymmetry (when unilateral, the orbit is displaced laterally and posteriorly with the underdevelopment of the orbital rim)
Sagittal	• Narrow dolichocephaly • Cranial index typically of 60–67% compared with the normal 76–78%
Lambdoid (can be unilateral or bilateral)	• Mastoid bulge of unaffected side, if unilateral • Ear on affected side is displaced in posterior and inferior directions

device is purely protective and is not meant to provide guidance of any skull development. Often, these devices are seen in children well past the age where a cranial molding is applicable, as well as in adults.

Equipment/Device

Once prescribed, CMHs are managed by orthotists who may use digital scanning technology to measure the fit and modify the CMH. CMHs can be full helmets or bands of a variety of colors and shapes. They most often have a hard outer shell with an adjustable soft material on the interior of the CMH.

Management

After a brief period of initiation (often less than one week), when helmets are worn for shorter intervals to assess for areas of excessive pressure, CMHs are recommended to be worn 23 hours a day. They require adjustments about every two weeks to accommodate the changing skull shape. In the time the helmet is off, the skin is assessed for evidence of excessive pressure, as exhibited by persistent redness. Children with conditions such as eczema, hemangiomas, or cranial shunt ports may require extra attention to avoid pressure sores.

The duration of CMH for positional plagiocephaly is dependent on the severity of the presentation, compliance, and response to helmeting. It may take four months or greater. It should be noted that if CMH is initiated earlier than six months of age, there may be a requirement for a second helmet, due to the rapid cranial growth that occurs in infants. Additionally, there is practice variation among prescribing providers as to when to initiate

CMHs. Insurance coverage for durable medical equipment varies; it may not be a covered expense. Lastly, though the final result of the CMH may be unpredictable, it is anticipated that there will be improvement in head shape for moderate or severe positional plagiocephaly after six months of age.

In some circumstances, CMH is recommended preoperatively for craniosynostosis. The treatment goal is to minimize the skeletal deformity in the preoperative period, since it has been noted that the deformity is typically progressive until surgical correction. Additionally, CMH has been used after endoscopic release of a single cranial suture to help "jump-start" the correction of the acquired skeletal deformity and to help normalize the skull shape. In this situation, length of use of the CMH may vary and could last as long as the second year of life.

Complications/Emergencies

Complications of CMH can include skin irritation and ulceration, eczema exacerbations, and, rarely, allergic contact dermatitis. More frequently encountered is noncompliance. If skin breakdown is encountered, helmet therapy is temporarily suspended to allow for wound healing. Meanwhile, the helmet is adjusted by the orthotic team to redistribute pressure to avoid further injury. If there are concerns for underlying tissue injury, the evaluating physician can safely remove the helmet for a better assessment, and then arrange for follow-up with the consultant provider.

Ear Molding

Introduction

Current literature cites an approximate incidence of 1 : 3800 newborns who have an ear malformation. There is a wide range of severity of malformations, from those that may affect the external ear only, to those associated with maldevelopment of inner ear structures and hearing loss. Ear molding devices (Figure 12.4) may be used in infancy to modify congenital ear deformities, which otherwise lead to misshapen external ears. This potentially could avert the need for surgical intervention later in life. Ear molding may be

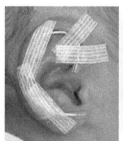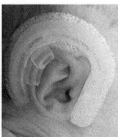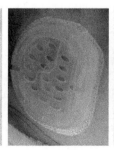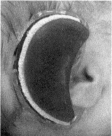

Figure 12.4 Various forms of ear molding from custom-fabricated (far left) to a variety of commercially available devices.

beneficial in helical rim deformities, protruding ears, cryptotia, constricted ears, or combination ear deformities. Ear molding devices, however, are not able to reconstruct missing portions of ear, as in microtia or anotia.

Indications

Ear molding takes advantage of the residual circulating maternal hormones in an infant to harness the pliability of the nascent ear cartilage. There are a range of custom or commercially available devices. Therapy is best initiated in the early days of life (within one week) for maximum efficacy. Most molding devices require some exposure to adhesives to maintain the device and thus harbor a risk of contact dermatitis.

Equipment/Device

Devices for ear molding may be custom-made from a variety of available products, such as covered surgical wire or commercially available molding devices. These typically consist of a base product placed on the scalp to allow fixation of conformers, or retractors, which promote a more optimal ear shape.

Management

These devices require reassessment of the skin and repositioning of the conformers approximately every two weeks. Therapy typically does not last longer than six weeks, though this is dependent on the age during the initiation, as older children may require longer duration to achieve adequate results. Children over the age of two months are at greater risk of intolerance of the molds due to their increased head movement and propensity to dislodge the device.

Complications/Emergencies

Ear molding devices are fairly well tolerated. Skin irritation, ulceration, and contact dermatitis are the most common complications. These should be managed with removal of the device, localized treatment with antibiotic ointment or lotion as needed, and reassessment for consideration of reapplication after the concern has been resolved.

Further Reading

1 Bialocerkowski, A.E., Vladusic, S.L., and Wei Ng, C. (2008). Prevalence, risk factors, and natural history of positional plagiocephaly: a systematic review. *Dev. Med. Child Neurol.* 50: 577–586.
2 Argenta, L.C., David, L.R., Wilson, J.A., and Bell, W.O. (1996). An increase in infant cranial deformity with supine sleeping position. *J. Craniofac. Surg.* 7: 5–11.
3 Kane, A.A., Mitchell, L.E., Craven, K.P., and Marsh, J.L. (1996). Observations on a recent increase in plagiocephaly without synostosis. *Pediatrics* 97: 877–885.

4 Mawji, A., Vollman, A.R., Hatfield, J. et al. (2013). The incidence of positional plagiocephaly: a cohort study. *Pediatrics* 132: 298–304.

5 Turk, A.E., McCarthy, J.G., Thorne, C.H., and Wisoff, J.H. (1996). The "back to sleep campaign" and deformational plagiocephaly: is there cause for concern? *J. Craniofac. Surg.* 7: 12–18.

6 Robinson, S. and Proctor, M. (2009). Diagnosis and management of deformational plagiocephaly. *J. Neurosurg. Pediatr.* 3: 284–295.

7 Xia, J.J., Kennedy, K.A., Teichgraeber, J.F. et al. (2008). Nonsurgical treatment of deformational plagiocephaly: a systematic review. *Arch. Pediatr. Adolesc. Med.* 162: 719–727.

8 Seruya, M., Oh, A.K., Taylor, J.H. et al. (2013). Helmet treatment of deformational plagiocephaly: the relationship between age at initiation and rate of correction. *Plast. Reconstr. Surg.* 131: 55e–61e.

9 Bartel-Friedrich, S. (2015). Congenital auricular malformations: description of anomalies and syndromes. *Facial Plast. Surg.* 31: 567–580.

13

Ear, Nose, and Throat Devices

Eva Delgado[1] and Adva Buzi[2,3]

[1] *Division of Emergency Medicine, Department of Pediatrics, Children's Hospital of Philadelphia, Philadelphia, PA, USA*
[2] *Division of Otolaryngology, Department of Surgery, Children's Hospital of Philadelphia, Philadelphia, PA, USA*
[3] *Perelman School of Medicine at the University of Pennsylvania, Philadelphia, PA, USA*

Introduction

Patients with injury, infection, dysfunction, or disease affecting the ears, nose, or throat may require an implantable device for either short- or long-term support of the underlying problem. This chapter will describe several devices put in place by, or in accordance with, the recommendations of otolaryngologists. The approach to device placement and management will be discussed, as well as how to tackle complications related to these devices that would prompt a patient to seek emergency care. Indications for immediate consultation with an otolaryngologist, versus expedited or routine referral for follow-up, will also be covered in each section.

Ear Devices

Several types of devices can be implanted in ears to improve drainage, reduce infection, facilitate hearing, or optimize appearance. The devices reviewed here will include myringotomy tubes, conventional hearing aids, middle ear implants, cochlear implants, bone-anchored hearing aids (BAHAs), and auricular prostheses.

Myringotomy Tubes

Indications

Myringotomy tubes (otherwise known as tympanostomy tubes) are commonly encountered implants. Figure 13.1 demonstrates the most common ("standard") myringotomy tubes used, while Figure 13.2 is a less commonly used "T-Tubes." Although implanted in

Emergency Management of the Hi-Tech Patient in Acute and Critical Care, First Edition. Edited by
Ioannis Koutroulis, Nicholas Tsarouhas, Richard J. Lin, Jill C. Posner, Michael Seneff, and Robert Shesser.
© 2021 John Wiley & Sons Ltd. Published 2021 by John Wiley & Sons Ltd.

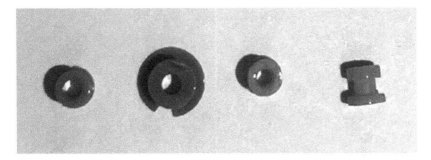

Figure 13.1 Myringotomy tubes – standard.

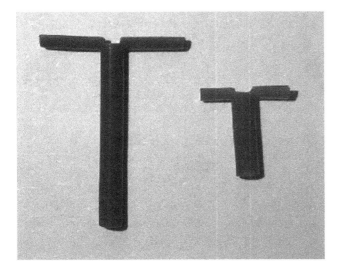

Figure 13.2 T-tubes.

both adult and pediatric patients, tympanostomy tube insertion is the most common pediatric ambulatory procedure in the US, with over 500 000 tubes inserted annually. Typically, these tubes are recommended for children diagnosed with chronic otitis media with effusion. This is the condition when middle ear fluid fails to respond to treatment for three months or longer and is associated with hearing difficulties. Children with recurrent acute otitis media (AOM) or children who have speech, language, or learning problems thought to be attributable to otitis media are also candidates for myringotomy tubes. Eustachian tube dysfunction (ETD) is another indication for these implants. ETD can continue into adulthood and can also result from nasopharyngeal cancer or radiation therapy in the area of the Eustachian tube.

Device Placement and Management

The purpose of myringotomy tubes is to equalize the pressure between the external environment and the middle ear space, bypassing the natural drainage of the middle ear through the Eustachian tube. They serve to improve ventilation of this space and relieve

Figure 13.3 Myringotomy tube in place.

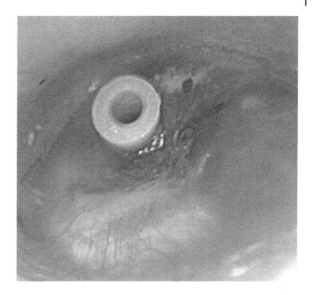

hearing loss due to chronic fluid retention. Tympanostomy tube insertion involves an incision of the tympanic membrane measuring 1/20 of an inch. Figure 13.3 shows a standard myringotomy tube placed in the tympanic membrane. This opening of the tubes may allow water into the middle ear, but the amount is so small that most otolaryngologists do not restrict bathing or swimming following tube insertion. The tubes inserted are usually for short term, that is, 6–18 months, and fall out on their own. Some tubes are intended for longer use and are designed with longer flanges below the tympanic membrane to keep them in place. The long-term tubes often need to be removed by an otolaryngologist.

Complications, Emergencies, and Consultation

A small amount of bleeding can happen shortly after tube placement, which is considered normal. Continued bleeding would be unusual and should prompt immediate evaluation by otolaryngology, as this might suggest injury to the jugular vein or carotid artery, which are very rarely found in an unusual location, or lying beneath dehiscent bone in the middle ear. Bleeding that occurs after the immediate postoperative period may be a tube granuloma. Present in 5–14% of patients, this granulation tissue may form in response to the tube itself, as this is a foreign material, or it may form in response to infection that triggers tissue destruction, fibrosis, angiogenesis, and obstruction. Ciprofloxacin/dexamethasone otic suspension is ideal for treatment of a granuloma since the steroid component inhibits continued proliferation and the antibiotic treats any potential infection. Patients with this presentation should be referred for close follow-up with an otolaryngologist.

Drainage from myringotomy tubes also may prompt presentation to an acute care setting. This drainage represents an infection. Treatment with antibiotic ear drops is the initial treatment of choice and is quite effective; oral antibiotics are of little added benefit unless treating a related systemic infection. If there is concern that drops will not be able to penetrate the drainage due to its amount or consistency, the provider can wick away some drainage with a cotton swab prior to starting treatment. The drops should demonstrate some improvement within 3–4 days, and drainage should completely resolve after the full 10-day course. An otolaryngologist should reassess the patient to help determine if there is any reason to follow a course of drops with oral antibiotics based on response.

Lastly, a patient with myringotomy tubes may present complaining of an extruded tube, as nearly 4% of tubes will extrude prematurely. The emergency care clinician may remove the myringotomy tube from the canal. If this is too difficult, the patient may be referred for outpatient otolaryngology follow-up.

Conventional Hearing Aids

Indications, Device Placement, and Management

Patients with mild to severe sensorineural hearing loss are candidates for conventional hearing aids (Figure 13.4), which typically sit behind (Figure 13.5) or within the ear. These hearing aids amplify sound using either analog or digital technology and direct the sound into the ear canal. There are several styles of hearing aids: behind-the-ear, in-the-ear, in-the-canal, and completely-in-the-canal. The type used is based on the degree of hearing loss, ear shape and size, battery life, and other patient preferences.

Complications, Emergencies, and Consultation

While some patients with hearing aids may seek care for general discomfort, some may also develop otitis externa as a result of the occlusive nature of some conventional hearing aids. Treatment of the infection with otic drops, such as ciprofloxacin/dexamethasone, is recommended. The use of the hearing aid should be discontinued until the infection has subsided.

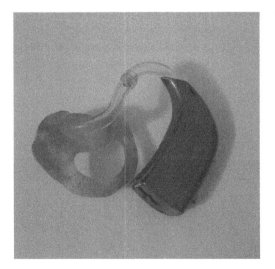

Figure 13.4 Conventional hearing aid.

Figure 13.5 Conventional hearing aid on patient.

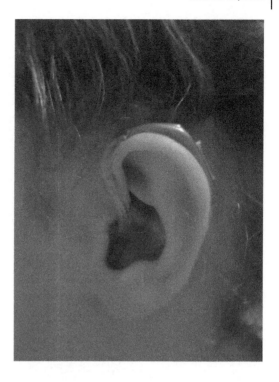

Further evaluation of the hearing aid, and decisions about temporary or long-term discontinuation of the device, should be made by an otolaryngologist in a follow-up visit.

Cochlear Implants

Indications and Device Placement

Cochlear implants are devices indicated for a child or adult with severe to profound sensorineural hearing loss and impaired speech comprehension. The indications for cochlear implantation are set and updated by the Food and Drug Administration. The implants consist of electrode arrays inserted into the cochlea where they stimulate the residual components of auditory neurons. External to the skull are key components: a microphone, a speech processor, and a transcutaneous power transmitter usually held in place by a magnet. An implanted receiver/stimulator, also magnetized to connect with the external components, is inserted into the temporal bone to decode a radio frequency signal and to transmit this to an internal cable that connects to the electrode array. Figure 13.6 is a schematic of a cochlear implant.

Management

The emergency care clinician should recognize that these devices are magnetized. A patient with cochlear implants cannot undergo magnetic resonance imaging (MRI) unless the devices can be made compatible. Should an emergent MRI be necessary, discussion with an otolaryngologist prior to the study is prudent.

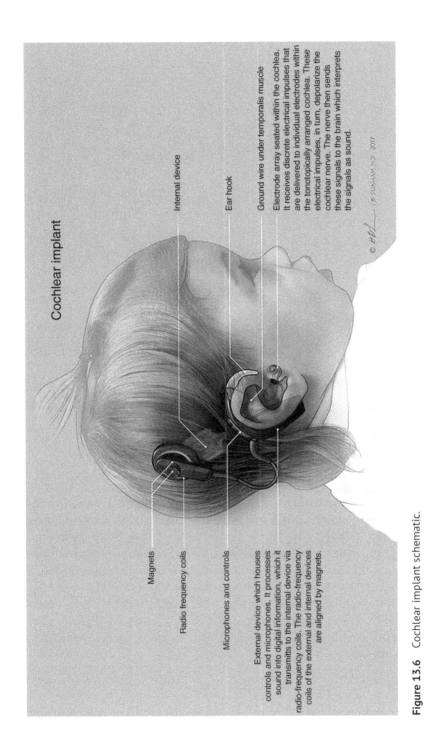

Cochlear implant

Internal device

Ear hook

Ground wire under temporalis muscle

Electrode array seated within the cochlea. It receives discrete electrical impulses that are delivered to individual electrodes within the tonotopically arranged cochlea. These electrical impulses, in turn, depolarize the cochlear nerve. The nerve then sends these signals to the brain which interprets the signals as sound.

Magnets

Radio frequency coils

Microphones and controls

External device which houses controls and microphones. It processes sound into digital information, which it transmits to the internal device via radio-frequency coils. The radio-frequency coils of the external and internal devices are aligned by magnets.

Figure 13.6 Cochlear implant schematic.

Complications, Emergencies, and Consultation

Infectious complications of cochlear implants can range from minor, local infections, to severe and invasive infections. In the immediate postoperative period, wound and device-related infections warrant emergent otolaryngology evaluation or immediate referral to the surgeon who performed the procedure. The treating provider must also be aware of the potential for bacterial meningitis in these patients. Patients with cochlear implants are at highest risk for bacterial meningitis in the two months immediately following surgery, but, even beyond that, they still remain at higher risk than the general population. Variables that may predispose to this increased risk include underlying ear-related anomalies, progressive complications of AOM, and even the actual type of implant. To mitigate these risks, otolaryngologists often elect to place myringotomy tubes prior to cochlear implants in patients with recurrent AOM. Comprehensive immunization is also indicated to prevent invasive pneumococcal disease.

In cochlear implant patients with AOM, infection may travel along the implant's electrodes from the middle ear to the inner ear. This may cause damage to the implant, damage to the nerve components that were still functional in the cochlea, or even infections such as mastoiditis or meningitis. Outpatient treatment of uncomplicated AOM with oral antibiotics, such as high-dose amoxicillin, may suffice, but inpatient intravenous therapy with cefotaxime or ceftriaxone may be warranted in some cases. Ill-appearing patients should undergo lumbar puncture to evaluate for bacterial meningitis. Other patients at higher risk for severe disease include immunocompromised or underimmunized patients. The management of these patients should be in close concert with otolaryngologists. In some cases, if tympanostomy tube placement was not done preoperatively, it may be necessary at this time.

Chronic indolent infections may require "explantation," or removal of the cochlear implant, though antibiotics are usually the first management strategy. These patients uncommonly present with acute infectious symptoms for emergency care. Follow-up with the otolaryngologist who manages the implant is paramount.

Recipients of cochlear implants may present with neurologic symptoms, including facial nerve palsy. Facial nerve injury may result from the surgical procedure, though this nerve is usually monitored carefully during the mastoidectomy and related phases of the procedure. If the facial nerve injury is minor, complete recovery is possible. Postoperative vestibular symptoms are also possible; more than one-third of patients will have vertigo or weakness that lasts for weeks to months before resolution. In elderly patients older than 70 years, vestibular symptoms may be even more long-standing. Depending on the patient's presentation and comorbidities, a comprehensive neurologic workup may be appropriate. Consultation with otolaryngology is again prudent to help determine the appropriate evaluation, disposition, and follow-up.

Device extrusion, in which the device becomes external to the scalp, is another potential complication with cochlear implants. Cochlear implants can create pressure on the skin flap that was created for its insertion, and this can lead to skin flap necrosis or skin breakdown from localized irritation, infection, or inflammation. Discussion with otolaryngology and potentially plastic surgery is warranted in these cases. If the device is still functional, the surgeons can plan for treatment of infection and repair of overlying tissues. Device extrusion is also possible following even minor head trauma, especially with the advent of cochlear implant magnets that are designed for easy removal to allow for MRI. As with device extrusion from necrosis or infection, repair of the overlying skin flaps by the treating surgeons is warranted.

Bone-Anchored Hearing Aids (BAHA)

Indications

A BAHA, as per the schematic in Figure 13.7, is a device implanted into the skull, which is ultimately integrated with the osteocytes to allow for direct bone conduction of sound. BAHAs are useful in cases of conductive hearing loss, but they can also be used in cases of mixed conductive and sensorineural hearing loss, or in severe unilateral sensorineural hearing loss. Patients with chronically draining ears, microtia (a congenital deformity where the pinna is underdeveloped) or other anatomical anomalies may be best suited to a BAHA.

Device Placement and Management

There are several types of BAHAs, with the main difference being related to the placement of the transducer in either a percutaneous or a transcutaneous position. In the percutaneous system, the transducer is connected to the mastoid via titanium fixtures that penetrate through the skin and are anchored into the skull. In the transcutaneous system, the transducer is made of two components that communicate with each other across thinned skin and are held into place by magnets. In this case, the internal transducer is anchored into the skull, underneath the skin, and the external portion sits outside the skin without penetrating it. Sound quality is better with the percutaneous option.

Complications, Emergencies, and Consultation

Newer surgical techniques and devices have improved engraftment, reduced infections, and decreased abutment dislodgements. (Past surgical approaches involved larger incisions, the use of skin flaps, and soft-tissue reduction procedures that are no longer necessary with the use of longer titanium abutments.) Dislodgements, however, still do occur and are more common in children. These are often due to trauma. Any concerns for dislodgement should prompt consultation with an otolaryngologist.

Patients with percutaneous BAHAs may present with concerns for soft-tissue overgrowth or skin infection. The implant site requires daily care to minimize the risk of infection. If a superficial cellulitis does occur, it may be treated with oral antibiotics active against common skin flora, such as cephalexin. Fortunately, reports of osteomyelitis are scarce and are seen mostly in immunocompromised hosts.

Patients with transcutaneous BAHAs often choose this type of approach as the external portion of the transducer is less obvious, so less cosmetically undesirable. Additionally, these sites do not require daily care. While the risk of infection is lower, these patients may

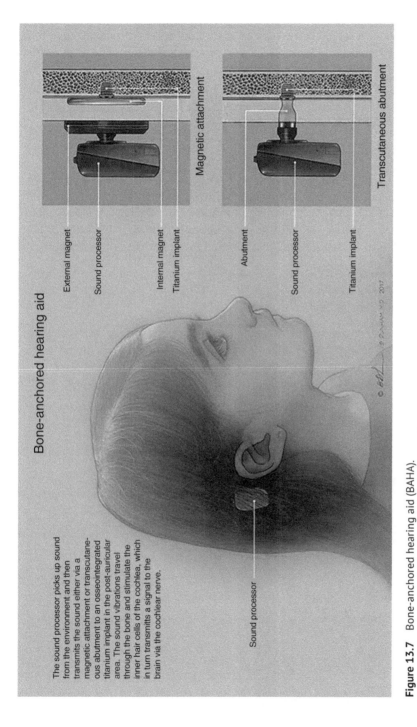

Bone-anchored hearing aid

The sound processor picks up sound from the environment and then transmits the sound either via a magnetic attachment or transcutaneous abutment to an osseointegrated titanium implant in the post-auricular area. The sound vibrations travel through the bone and stimulate the inner hair cells of the cochlea, which in turn transmitts a signal to the brain via the cochlear nerve.

Sound processor

External magnet
Sound processor
Internal magnet
Titanium implant

Magnetic attachment

Abutment
Sound processor
Titanium implant

Transcutaneous abutment

Figure 13.7 Bone-anchored hearing aid (BAHA).

present with discomfort from the pressure of a too-high magnetic setting where the device attaches to the skull (via magnets).

A newer type of bone conduction implant places the transducer permanently under the skin and aims for better outward appearance, as well as better sound transmission. Insertion is complicated, so these are not yet commonly seen.

Auricular Prosthesis

Indications and Device Placement

Patients with microtia, other auricular malformations, or auricular damage are candidates for auricular prostheses. Figure 13.8 demonstrates the medial and Figure 13.9, the external surfaces of auricular prostheses. Typically, these devices are adhered to the skull analogously to percutaneous BAHAs and undergo osseointegration as well. Unlike the BAHA, the prosthesis abutment is shaped a bit differently, and the device needs to be anchored in two places.

Complications, Emergencies, and Consultation

The percutaneous nature of the implant again makes skin infection a potential complication, but these implants seem to be slightly less susceptible to infection than BAHAs. Infections occur more commonly in children. As above, superficial skin infections may be treated with cephalexin. Urgent outpatient follow-up with the surgeon who inserted the implant is recommended.

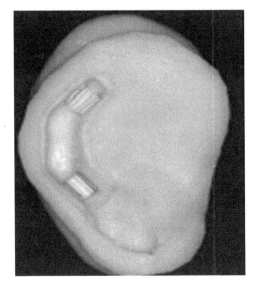

Figure 13.8 Auricular prosthesis (medial view).

Figure 13.9   Auricular prosthesis (external surfaces).

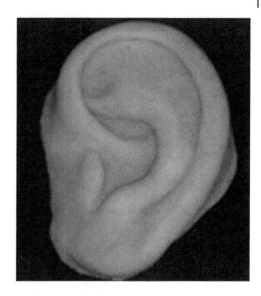

Nasal Devices

Devices are inserted or implanted into the nose to stop bleeding, enhance breathing, or allow for the maintenance of normal nasal drainage. Septal buttons and sinus stents are devices that are fitted and implanted by an otolaryngologist. In contrast, nasal packing is often inserted by an emergency care provider in order to manage acute epistaxis. It is worthwhile to review the materials, indications, and insertion techniques, as well as the potential complications that may result from nasal packing. Management concerns and possible complications of septal buttons and sinus stents will be covered in the latter portion of this section.

Nasal Packing

Indications
Epistaxis is a common chief complaint, especially in very young and very old patients. In children, this is often due to local causes such as habitual nose picking or nasal dryness. Trauma is one of the most common causes of epistaxis in all age groups, though systemic illness and disease contribute as well.

Initial management should begin with a nasal exam. Perhaps most important is to identify the source of bleeding, as anterior and posterior bleeds require different management. The patient should lean forward (not back), and blow the nose to remove clots to allow for better visualization of the bleeding source. Manual digital pressure applied to the sides of the nose, toward the septum, at the tip of the nose, is often effective in achieving hemostasis. A topical vasoconstrictor can be also be used for effective hemostasis. As the use of a nasal speculum allows for an even better internal nasal exam, a topical anesthetic helps to alleviate the discomfort. Children may also benefit from or need medication for anxiolysis, restraints, and the assistance of child life specialists.

Most anterior bleeding, especially in children, occurs at Kiesselbach's plexus, an area located at the anteroinferior portion of the caudal septum. Bleeding, ulceration, or erosion at this site usually suggests this area as the culprit. While most of these bleeds are responsive to manual pressure and vasoconstrictors, cauterization by a trained provider may be necessary. When it is difficult to locate the exact source of a presumed anterior bleed, or if bleeding recurs, nasal packing may be necessary. Minor bleeding may be stopped by an absorbable packing that helps clotting; this avoids the need for later removal. More significant bleeding warrants insertion of removable packing material to achieve hemostasis, as well as to prevent dryness and to protect from further trauma.

Device Placement

There are many types of packing materials: an anterior packing gauze, simple nasal tampons (Figure 13.10), and nasal tampons with balloon catheters (Figure 13.11). Coating the packing material with antibiotic ointment (unless already lubricated or otherwise

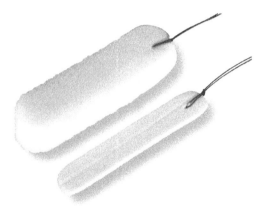

Figure 13.10 Nasal tampons. (*Source:* Reprinted with the permission of Medtronic, Inc. © 2017).

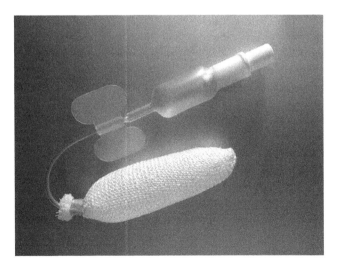

Figure 13.11 Nasal tampons with balloon catheters. (*Source:* Rapid Rhino, image courtesy of Smithe & Nephew Inc.)

contraindicated by the manufacturer) can aid in lubricating the device and may also prevent infection. The fit of the device to the nasal cavity is paramount. Gauze should be measured to twice the length of the nasal cavity, while the nasal tampon should be measured alongside the nose and cut to fit if necessary.

Using a nasal speculum to visualize the floor of the nasal cavity, the proceduralist can insert the device with forceps. Some brands of tampons have syringe-like applicators that obviate the need for forceps. Gauze should be inserted in segments. A tampon requires the moisture from the nose, or from added normal saline to expand to achieve hemostasis. A balloon catheter nasal tampon requires the balloon to be inflated to occlude the nasal cavity properly. Each of these systems is secured to the cheek. Children may require anxiolysis and/or sedation for this procedure.

If bleeding is not controlled following the application of anterior packing, it is possible that the patient is experiencing a posterior bleed. Posterior bleeds are problematic, as hemostasis is more difficult to achieve. Placement of a posterior pack is possible, but children will likely require procedural sedation and consultation with an otolaryngologist.

A Foley catheter may be used in some cases of refractory bleeds. After the Foley catheter is inserted through the nares, the balloon is inflated with water, and then the catheter is retracted into a stable position. Dual balloon packs designed for this purpose can be inserted similarly: the posterior balloon is inflated halfway, then pulled anteriorly, and then inflated further. Once the posterior balloon is in good position, the anterior balloon is inflated to keep the entire device in place. In an awake patient, the degree of inflation depends on patient comfort.

Management

Anterior packing should ideally stay in place for two to five days in order to avoid re-bleeding, while minimizing the risks of infection and tissue destruction associated with prolonged nasal foreign body retention. Antibiotics (amoxicillin-clavulanate) are commonly prescribed after the insertion of anterior nasal packing. A recent study, however, demonstrated similar outcomes in patients with and without antibiotics. Close follow-up with an otolaryngologist should be arranged.

Most posterior nasal packing is left in place for 72–96 hours. These patients usually warrant admission. Broad-spectrum antibiotics are used to prevent toxic shock syndrome and sinusitis. Intravenous hydration is usually necessary, as the device may cause dysphagia and limit oral intake. Children and adults with comorbidities (increased risk for hypoventilation in the setting of this iatrogenic obstruction) may warrant admission to an intensive care unit for even closer monitoring.

Complications, Emergencies, and Consultation

Nasal packing may lead to otitis media, bacterial sinusitis, and even toxic shock syndrome. Infectious symptoms in a patient presenting to emergency care with anterior packing in place warrant removal of the nasal packing and inspection for both signs of local infection and bleeding. Anterior packing can also block drainage of the paranasal sinuses and the nasolacrimal ducts and may even cause blood to leak into the eye. Other complications of anterior nasal packing include the potential damage it can cause to nasal skin, mucosa, cartilage, or even bone. All of the aforementioned complications may warrant consultation with an otolaryngologist.

Posterior packing creates a more significant obstruction in the sinuses, thereby increasing the infection risk and the potential for tissue destruction. The posterior packing can also cause vagal nerve stimulation, which can trigger bradycardia or bronchoconstriction. These devices may impede normal breathing enough to lead to hypercapnia and/or hypoxia. Other airway-related risks include asphyxiation and aspiration, should the packing become dislodged in the oropharynx. Patients with posterior nasal packing who presents with potential complications should prompt urgent otolaryngology consultation.

Septal Buttons

Indications/Management

A septal button (Figure 13.12) is a device inserted to occlude a septal perforation. Patients with septal perforations suffer from frequent crusting, epistaxis, and whistling sounds on inhalation. The use of a silicone button, especially one that is custom-made to fit the opening, can relieve the majority of these symptoms. Some patients find the buttons uncomfortable or difficult to insert. Consequently, they may remove/discontinue their use.

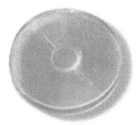

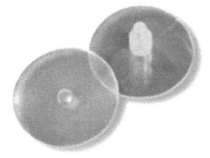

Figure 13.12 Septal button. (*Source:* Reprinted with the permission of Medtronic, Inc. © 2017.)

Complications, Emergencies, and Consultation

There are case reports of dislodged buttons that migrate posteriorly; urgent ear, nose, and throat (ENT) consultation may be necessary to assist with removal. Older versions of these buttons were not custom-made, were reported to cause irritation, and even pose a risk for aspiration. Infection is theoretically possible since this is a foreign body, but the literature does not support this, perhaps because patients are instructed to monitor and remove the device for necessary cleaning. Patients who are experiencing discomfort or who have difficulty in removing the device may be referred to ENT nonurgently, so long as there is not imminent risk of accidental dislodgement or aspiration.

Sinus Stents

Indications

Endoscopic sinus surgery is a common procedure for chronic rhinosinusitis, nasal polyp disease, tumors, and trauma. Sinus stents (Figure 13.13) are sometimes inserted into the middle meatus, extending into the ethmoid, or into the frontal sinus and frontal recess to help minimize scarring and obstruction from blood, mucous, or fibrin.

Device Placement and Management

The stents were once made of hard plastic, but now are more commonly made of flexible silicone. They may be removed a month to a year or more postoperatively. There is a newer type of stent that is made of a bioabsorbable steroid-eluting material that seems to reduce inflammation and promote patency better.

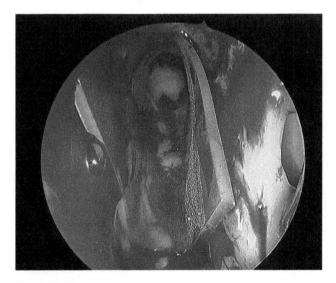

Figure 13.13   Sinus stent.

Complications, Emergencies, and Consultation

As these stents are foreign bodies, one possible complication is infection. There is some evidence that patients with chronic rhinosinusitis may harbor bacterial biofilms that may be transferred to the stents. Since these syncytia of bacteria are resistant to systemic antibiotics, stent removal may be necessary to manage chronic infection, especially given the remote but real possibility of toxic shock syndrome. Removal versus a trial of local or systemic antibiotics should be discussed with an otolaryngologist, as the surgeon must weigh the risks of stent removal with the risks of infection. Newer stents designed to elute antibiotics may help to mitigate this issue in the future.

Another possible complication of stents placed following endoscopic sinus surgery is obstruction, since granulation tissue may form across the opening. Obstructed stents warrant urgent ENT removal. Rarely, stents may migrate or become dislodged, making them aspiration risks, which warrant emergent removal. The emergency care clinician may be able to do his under direct visualization (with a head lamp). However, deeply migrated stents, or concerns that a portion of the stent may have broken off, should prompt emergent consultation with an otolaryngologist.

Nasolacrimal Duct Stents

Indications

Nasolacrimal duct stents (Figure 13.14) are often placed to treat nasolacrimal duct obstruction that has not responded to massage, probing, or other techniques. This obstruction is most commonly seen in infants and is typically a congenital anatomic issue. Older children and adults may suffer from nasolacrimal duct obstruction as well, but the cause is usually inflammatory. Regardless of the etiology, continued tearing may lead to repeated infection due to lack of adequate drainage. Infants with persistent obstruction may be at increased risk for developing amblyopia.

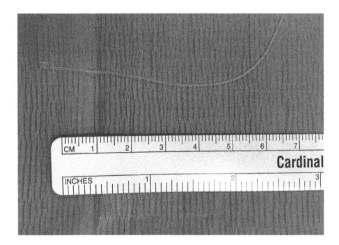

Figure 13.14 Nasolacrimal duct stent.

Figure 13.15 Nasolacrimal duct stent in the punctum of medial canthus.

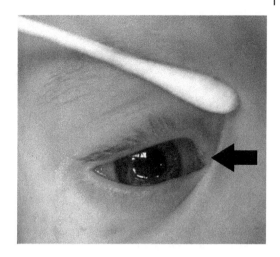

Device Placement and Management

The stents used to treat this problem are most commonly made of polyurethane or silicone. They are maintained in place for two to six months depending on patient age and indication. The stents are placed by an ophthalmologist into the puncta of the eyes, which are located at the medial canthus (Figure 13.15). The stent exits through the nasolacrimal duct in the nose, sometimes with a suture to hold it in place.

Complications, Emergencies, and Consultation

Complications that would warrant urgent consultation with an ophthalmologist for early removal would include partial dislodgement, corneal or conjunctival abrasion, granuloma formation, or other obstructions.

Throat

Oropharyngeal devices are relatively uncommon; most are designed to relieve symptoms associated with obstructive sleep apnea (OSA).

Palatal Implants

Indications and Device Placement

Palatal implants are indicated for OSA symptoms that have not responded to medical therapies. These implants consist of three small polyester devices, which are shaped like short rods. They are inserted into the soft palate, just posterior to the juncture with the hard palate. This provides rigidity to the soft palate and allows for less airway resistance. When functioning properly, these devices should not be visible on routine examination of the oropharynx. While some initial discomfort is expected after device placement, most of these symptoms resolve shortly following implantation. Transient complaints about speech and swallowing are also common.

Complications, Emergencies, and Consultation

Implant extrusion, while bothersome, is only an emergency if aspiration is a risk. As long as the implant is fully removed and has no potential for aspiration, the role of the emergency care provider is to offer outpatient referral to ENT for consideration of reimplantation. Abscess formation under the implant is an exceedingly rare complication. Antibiotics and consultation with otolaryngology for possible abscess drainage (and implant removal) is indicated.

Further Reading

Ear

1 Rosenfeld, R., Schwartz, S., Pynnonen, M. et al. (2013). Clinical practice guideline: tympanostomy tubes in children. *Otolaryngology – Head and Neck Surgery* 149 (IS): S1–S35.
2 Roland PS, Dohar JE, Lanier BJ, et al. Topical ciprofloxacin/dexamethasone otic suspension is superior to ofloxacin otic solution in the treatment of granulation tissue in children with acute otitis media with otorrhea through tympanostomy tubes. *Otolaryngol – Head Neck Surgery* 2004 Jun; 130(6):736–41.
3 Kay, D.J., Nelson, M., and Rosenfeld, R.M. (2001 Apr). Meta-analysis of tympanostomy tube sequelae. *Otolaryngol – Head Neck Surgery* 124 (4): 374–380.
4 Palmer, C. (2009 Nov). A contemporary review of hearing aids. *The Laryngoscope* 119 (11): 2195–2204.
5 Schaefer, P. and Baugh, R.F. (2012 Dec). Acute otitis externa: an update. *American Family Physician* 86 (11): 1055–1062. Review.
6 Wilson and Dorman (2008 Aug). Cochlear implants: a remarkable past and a brilliant future. *Hearing Research* 242 (1–2): 3–21.
7 Rubin, L.G., Papsin, B., and Committee on Infectious Diseases and Section on Otolaryngology-Head and Neck Surgery (2010 Aug). Cochlear implants in children: surgical site infections and prevention and treatment of acute otitis media and meningitis. *Pediatrics* 126 (2): 381–391.
8 Yawn, R., Hunter, J.B., Sweeney, A.D., and Bennett, M.L. (2015 Apr). Cochlear implantation: a biomechanical prosthesis for hearing loss. *F1000 Prime Reports* 7: 45.
9 Geraghty, M., Fagan, P., and Moisidis, E. (2014 Jul). Management of cochlear implant device extrusion: case series and literature review. *The Journal of Laryngology Otology* 128 (Suppl 2): S55–S58.
10 Yun, J., Colburn, M., and Antonelli, P. (2005 Aug). Cochlear implant magnet displacement with minor head trauma. *Otolaryngology – Head and Neck Surgery* 133 (2): 275–277.
11 Hakansson, B., Tjellstrom, A., and Carlsson, P. (1990 Apr). Percutaneous vs. transcutaneous transducers for hearing by direct bone conduction. *Otolaryngology – Head Neck Surgery* 102 (4): 339–344.
12 Shirazi, M.A., Marzo, S.J., and Leonetti, J.P. (2006 Feb). Perioperative complications with the bone-anchored hearing aid. *Otolaryngology – Head and Neck Surgery* 134 (2): 236–239.
13 Edminston, R.C., Aggarwal, R., and Green, K.M. (2015 Oct). Bone conduction implants – a rapidly developing field. *The Journal of Laryngology Otology* 129 (10): 936–940.

14 Tzortzis S, Tzifa K, Tikka T, et al. A ten-year review of soft tissue reactions around percutaneous titanium implants for auricular prosthesis. *Laryngoscope*. 2015 Aug; 125(8): 1934–9.

Nose

15 Bequignon, E., Teissier, N., Gauthier, A. et al. (2016 Aug 19). Emergency department care of childhood epistaxis. *Emergency Medicine Journal* 0: 1–6. Epub https://doi.org/10.1136/emermed-2015-205528.

16 Delgado, E. and Nadel, F. (2016). Epistaxis. In: *Fleisher & Ludwig's Textbook of Pediatric Emergency Medicine* (eds. Shaw and Bachur), 149–152. Philadelphia: Wolters Kluwer.

17 Mittiga, M. and Ruddy, R. (2016. E-book chapter). Procedures: nasal packing: anterior and posterior. In: *Fleisher & Ludwig's Textbook of Pediatric Emergency Medicine* (eds. Shaw and Bachur), 141. Philadelphia: Wolters Kluwer.

18 Riviello, R. and Brown, N.A. (2010). Otolaryngologic procedures. In: *Clinical Procedures in Emergency Medicine* (eds. Roberts and Hedges), 1199–1209. Philadelphia: Saunders Elsevier.

19 Cohn, B. (2015 Jan). Are prophylactic antibiotics necessary for anterior nasal packing in epistaxis? *Annals of Emergency Medicine* 65 (1): 109–111.

20 Zaoui, K., Schneider, M.H., Neuner, O., and Federspil, P.A. (2016 Dec). Prosthetic treatment of nasal septal perforations: results with custom-made silicone buttons. *HNO* 64 (12): 897–904.

21 Blind, H. and Berggren (Jan 2009). Treatment of nasal septal perforations with a custom-made prosthesis. *European Archives of Oto-Rhino-Laryngology*. 266 (1): 65–69.

22 Hunter B, Silva S, Youngs R, et al. Long-term stenting for chronic frontal sinus disease: case series and literature review. *The Journal of Laryngology & Otology*. 2010 Nov; 124 (11):1216–1222.

23 Murr AH, Smith TL, Hwang PH, et al. Safety and efficacy of a novel bioabsorbable steroid-eluting sinus stent. *International Forum Allergy and Rhinology* 2011 Jan-Feb;1(1): 23–32. 1/2011.

24 Perloff, J.R. and Palmer, N.J. (2004 Nov-Dec). Evidence of bacterial biofilms on frontal recess stents in patients with chronic rhinosinusitis. *Americal Journal of Rhinology* 18 (6): 377–380.

25 Bednarski, K.A. and Kuhn, F.A. (2009 Oct). Stents and drug-eluting stents. *Otolaryngologic Clinics of North America* 42 (5): 857–866.

26 Schnall, B. (2013 Sept). Pediatric nasolacrimal duct obstruction. *Current Opinion in Ophthalmology* 24 (5): 421–424.

Throat

27 Neruntarat, C. (2011 Jul). Long-term results of palatal implants for obstructive sleep apnea. *European Archives of Otolaryngology* 268 (7): 1077–1080.

Section IV

CNS Devices

14

Cerebral-ventricular Shunts

Panagiotis Kratimenos[1,2], Angela Burd[3], and Chima Oluigbo[2,4]

[1] Division of Neonatal-Perinatal Medicine, Children's National Hospital, Washington, DC, USA
[2] George Washington University School of Medicine and Health Sciences, Washington, DC, USA
[3] Hospital Medicine Division, Children's National Hospital, Washington, DC, USA
[4] Department of Neurosurgery, Children's National Hospital, Washington, DC, USA

Introduction

Cerebral shunts are commonly used for the treatment of hydrocephalus and prevention of increased intracranial pressure (ICP). Hydrocephalus can be categorized as congenital or acquired, or by the ability of the cerebrospinal fluid (CSF) to drain through the ventricular system. Communicating hydrocephalus refers to the absence of obstruction of CSF drainage; noncommunicating hydrocephalus refers to an obstruction of CSF drainage (e.g. cerebral aqueductal stenosis due to a brain tumor).

Equipment/Device

In general, cerebral shunts share common characteristics and parts:

- An inflow catheter (proximal draining) communicates with an outflow (distal draining) catheter under the control of a valve that regulates pressure (differential pressure valves) or controls flow (flow-regulated valves) (Figure 14.1a).
- Based on the location of the drainage, shunts can be ventriculoperitoneal (VP, draining into the peritoneal cavity), ventriculoatrial (VA, draining into the right atrium of the heart), ventriculopleural (VPL, draining into the pleural cavity), or lumboperitoneal (LP, connecting the lumbar subarachnoid space to the peritoneal cavity.

  Three basic valve designs are available (Figure 14.1b):

- Slit valves: Characterized by a cut (slit) in the wall of the end of the distal catheter. Fluid pressure within the lumen of the catheter, if sufficient, will open the slit and allow CSF to flow out of the catheter.
- Diaphragm valves: A flexible membrane (diaphragm) moves in response to pressure differences. They involve the deflection of a silicone membrane in response to pressure in order to allow flow of CSF.

Emergency Management of the Hi-Tech Patient in Acute and Critical Care, First Edition. Edited by
Ioannis Koutroulis, Nicholas Tsarouhas, Richard J. Lin, Jill C. Posner, Michael Seneff, and Robert Shesser.
© 2021 John Wiley & Sons Ltd. Published 2021 by John Wiley & Sons Ltd.

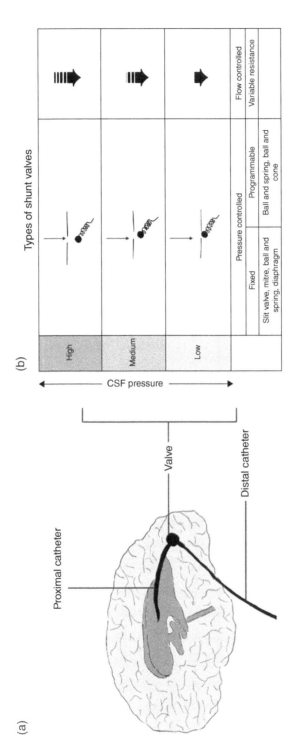

Figure 14.1 Common characteristics of (a) VP shunts and (b) types of valves.

- Spring-loaded, ball-in-cone valves: These valves incorporate a metallic coiled or flat spring that applies a calibrated force to a ball manufactured from a synthetic ruby located in a cone-shaped orifice.

Indications

The overwhelming indication for shunts is CSF diversion for hydrocephalus of various etiologies. The discussion of the causes of hydrocephalous is beyond the scope of this chapter.

Complications/Emergencies

Cerebral shunts are associated with a number of complications often requiring urgent medical attention (Table 14.1). In children, the shunt failure rate two years after implantation has been estimated to be as high as 50%. Consequently, shunt complications should always be excluded for symptomatic patients with a shunt. In general, the possible shunt complications that may result in presentation to the emergency room are shunt obstruction (also known as shunt failure or shunt malfunction) and infection.

Shunt Obstruction

Shunt failure is unpredictable in its timing but can lead to death if not diagnosed and treated immediately. It results in the progressive accumulation of CSF and subsequent increase in ICP, causing the clinical manifestations and implications seen in shunt failure. Unresolved severe intracranial hypertension may cause rostro-caudal brainstem herniation and death. The most common obstructed portion of the shunt is the proximal (ventricular) catheter, followed by the shunt valve apparatus and the distal shunt catheter, respectively. Key signs and symptoms suggesting shunt obstruction are included in Table 14.1.

Shunt Infection

Shunt infection involves colonization and active infection of the implanted shunt by microorganisms. This results in systemic manifestations of inflammation and infection and potentially life-threatening complications like encephalo-meningitis and brain abscesses.

The timing of clinical presentation is an important factor to consider when ruling out shunt infection. Shunt infections typically occur in the initial weeks and months following shunt implantation. Although the incidence of shunt infection falls significantly six months after implantation, shunt infections have been known to manifest beyond this time.

The clinical manifestation of shunt infections can be fairly nonspecific. A history of recent shunt implantation or shunt revision is important, as it may be suggestive of a shunt infection. Key concepts regarding presentation of shunt infection are shown in Table 14.1.

Table 14.1 Common presentation of shunt problems by age group.

	Shunt malfunction	Shunt infection	Shunt overdrainage
Headache	±7	±7	7
Head enlargement	+±		
Apnea	+	+	
Bradycardia	±7	±7	
Irritability	+±7	+±7	
Lethargy/sleepiness	+±7	+±7	
New seizures or change in pattern	+±7	+±7	7
Fever		+±7	
Eye deviation	+		
Papilledema	±7		
Vision changes (blurry, gaze palsies, strabismus)	±7		
Difficulty in speaking	±7		
Loss of coordination or balance	±7		
Ataxia	±7		
Loss of milestones	+±		
Decline in academic performance	7		
Nausea/vomiting	±7		7
Swelling along shunt tract or site	+±7	+±7	
Erythema along shunt site	+±7	+±7	
Drainage or odor from shunt site	+±7	+±7	
Ascites or intra-abdominal mass (pseudocyst)		+±7	
Respiratory compromise	+±7	+±7	

+, infants; ±, toddlers; 7, children and adults

Consultations and Management

The evaluation of a patient with suspected shunt malfunction is time-sensitive and should include thorough history, physical exam of the patient, and imaging (Figure 14.2).

Briefly, one should pay attention to the following:

- Location of shunt (VP, VA, VPL, or LP).
- Timing of presentation including date of shunt implantation and revision shunt surgeries.
- Type of shunt valve including whether the shunt is programmable or fixed pressure (nonprogrammable). For programmable shunt valves, confirm the last setting of the shunt valve.

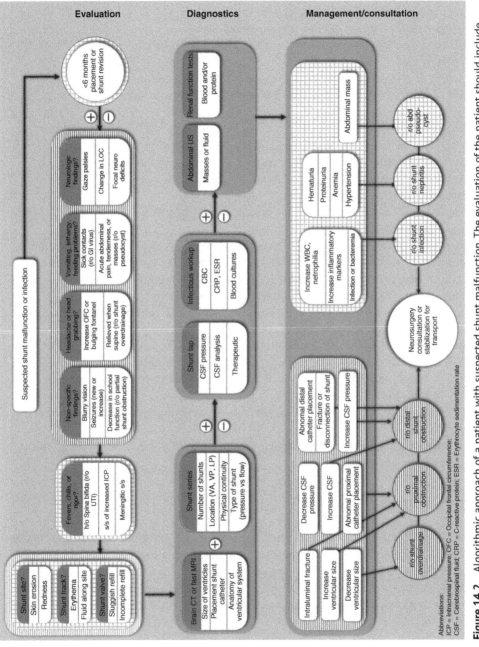

Figure 14.2 Algorithmic approach of a patient with suspected shunt malfunction. The evaluation of the patient should include thorough history, physical exam of the patient, and imaging.

Abbreviations:
ICP = Intracranial pressure; OFC = Occipital frontal circumference;
CSF = Cerebrospinal fluid; CRP = C-reactive protein; ESR = Erythrocyte sedimentation rate

- History of headache, head holding, vomiting, lethargy, irritability, gaze palsies, seizures (new onset or increase in baseline frequency), fevers, or depression in level of consciousness.
- In infants, the state of and/or changes in fontanel.
- Symptoms associated with prior shunt malfunction(s).
- History of nonspecific complaints such as declining efficiency in work or school or blurry vision.
- History of gradual acceleration of head growth across percentiles.
- History of urinary tract infections, especially in children with spina bifida.

Thorough general and neurological examination is essential including:

- Vital signs including temperature and hemodynamic stability.
- Current and trend of head circumference across growth percentiles (infants).
- Anterior fontanel and evidence of sutural splaying (infants).
- Signs and symptoms of meningitis.
- Neurological examination (level of consciousness, presence of gaze palsies, pupillary size and reactivity, and any focal neurological deficit).
- Shunt site palpation (to exclude breaks or disconnections) and inspection for erythema, skin erosion, exposure of shunt tubing, or fluid collections. A streaky erythema along the shunt tubing may suggest infection. Fluid collection along the shunt tract may signify shunt infection, obstruction, shunt fracture, or disconnection.
- Assessment of the shunt valve for emptying and rapid refilling by depressing and releasing the refillable chamber to evaluate patency of the proximal shunt tubing. A shunt valve that is sluggish or does not refill may indicate a complete or partial proximal shunt obstruction or a small collapsed ventricle. Brain imaging is useful to assess for ventricular size to differentiate between possible shunt obstruction versus collapsed ventricle.
- Current setting of shunt valve (programmable valves) using shunt valve programmer (if available).
- Abdominal exam for abdominal tenderness or a palpable abdominal mass to rule out abdominal pseudocyst or abscess.

Head Imaging

Radiological imaging either by computed tomography (CT) or by fast magnetic resonance imaging (MRI) is vital to the diagnosis of shunt malfunction. The ability to compare recently obtained brain imaging to previous "baseline" brain imaging with a functioning shunt is extremely useful to appreciate a relative mild increase in ventricular size that supports the diagnosis of a shunt obstruction. Brain imaging by CT scans or MRI are useful in identifying the:

- Size of the ventricles, a surrogate marker for the presence and degree of accumulation of CSF in the ventricles
- Position of the shunt catheter relative to the ventricles to confirm that the proximal ventricular catheter is well placed within the ventricles

- Anatomy of the ventricular system in detail such as multiloculated ventricles in complex hydrocephalus, which may have multiple draining catheters and also a "slit," or overly decompressed ventricle

An institution without MRI scanning availability should not delay the investigation of a sick and unstable patient with a potential shunt malfunction to avoid a CT scan.

Shunt Radiographic Series

The shunt series is a vital part of the radiological assessment of a shunt and should be obtained in most if not all shunt assessments. It consists of multiple planar x-rays of the skull, neck, chest, and abdomen depicting the entire length of the shunt system. At a glance, it confirms the number, location, and physical continuity of the shunt system. It may show the presence of additional components of the shunt system such as reservoirs and antiphon devices. Knowledge of this "shunt anatomy" is vital in situations in which the shunt was implanted at another institution with limited access to the records from that other institution. It can easily identify a fractured or disconnected shunt catheter.

For a ventricular atrial shunt, the shunt series can show the location of the distal catheter tip relative to the right atrium on the chest radiograph. The skull films will demonstrate the type of shunt valve (if this is known) based on the characteristic radiological appearance of each shunt valve. In the case of programmable shunt valves, it may confirm the present setting of that shunt valve.

Abdominal Ultrasound

Occasionally, abdominal ultrasonography may be indicated in the investigation of shunt malfunction due to the formation of an abdominal pseudocyst around the intra-abdominal part of the shunt.

Shunt Tap

The shunt tap is an invasive investigation for shunt malfunction. It involves gaining percutaneous needle access to the refillable chamber of the shunt valve (or additional reservoir when present) to aspirate fluid from the chamber. With a non-collapsed ventricle and a shunt with a functioning proximal catheter, fluid should be easily aspirated from the chamber. This level of intervention is usually undertaken by the neurosurgical personnel but is not technically challenging to any clinician with a good understanding of the various shunt components and the location of the refillable shunt chamber.

The shunt tap must be performed with strict aseptic technique to prevent introducing infection. It should also be deliberate, as frequent shunt taps increase the risk of shunt infections. CSF pressure may be assessed using a manometer during the tap. This is important in distal shunt malfunctions where there may be easy aspiration of fluid from the chamber since the proximal shunt catheter is patent. The absence of distal catheter flow results in CSF accumulation and increased intracranial CSF pressure.

The shunt tap may also be used in a therapeutic manner for the temporary drainage of CSF (typically in patients with distal catheter malfunction), pending definitive surgical intervention with shunt revision. The fluid aspirated from a shunt tap can be sent for microbiological analysis to detect the presence of CSF or shunt infection. Microbiological CSF fluid analysis includes:

- CSF cell count and differential,
- protein and glucose levels,
- Gram stain for presence of organisms, and
- aerobic and anaerobic blood cultures and assessment of antibiotic sensitivity.

Many cases of cryptic delayed presentation of shunt infection have been resolved by a shunt tap and microbiological assessment of the aspirated CSF.

Ancillary Investigations

A complete blood count may indicate raised white cell count and neutrophilia in shunt infections. Other inflammatory markers that may be raised in this situation include C-reactive protein and erythrocyte sedimentation rate levels. Blood culture may be obtained for patients with suspected shunt infection and bacteremia. Finally, renal function tests should be ordered for patients with a suspected infected VA (ventriculoatrial) shunt to exclude the diagnosis of the shunt nephritis syndrome.

Further Reading

1 Abode-Iyamah, K.O., Khanna, R., Rasmussen, Z.D. et al. (2016). Risk factors associated with distal catheter migration following ventriculoperitoneal shunt placement. *J. Clin. Neurosci.* 25: 46–49. https://doi.org/10.1016/j.jocn.2015.07.022.

2 Akhtar, N., Khan, A.A., and Yousaf, M. (2015). Experience and outcome of ventricular-atrial shunt: a multi centre study. *J. Ayub Med. Coll. Abbottabad* 27 (4): 817–820.

3 Bir, S.C., Konar, S., Maiti, T.K. et al. (2016). Outcome of ventriculoperitoneal shunt and predictors of shunt revision in infants with posthemorrhagic hydrocephalus. *Childs Nerv. Syst.* 32 (8): 1405–1414. https://doi.org/10.1007/s00381-016-3090-6.

4 Blakeney, W.G. and D'Amato, C. (2015). Ventriculoperitoneal shunt fracture following application of halo-gravity traction: a case report. *J. Pediatr. Orthop.* 35 (6): e52–e54. https://doi.org/10.1097/BPO.0000000000000510.

5 Ghritlaharey, R.K., Budhwani, K.S., Shrivastava, D.K., and Srivastava, J. (2012). Ventriculoperitoneal shunt complications needing shunt revision in children: a review of 5 years of experience with 48 revisions. *Afr. J. Paediatr. Surg.* 9 (1): 32–39. https://doi.org/10.4103/0189-6725.93300.

6 Jorgensen, J., Williams, C., and Sarang-Sieminski, A. (2016). Hydrocephalus and ventriculoperitoneal shunts: modes of failure and opportunities for improvement. *Crit. Rev. Biomed. Eng.* 44 (1–2): 91–97. https://doi.org/10.1615/CritRevBiomedEng.2016017149.

7 Khalil, A., Caric, V., Papageorghiou, A. et al. (2014). Prenatal prediction of need for ventriculoperitoneal shunt in open spina bifida. *Ultrasound Obstet. Gynecol.* 43 (2): 159–164. https://doi.org/10.1002/uog.13202.

8 Kitagawa, H., Seki, Y., Nagae, H. et al. (2013). Valved shunt as a treatment for obstructive uropathy: does pressure make a difference? *Pediatr. Surg. Int.* 29 (4): 381–386. https://doi. org/10.1007/s00383-012-3249-5.

9 Mizrahi, C.J., Spektor, S., Margolin, E. et al. (2016). Ventriculoperitoneal shunt malfunction caused by proximal catheter fat obstruction. *J. Clin. Neurosci.* 30: 120–123. https://doi.org/10.1016/j.jocn.2015.11.029.

10 Nikas, D.C., Post, A.F., Choudhri, A.F. et al. (2014). Pediatric hydrocephalus: systematic literature review and evidence-based guidelines. Part 10: change in ventricle size as a measurement of effective treatment of hydrocephalus. *J. Neurosurg. Pediatr.* 14 (Suppl 1): 77–81. https://doi.org/10.3171/2014.7.PEDS14330.

11 Pikis, S., Cohen, J.E., Shoshan, Y., and Benifla, M. (2015). Ventriculo-peritoneal shunt malfunction due to complete migration and subgaleal coiling of the proximal and distal catheters. *J. Clin. Neurosci.* 22 (1): 224–226. https://doi.org/10.1016/j.jocn.2014.08.005.

12 Reddy, G.K., Bollam, P., and Caldito, G. (2014). Long-term outcomes of ventriculoperitoneal shunt surgery in patients with hydrocephalus. *World Neurosurg.* 81 (2): 404–410. https://doi.org/10.1016/j.wneu.2013.01.096.

13 Sankpal, R., Chandavarkar, A., and Chandavarkar, M. (2011). Safety of laparoscopy in ventriculoperitoneal shunt patients. *J. Gynecol. Endosc. Surg.* 2 (2): 91–93. https://doi.org/ 10.4103/0974-1216.114082.

14 Singh, D., Saxena, A., Jagetia, A. et al. (2012). Endoscopic observations of blocked ventriculoperitoneal (VP) shunt: a step toward better understanding of shunt obstruction and its removal. *Br. J. Neurosurg.* 26 (5): 747–753. https://doi.org/10.3109/02688697. 2012.690908.

15 Tamber, M.S., Klimo, P. Jr., Mazzola, C.A. et al. (2014). Pediatric hydrocephalus: systematic literature review and evidence-based guidelines. Part 8: management of cerebrospinal fluid shunt infection. *J. Neurosurg. Pediatr.* 14 (Suppl 1): 60–71. https://doi.org/10.3171/2014.7. PEDS14328.

16 Thiong'o, G.M., Luzzio, C., and Albright, A.L. (2015). Ventriculoperitoneal shunt perforations of the gastrointestinal tract. *J. Neurosurg. Pediatr.* 16 (1): 36–41. https://doi. org/10.3171/2014.11.PEDS14347.

17 Wiwanitkit, V. (2012). Endoscopic observations of blocked ventriculoperitoneal (VP) shunt. *Br. J. Neurosurg.* 26 (5): 784. https://doi.org/10.3109/02688697.2012.707705.

18 Yuh, S.J. and Vassilyadi, M. (2012). Management of abdominal pseudocyst in shunt-dependent hydrocephalus. *Surg. Neurol. Int.* 3: 146. https://doi. org/10.4103/2152-7806.103890.

15

Initial Evaluation and Management of Patients with Neurosurgical Devices

Peter J. Madsen[1,3], Chariton Moschopoulos[2], and Benjamin C. Kennedy[1,3]

[1] *Department of Neurosurgery, Perelman School of Medicine at the University of Pennsylvania, Philadelphia, PA, USA*
[2] *Division of Neurology, Boston Children's Hospital, Harvard Medical School, Boston, MA, USA*
[3] *Division of Neurosurgery, Children's Hospital of Philadelphia, Philadelphia, PA, USA*

Introduction

Over the course of the past few decades, the field of neurosurgery has evolved into one that heavily utilizes various devices for the treatment of central and peripheral nervous system disorders, such as hydrocephalus, movement disorders, chronic pain, epilepsy, and spasticity. This explosion in device use virtually guarantees that all clinicians will encounter both pediatric and adult patients who are dependent upon these technologies and who may be experiencing complications of their device. Therefore, it would be helpful for clinicians to familiarize themselves with this wide range of neurosurgical devices in the hopes of providing swift, appropriate care to these patients. This chapter addresses a variety of devices, including neuromodulatory devices such as deep brain stimulators and spinal cord stimulators (SCSs), and intrathecal infusion pumps. Each category has its own unique indications, potential complications, and salient points about device management with which a clinician should become familiar. Of critical importance are those situations in which device-related complications may have profound impact on patient outcomes and if managed improperly can lead to significant morbidity or mortality. This chapter should serve as a guide to clinicians during these situations, helping to optimize patient outcomes in this frequently challenging patient population.

Neuromodulatory Devices

The class of devices that are intended to modulate the function of the brain, spinal cord, or peripheral nerves can be considered neuromodulatory devices. It is a group of devices that has expended greatly in prevalence over the past 15 years, with a growing number of indications and acceptance into treatment algorithms. In general, the goal of a neuromodulatory device is to deliver electric current to a nerve or group of neurons (either in the peripheral or central nervous system) in order to alter the behavior of a neural network or pathway that is presumed to be dysfunctional. Multiple different pathways can be targeted by various devices and include those involved with motor function, coordination, pain, or seizure generation. Indications for neuromodulatory devices are expanding at a significant rate, but a few of the most common devices, as well as their typical indications and complications, are described below.

Deep Brain Stimulators

Indications and Device Description

Deep brain stimulation (DBS) has gained wide acceptance in the treatment of certain neurological disorders. Strong clinical data have demonstrated the efficacy of DBS in the treatment of movement disorders, such as Parkinson's disease (PD), essential tremor, and dystonia, as well as psychiatric conditions, such as obsessive–compulsive disorder. It is being investigated or in early clinical use in diseases such as depression, Alzheimer's disease, and obesity. In general, this device consists of an electrode or multiple electrodes (typically one electrode on each side) that have been precisely inserted into a deep subcortical or cortical structure and connected to a lead that tunnels posteriorly behind the ear and down the neck to the chest wall where it attaches to the implantable pulse generator (IPG) (Figure 15.1). The location within the brain of the stimulating electrode is dependent upon which disease is being treated. Common targets include the subthalamic nucleus, various nuclei of the thalamus, globus pallidus, substantia nigra, and cingulate gyrus. Following device insertion, electrical stimulation can be given to the target location. The stimulation can be modulated in a number of ways to either improve the effect of stimulation or minimize off-target side effects. This is typically done by the patient's treating neurologist. Electrical stimulation is generated by the IPG and battery power associated with the device. Historically, the most common battery in an IPG is a nonrechargeable battery capable of lasting two to four years, but batteries that require daily recharging have more recently been utilized, but can last up to nine years before needing replacement. The device is periodically interrogated by the patient's managing neurologist to assess the battery life.

A common question regarding DBS systems that arises is that of magnetic resonance imaging (MRI) compatibility. If an MRI is performed on a patient with an incompatible device, complications of this scenario include the generation of thermal energy capable of damaging tissue and unwanted movement of ferromagnetic portions of the implanted devices. The ability to obtain an MRI will depend greatly on the specific device implanted. Some devices are completely incompatible with MRI, some allow for only MRI of the brain or head, some impose restrictions on magnet strength, while some have limited or no restrictions. These scenarios have been grouped into categories as defined by international safety standard working groups and include MR Unsafe, MR Safe, and MR Conditional. Devices are categorized into these groups, and their designation is available in their accompanying documentation. Medtronic, a very common producer of DBS hardware, has a number of devices currently on the market or historically implanted. MRI compatibility of their devices varies significantly. After identifying the make and model of device, a clinician can determine MRI eligibility of a Medtronic device using online tools provided by Medtronic, but the ultimate determination should be made in coordination with a device

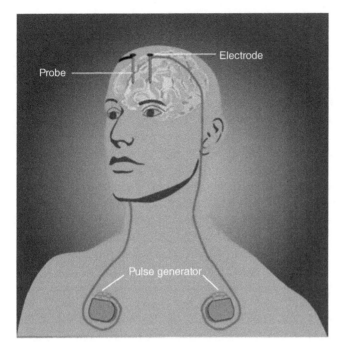

Figure 15.1 Schematic diagram for a deep brain stimulation implant. Electrode probes or leads are inserted into various brain structures and connected to extension wires that tunneled under the skin to combined pulse generators and batteries that are placed in the subcutaneous tissues in the anterior chest wall.

representative from the company who is very familiar with device compatibility. St. Jude Medical (now Abbott) now also has a DBS device available, but this device has been designated MR Unsafe.

Complications and Management

Complications can be divided into those that occur in the immediate postoperative period and those that occur in a more delayed fashion. Infection is the most common complication of the procedure, with a reported rate of around 5%. Signs and symptoms of infection include fever, erythema or pain at incision sites or along lead tracts, swelling at surgical sites, and discharge from incisions. Neurologic changes, such as altered mental status or focal neurologic deficits, can also occur if the infection has extended into the intracranial space. Infection in these patients can result in serious neurologic complications, so an urgent neurosurgical consult is recommended for evaluation of the patient if any neurologic signs or symptoms are present. Initial evaluation of a patient for possible infection should include basic infectious labs complete blood count (CBC), erythrocyte sedimentation rate (ESR), and C-reactive protein (CRP), blood cultures, and a helical computed tomography (HCT) with and without contrast. If there is still concern for intracranial infection (cerebritis or abscess), an MRI of the brain with contrast may be warranted for further evaluation if the device is MRI compatible.

Complications that occur more often in the long term rather than in the immediate postoperative period include skin erosion with exposed hardware, lead fracture or migration, device malfunctions such as battery depletion, and side effects of overstimulation. Skin breakdown occurs at a rate of approximately 1–2% and can occur at any time following insertion. Typically, it occurs at sites of prominent hardware or thin skin, such as on the scalp or behind the ear. The site may or may not have evidence of associated infection (i.e. erythema, drainage, pus, and warmth). Evaluation of the patient with exposed hardware should include labs for infectious workup (especially ESR and CRP to evaluate for chronic inflammation associated with an indolent infection). Neurosurgical consult should be sought for a thorough inspection of the site to determine if there is active infection and explant needs to be considered or if simple skin closure can be performed with or without rerouting of the device away from the site of skin breakdown. Fracture of the lead or extension wires as well as lead migration can occur at any time during the lifetime of the device and is often accompanied by acute return of the patient's neurologic symptoms. This occurs in around 1% of patients. Radiographs of the path of the device (skull, neck, and chest) are useful to identify the site of fracture along the lead or wires. MRI, in patients with compatible devices, is also useful to compare the position of the lead to its desired location on postoperative imaging. Surgical revision of the device is required in these instances to replace fractured hardware or reposition the lead in the desired location.

Device malfunctions and related technical complications are relatively rare but can occur when the battery is allowed to deplete. In situations where there is concern for device malfunction, the patient's neurologist is often able to interrogate the device to determine the battery and device status. A patient or family member may also be capable of interrogating the device, but a representative for the device manufacturer should be called to give an official assessment of the device if the neurologist is unable to perform definitive interrogation. In the case of an abrupt device malfunction, such as a battery depletion, the patient can experience significant return of their symptoms, such as severe rigidity or dystonia. This acute change can be dangerous and may lead to an emergent scenario where severe rigid dystonia can make breathing difficult. This complication is often best managed in coordination with the patient's neurologist, and they should be urgently consulted if significant symptoms are present. In this situation, their medications can often be titrated or new ones added to temporarily overcome the symptoms. A patient may require urgent battery replacement in the case of a depleted battery, but this should be performed after any symptoms are stabilized medically.

Spinal Cord Stimulators

Indications and Device Description

Spinal cord stimulators (SCSs) represent another subset of neuromodulatory devices that have become increasingly prevalent in recent years, becoming more commonly used in the treatment of chronic pain syndromes, such as neuropathic pain and failed back surgery syndrome (FBSS). Evidence for efficacy and safety of SCS exists for patients with FBSS who have predominantly leg pain symptoms as well as those with neuropathic pain associated with complex regional pain syndrome. Although manufactured by a number of device companies, SCSs generally consist of a combined IPG and battery typically implanted in the subcutaneous tissues of the posterolateral or anterolateral abdominal wall, extension wires that extend from the IPG, and leads that attach to the extension wires. The leads are tunneled under the skin and into spinal canal and can either be inserted into the thecal sac and directed superiorly to lay dorsal to the spinal cord in the subarachnoid space or, more commonly, directed superiorly in the epidural space to avoid complications that come with intradural insertion, mainly CSF leak. The leads tend to lie over the dorsal columns of the mid or lower thoracic spine, but they can be placed in higher locations if the pain being treated is associated with a higher spinal cord level. Two different types of leads are commonly used: percutaneously insertable cylindrical leads or wider paddle-type leads that require a small laminectomy for insertion. Patients will typically undergo temporary lead insertion during a trial period to determine whether a permanent system should be placed if they receive benefit during the trial period. Although the exact mechanism of pain relief is poorly understood, an SCS is thought to work by interrupting the usual pain signals that pass through the spinal cord, leaving patients with paresthesia or other altered sensation rather than pain. Newer advances in SCS technology utilize alternative stimulation frequencies and targets, but the basics regarding evaluation and management of these patients when issues arise remain quite similar.

Complications and Management

The overall complication rate for SCS implantation derived from multiple reviews is approximately 35%. These can be divided into problems at arise in the immediate postoperative period, such as infection, CSF leak, hematoma, or seroma at the IPG site, and those that occur more remotely from surgery, such has hardware migration or malfunction. The mean infection rate in the literature is approximately 2.5–5% and is most commonly caused by skin flora such as staphylococcal species. Signs and symptoms of infection include erythema, discharge, dehiscence, and fluctuance at the wound site as well as systemic symptoms of infection. Rarely, infection can spread to the central nervous system and lead to signs and symptoms of meningitis, but this tends to only occur when the CSF space was entered at the time of surgery. Evaluation of a patient with presumed SCS infection should include laboratory tests for infection (CBC, ESR, CRP, etc.). Wounds should also be evaluated for the presence of any exposed hardware. If a collection in present, ultrasound examination can be useful to assess for loculations or other signs that might suggest infection of a collection. Management of an SCS infection will depend upon the extent of infection. Superficial wound infections can often be managed with a course of oral antibiotics, but deeper infections, dehiscing wounds, exposed hardware, or infected collections will likely require surgical wound exploration and likely removal of hardware. Antibiotic treatment should be directed by microbial culture sensitivities and specificities, but antibiotic coverage should be started immediately after obtaining cultures. As another complication of immediate postoperative period, CSF leak can occur in cases of intradural lead placement or following placement of epidural leads where the dura was violated during the procedure. In cases of CSF leak, infection should be ruled out with laboratory testing and examination. Prophylactic antibiotics are often used to prevent the development of meningitis until the CSF leak can be stopped. Patients with CSF leak from a lumbar insertion site should be on bedrest with the head of bed flat. The leak can often be stopped by oversewing the skin at the leak site, but more extensive surgery or even hardware removal may be required to repair a leak. Postoperative hematoma and seromas can also occur at the IPG site following surgery. Infection should also be ruled out in these patients as described above. Ultrasound can be of use in this situation to define a simple or complex collection. Surgical drainage is typically not required unless there is evidence of superimposed infection.

Long-term complications of SCS, such as hardware migration and malfunction, are relatively common and occur in approximately 5–15% of patients. Lead migration occurs when the leads move from their desired position in the epidural or intradural space, affecting the desired efficacy of the stimulation. Patients may notice a change in the location of their induced paresthesia or loss of pain control. If suspected, lead migration should be confirmed with imaging, typically with an anteroposterior radiograph that can be compared to a postoperative film that shows the desired lead location. Reprogramming of the device can sometimes account for a migration, but considerable migration of the lead may necessitate a surgical revision of the SCS. Another cause of a sudden change in the induced paresthesia can be due to a fracture in the extension wires or leads or failure of the IPG/battery. A radiograph should be obtained to identify a break in the wires or lead, and if a fracture is found, surgical revision of the device can be planned. A suspected malfunction of the device should be interrogated using the handheld programmer, which often requires assistance from a representative of the device manufacturer. Interrogation may reveal a depleted battery or other dysfunction that may require battery replacement or device revision. During the period of device malfunction, patients may experience a return of significant pain and will likely require increases to their systemic analgesia often in coordination with their pain medicine specialist.

Vagus Nerve Stimulators

Indications and Device Description

Vagus nerve stimulators (VNSs) are neuromodulatory devices used to reduce seizure frequency in patients with medically refractory epilepsy through direct electrical stimulation of the vagus nerve in the neck. Originally approved for patients over the age of 12 years with partial onset seizures refractory to medical management, the therapy has been extended to younger age groups and patients with various seizure semiologies. In some studies, VNS appears to be more effective in reducing seizure frequency for generalized epilepsy syndromes, such as Lennox Gastaut syndrome, than in partial epilepsy syndromes for which it was originally approved. Although the definitive mechanism of action is unclear, VNS, by way of activating afferent pathways of the vagus nerve, is thought to modulate multiple brain nuclei and the limbic circuit to affect seizure pathways. VNS is also currently used or under investigation for conditions other than epilepsy, such as depression, traumatic brain injury, headache, chronic pain disorders, and inflammatory disorders thought to be mediated by the autonomic nervous system, such as asthma and inflammatory bowel disease.

A VNS consists of a combined IPG and battery and a combined extension wire with coiled leads for placement on the nerve. The IPG/battery is implanted in the subcutaneous tissue of the left anterior chest wall, and wires are tunneled into to the left side of the neck where the coiled ends of the leads are wrapped around the vagus nerve in the carotid sheath (Figure 15.2). The IPG can be programmed and interrogated using a wireless, handheld device. Currently, the vast majority of VNS devices implanted in the US are manufactured by Cyberonics, Inc. Of note, MRI can be performed in patients with the VNS device manufactured by Cyberonics as long as their guidelines are followed, which can be found on the device manufacturer's website. In general, MRI can be performed as long as the lead and pulse generator are not included in the field being imaged.

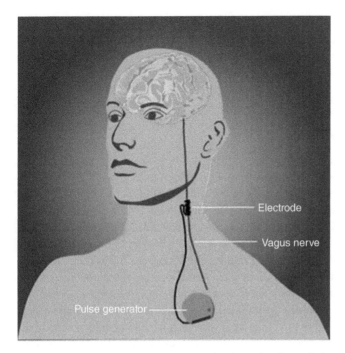

Figure 15.2 Diagram of a vagus nerve stimulator. An electrode is wound around the vagus nerve in the neck, and the lead is tunneled under the skin to a pulse generator that is placed subcutaneously over the chest wall.

Complications and Management

Complications of VNS devices are rare. Infection occurs in approximately 1% of patients and is diagnosed and managed similarly to other neuromodulatory devices with the exception that the device is not in communication with the central nervous system (CNS), so there is no risk of meningitis. Malfunction of the device is extremely rare, but fracture of the lead or extension wire can occur and should be investigated with radiographs if suspected. Patients presenting with an increase in seizure frequency over a period of time should be investigated for hardware malfunction through interrogation of the device by the patient's neurologist or a device manufacturer representative. Interrogation can identify a depleted battery, a break in the circuit, or other problems with the device. Side effects of stimulation can occur in up to 28% of patients and include hoarseness, shortness of breath, and headache. These tend to be transient and can be improved by adjusting stimulation parameters in coordination with the patient's neurologist and a device manufacturer representative.

Other Peripheral Nerve Stimulators

Currently, there exist multiple other types of peripheral nerve stimulators for various disorders – occipital nerve stimulators for headache and migraine, sacral nerve stimulators for neurogenic bladder, and hypoglossal nerve stimulators for obstructive sleep apnea – with other sites and disorders still under investigation. The principles of evaluating and managing these patients are similar to what has been described above. Infection is a common concern in the immediate postoperative period, and acute changes in the effect of stimulation should be investigated using imaging to diagnose a fracture in a lead or extension wire or a migration of the lead from its intended stimulation site.

Intrathecal Infusion Pumps

Indications and Device Description

A final category of neurosurgical devices is the intrathecal infusion pump. In general, the purpose of this device is to continuously deliver an infusion of a drug into the intrathecal space for the treatment of various chronic conditions. Examples of conditions that are treated with this device include spasticity and chronic pain. Intrathecal infusion of the gamma aminobutyric acid (GABA) receptor agonist baclofen has shown efficacy in the treatment of spasticity and dystonia secondary to disorders such as cerebral palsy, multiple sclerosis, spinal cord injury, and traumatic brain injury. Intrathecal infusion of opioids, typically morphine, can be utilized in a palliative fashion for cancer-associated pain or for severe cases of chronic noncancer pain.

Intrathecal infusion pumps comprise a combined pump and reservoir for storage of the drug, which is typically implanted in the posterior, posterolateral, or anterolateral abdominal subcutaneous tissues. A catheter travels from the pump under the skin to the lower back where it has been inserted into the thecal sac. Following the initial implantation, patients require refills of the reservoir with the drug. Frequency of refilling can vary depending on the medication being delivered, its concentration, and the infusion rate. Pump refills can typically be performed by the patient's pain specialist or neurologist through percutaneous injection.

Complications and Management

Complications of intrathecal infusion pumps are similar to other device complications with some caveats. Infection in the postoperative period following device insertion has been reported to occur in approximately 3–27% of patients with baclofen pumps and 3–9% of patients with intrathecal pain pumps. Rates of infection for baclofen pumps tend to be higher because they are more often inserted in children and patients with significant comorbidities associated with their underlying spasticity disorders. Wound infections are most common in the first month after implantation or revision of the device, but because these devices require frequent refilling, infections can occur following percutaneous access of the device for refilling. Signs and symptoms of infection are similar to other device infections, and staphylococcal species are again the most common causative organisms. Given that these devices terminate in the intrathecal space, there is a risk of central nervous system infection, so prompt identification and management of wound infections are important to avoid more serious infections. If there is concern for a device infection, imaging should be obtained to determine the extent of the infection and to identify any fluid collections that can be aspirated for bacterial culture. Ultrasound can often be useful for this, but CT scan of the site may be required to determine the depth of the infection. Superficial wound infections can often be treated with a course of intravenous or oral antibiotics, but deeper infections and infections of the device pocket typically require explant of the device and extensive antibiotic treatment prior to its replacement.

Intrathecal infusion pumps are also prone to a number of issues unique to this device category. At the time of reservoir refill, there is a risk of missing the device and inadvertently injecting the drug into its subcutaneous pocket, referred to as a "pocket fill." This has been reported to occur rarely, in about 1 in every 10 000 refills, but depending on the drug being delivered, it can be a fatal complication. Complications of a pocket fill include systemic overdose of the medication due to exposure to a large volume of the drug as well as delayed withdrawal from the drug or prolonged underdosing because it was not injected into the pump.

Overdose should be identified quickly and general supportive measures undertaken immediately. In the case of narcotic overdose, naloxone should be administered and titrated. The device should also be urgently interrogated by the physician managing the device, which typically involves aspirating the pump to determine the amount of drug in the pump versus the amount that was injected at the time of refill. Any discrepancy would represent the amount of drug injected into the pocket. During the management of this situation, the pump should be turned off and emptied, and the infusion should only resume once the effects of the inadvertently injected drug have worn off. Programming errors can also result in improper drug delivery, giving too much or too little, leading to overdose or withdrawal symptoms. Interrogation of the device by either the specialist managing the infusion or device manufacturer representative is required to determine and correct the error. Supportive therapies for either overdose or withdrawal symptoms may be required until the error can be corrected.

Intrathecal infusion pumps can have abrupt failures for a number of reasons. Symptoms of failure will depend on the medication being infused but can include subtle symptoms of reduced dose delivery (increase in pain or spasticity) or acute opioid or baclofen withdrawal (discussed further below). Causes of pump failure include fracture of the catheter, migration of the catheter out of the intrathecal space, and acute mechanical malfunction of the pump. Catheter fracture and migration should be ruled out by obtaining radiographs of the system and comparing them to postoperative images that show the device in its desired location. Occasionally, CT imaging is required to more closely inspect the course of the catheter to assess for fractures or malposition. Acute mechanical failure of the pump is quite rare, especially in newer models, and occurs in only about 2.5% of patients. During interrogation of the system at the time of suspected malfunction, the device may provide feedback that can guide in this diagnosis. One useful test of the device is a that of pump aspiration. Most pump models have a side port that connects directly with the intrathecal catheter. A trained clinician can use the port to aspirate the system, and if free flow of cerebrospinal fluid (CSF) is obtained, then the system is presumed to be in continuity with the intrathecal space. Inability to aspirate would indicate a discontinuity in the system and need for surgical evaluation and possible replacement.

A unique and potentially life-threatening complication of intrathecal baclofen pumps (ITB pumps) is that of acute baclofen withdrawal. Abrupt disruptions in the delivery of baclofen in patients with chronic exposure to the drug can lead to very serious withdrawal complications. These symptoms can be varied and include rebound spasticity, rigidity, altered mental status, autonomic instability, organ failure, seizures, and even progression to coma and death if not recognized and treated. Concern for baclofen withdrawal should lead to an immediate investigation of the pump to determine if there has been a malfunction or other error, including radiographs to look for fractures or malposition of the catheter, interrogation of the pump by the managing clinician or device manufacturer representative, and even a pump aspiration by a trained clinician. Clinicians should also emergently administer baclofen to counteract the withdrawal symptoms and prevent further decline. Aggressive supportive measures, such as airway management and vasopressor support, may be required. The following algorithms describe a step-by-step approach to patients with baclofen pump complications.

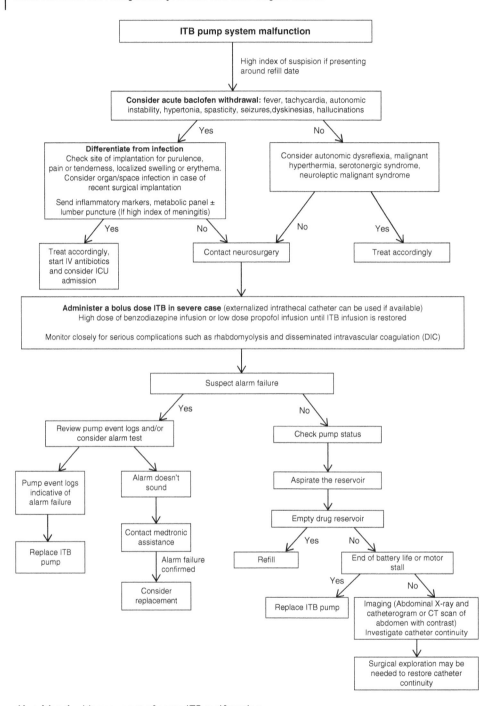

Algorithm 1   Management of acute ITB malfunction.

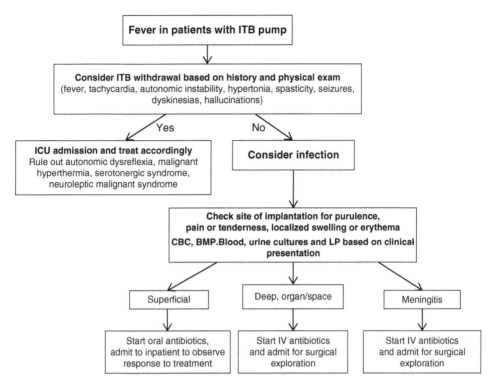

Algorithm 2 Management of fever in patients with ITB.

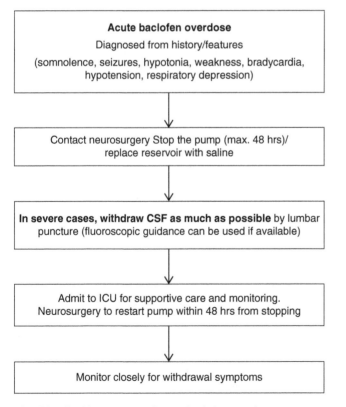

Algorithm 3 Management of acute baclofen overdose.

Further Reading

1 The International Society for Pediatric Neurosurgery. The ISPN Shunt Guide [Internet]. [cited 2017 Dec 6]. Available from: https://www.ispn.guide/hydrocephalus-and-other-anomalies-of-csf-circulation-in-children/the-ispn-shunt-guide

2 Tervonen, J., Leinonen, V., Jääskeläinen, J.E. et al. (2017). Rate and risk factors for shunt revision in pediatric patients with hydrocephalus-a population-based study. *World Neurosurg.* 101: 615–622.

3 Reddy, G.K., Shi, R., Nanda, A., and Guthikonda, B. (2011). Obstructive hydrocephalus in adult patients: the Louisiana State University Health Sciences Center-Shreveport experience with ventriculoperitoneal shunts. *World Neurosurg.* 76 (1–2): 176–182.

4 Stone, J.J., Walker, C.T., Jacobson, M. et al. (2013). Revision rate of pediatric ventriculoperitoneal shunts after 15 years. *J. Neurosurg. Pediatr.* 11 (1): 15–19.

5 Wong, J.M., Ziewacz, J.E., Ho, A.L. et al. (2012). Patterns in neurosurgical adverse events: cerebrospinal fluid shunt surgery. *Neurosurg. Focus* 33 (5): E13.

6 Pindrik, J., Huisman, T.A.G.M., Mahesh, M. et al. (2013). Analysis of limited-sequence head computed tomography for children with shunted hydrocephalus: potential to reduce diagnostic radiation exposure. *J. Neurosurg. Pediatr.* 12 (5): 491–500.

7 Wallace, A.N., Vyhmeister, R., Bagade, S. et al. (2015). Evaluation of the use of automatic exposure control and automatic tube potential selection in low-dose cerebrospinal fluid shunt head CT. *Neuroradiology* 57 (6): 639–644.

8 O'Neill, B.R., Pruthi, S., Bains, H. et al. (2013). Rapid sequence magnetic resonance imaging in the assessment of children with hydrocephalus. *World Neurosurg.* 80 (6): e307–e312.

9 Desai, K.R., Babb, J.S., and Amodio, J.B. (2007). The utility of the plain radiograph "shunt series" in the evaluation of suspected ventriculoperitoneal shunt failure in pediatric patients. *Pediatr. Radiol.* 37 (5): 452–456.

10 Ouellette, D., Lynch, T., Bruder, E. et al. (2009). Additive value of nuclear medicine shuntograms to computed tomography for suspected cerebrospinal fluid shunt obstruction in the pediatric emergency department. *Pediatr. Emerg. Care* 25 (12): 827–830.

11 Poca, M.A. and Sahuquillo, J. (2005). Short-term medical management of hydrocephalus. *Expert Opin. Pharmacother.* 6 (9): 1525–1538.

12 Kestle, J.R.W., Riva-Cambrin, J., Wellons, J.C. et al. (2011). A standardized protocol to reduce cerebrospinal fluid shunt infection: the hydrocephalus clinical research network quality improvement initiative. *J. Neurosurg. Pediatr.* 8 (1): 22–29.

13 Conen, A., Walti, L.N., Merlo, A. et al. (2008). Characteristics and treatment outcome of cerebrospinal fluid shunt-associated infections in adults: a retrospective analysis over an 11-year period. *Clin. Infect. Dis.* 47 (1): 73–82.

14 Arnell, K., Cesarini, K., Lagerqvist-Widh, A. et al. (2008). Cerebrospinal fluid shunt infections in children over a 13-year period: anaerobic cultures and comparison of clinical signs of infection with Propionibacterium acnes and with other bacteria. *J. Neurosurg. Pediatr.* 1 (5): 366–372.

15 Tamber, M.S., Klimo, P., Mazzola, C.A. et al. (2014). Pediatric hydrocephalus: systematic literature review and evidence-based guidelines. Part 8: management of cerebrospinal fluid shunt infection. *J. Neurosurg. Pediatr.* 14 (Suppl. 1): 60–71.

16 Ros, B., Iglesias, S., Martín, Á. et al. (2017). Shunt overdrainage syndrome: review of the literature. *Neurosurg. Rev.* 41 (4): 969–981.

17 Baird, L.C., Mazzola, C.A., Auguste, K.I. et al. (2014). Pediatric hydrocephalus: systematic literature review and evidence-based guidelines. Part 5: effect of valve type on cerebrospinal fluid shunt efficacy. *J. Neurosurg. Pediatr.* 14 (Suppl. 1): 35–43.

18 Kalyvas, A.V., Hughes, M., Koutsarnakis, C. et al. (2017). Efficacy, complications and cost of surgical interventions for idiopathic intracranial hypertension: a systematic review of the literature. *Acta Neurochir.* 159 (1): 33–49.

19 Wang, V.Y., Barbaro, N.M., Lawton, M.T. et al. (2007). Complications of lumboperitoneal shunts. *Neurosurgery* 60 (6): 1045–1048; discussion 1049.

20 Isik, N., Elmaci, I., Isik, N. et al. (2013). Long-term results and complications of the syringopleural shunting for treatment of syringomyelia: a clinical study. *Br. J. Neurosurg.* 27 (1): 91–99.

21 Miocinovic, S., Somayajula, S., Chitnis, S., and Vitek, J.L. (2013). History, applications, and mechanisms of deep brain stimulation. *JAMA Neurol.* 70 (2): 163–171.

22 Youngerman, B.E., Chan, A.K., Mikell, C.B. et al. (2016). A decade of emerging indications: deep brain stimulation in the United States. *J. Neurosurg.* 125 (2): 461–471.

23 Thornton, J.S. (2017). Technical challenges and safety of magnetic resonance imaging with in situ neuromodulation from spine to brain. *Eur. J. Paediatr. Neurol.* 21 (1): 232–241.

24 Medtronic. MRI SureScan for Clinicians | Medtronic [Internet]. [cited 2018 Apr 18]. Available from: https://professional.medtronic.com/mri/surescan-mri-clinicians/index.htm#.Wte0rtPwZ24

25 St. Jude Medical. St. Jude Medical Device Manuals [Internet]. [cited 2018 Apr 18]. Available from: https://manuals.sjm.com

26 Jitkritsadakul, O., Bhidayasiri, R., Kalia, S.K. et al. (2017). Systematic review of hardware-related complications of deep brain stimulation: do new indications pose an increased risk? *Brain Stimul.* 10 (5): 967–976.

27 Fenoy, A.J. and Simpson, R.K. (2012). Management of device-related wound complications in deep brain stimulation surgery. *J. Neurosurg.* 116 (6): 1324–1332.

28 Verrills, P., Sinclair, C., and Barnard, A. (2016). A review of spinal cord stimulation systems for chronic pain. *J. Pain Res.* 9: 481–492.

29 Bendersky, D. and Yampolsky, C. (2014). Is spinal cord stimulation safe? A review of its complications. *World Neurosurg.* 82 (6): 1359–1368.

30 Hoelzer, B.C., Bendel, M.A., Deer, T.R. et al. (2017). Spinal cord stimulator implant infection rates and risk factors: a multicenter retrospective study. *Neuromodulation* 20 (6): 558–562.

31 Amar, A.P. (2007). Vagus nerve stimulation for the treatment of intractable epilepsy. *Expert Rev. Neurother.* 7 (12): 1763–1773.

32 Boon, P., Raedt, R., de Herdt, V. et al. (2009). Electrical stimulation for the treatment of epilepsy. *Neurotherapeutics* 6 (2): 218–227.

33 Yuan, H. and Silberstein, S.D. (2016). Vagus nerve and vagus nerve stimulation, a comprehensive review: part III. *Headache* 56 (3): 479–490.

34 Cyberonics, Inc. MRI Guidelines for VNS Therapy [Internet] 2014 [cited 2018 Nov 23]. Available from: http://www.cardion.cz/data/mri-kompatibilita/vns-terapie.pdf

35 Woolf, S.M. and Baum, C.R. (2017). Baclofen pumps: uses and complications. *Pediatr. Emerg. Care* 33 (4): 271–275.

36 Hayek, S.M., Deer, T.R., Pope, J.E. et al. (2011). Intrathecal therapy for cancer and non-cancer pain. *Pain Physician* 14 (3): 219–248.

37 Saulino, M., Anderson, D.J., Doble, J. et al. (2016). Best practices for intrathecal baclofen therapy: troubleshooting. *Neuromodulation* 19 (6): 632–641.

38 Malheiro, L., Gomes, A., Barbosa, P. et al. (2015). Infectious complications of intrathecal drug administration systems for spasticity and chronic pain: 145 patients from a tertiary care center. *Neuromodulation* 18 (5): 421–427.

39 Prager, J., Deer, T., Levy, R. et al. (2014). Best practices for intrathecal drug delivery for pain. *Neuromodulation* 17 (4): 354–372; discussion 372.

40 Cancer Research UK. Diagram showing a brain shunt [Internet]. 2014 [cited 2017 Dec 5]. Available from: https://upload.wikimedia.org/wikipedia/commons/c/c7/Diagram_showing_a_brain_shunt_CRUK_052.svg

41 Lynch PJ. Ommaya reservoir [Internet]. 2008 [cited 2017 Dec 7]. Available from: https://commons.wikimedia.org/wiki/File:Ommaya_01.png

42 The National Institute of Mental Health. Deep brain stimulation [Internet]. 2016 [cited 2017 Dec 5]. Available from: https://www.nimh.nih.gov/health/topics/brain-stimulation-therapies/brain-stimulation-therapies.shtml

43 The National Institute of Mental Health. Vagal Nerve Stimulation [Internet]. 2016 [cited 2017 Dec 5]. Available from: https://www.nimh.nih.gov/health/topics/brain-stimulation-therapies/brain-stimulation-therapies.shtml

Section V

Miscellaneous Devices

16

Ophthalmic Devices

Marlet Bazemore[1,3] and William P. Madigan[1,2,3]

[1] Division of Ophthalmology, Children's National Hospital, Washington, DC, USA
[2] Uniformed Services University of the Health Sciences, Bethesda, MD, USA
[3] George Washington University School of Medicine and Health Sciences, Washington, DC, USA

Introduction

There are several ophthalmic devices that may be implanted in and around the eye. An awareness of this therapeutic hardware will prevent unwitting damage to their function or unnecessary investigation as to their provenance. For the emergency room physician, the purpose of this review is not to provide an algorithm of malfunction management, as their function may not be assessed adequately in the emergency room setting. Knowledge of these devices, placement, and purpose, however, is important to prevent iatrogenic injury during examination and can be useful in understanding what requires ophthalmic referral.

Eyelid

Conditions of the eye, lids, or orbit may lead to ocular surface exposure when either the eye becomes proptotic or the lid tissue is missing or dysfunctional.

Examples of conditions leading to proptosis may include thyroid eye disease, intraorbital tumor, and syndromes causing shallow orbits (as in Crouzon syndrome). In some instances, the condition may be ameliorated with a *tarsorrhaphy* (usually lateral but can also be medial), in which the margins of the eyelid are sewn together to reduce the size of the interpalpebral fissure and provide better corneal coverage. These can be rather easily torn open with only moderate pressure, if they are not identified or treated gently.

Cranial nerve VII palsy (Bell's palsy) may leave permanent eyelid dysfunction, leading to poor eyelid protection of the cornea. In some instances, a wafer-thin *gold eyelid implant* may be inserted below the skin of the upper eyelid to provide additional weight to the upper eyelid. Gravity acting on the gold weight creates mild mechanical ptosis, resulting in better coverage of the cornea.

Nasolacrimal Duct (NLD)

Nasolacrimal Duct (NLD) function is frequently degraded for a variety of reasons such as congenital membrane obstruction, acquired stenosis, or traumatic injury. Often, the repair will require placement of a *silicone tube* through the eyelid puncta and down the NLD into the area of the nose below the inferior turbinate and in the lateral nares. This tube is 1 mm in diameter and is visible as a clear solid core tube in the medial canthal angle. At times, the tubing may cheesewire through the eyelid margins along the course of the canaliculus and thus disappear from view in the medial canthal angle, though it is still present on a deeper level in the tear sac. At other times, when manipulated inadvertently by the patient, a loop of tubing may become visible on the nasal conjunctiva between the upper and lower puncta, visible over the nasal conjunctiva and perhaps the cornea (Figure 16.1). In such a case, ophthalmic ointment may be given to prevent ocular surface irritation, and referral is warranted to the surgeon who placed it, for either replacement or removal.

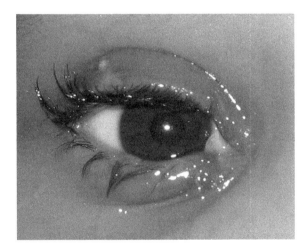

Figure 16.1 Visible loop of tubing.

Frequently, the silicone tubing is imbricated in a 3–5 mm diameter *soft white silicone sponge*, which will be found inside the nose and which serves to anchor the silicone tubing in the correct anatomic location for several months while the NLD heals with an open lumen. After three to six months, these devices are then removed. This sponge is not infrequently identified in the emergency room as an intranasal foreign body and, if not recognized as a medical device, attempts may be made to remove it, leading to significant injury to the NLD.

Sometimes, complete reconstruction of the NLD system is required and a conjunctival-dacryocystorhinostomy is performed. In the postoperative period, there may be silicone tubing extending into the nose with associated silicone sponge as mentioned above, but there is also a permanent (removable only for cleaning) *pyrex horn-shaped tube* in the medial canthal area, which drains tears from the fornix into the reconstructed tear sac and thus into the nose.

Orbit

In the case of enucleation, the volume of the globe must be replaced to ensure adequate orbital volume. This is typically accomplished with a *silicone ball* (20 mm average diameter) or a rounded *hydroxyapatite (coral) implant*. In the case of the silicone ball, the device is completely covered by orbital fat, muscle, and conjunctiva; a *prosthetic faceplate (or shell)* is painted to resemble an eye and sits between the fornices over the healthy conjunctiva. This prosthetic is easily removed for cleaning and inspection of the orbit underneath.

In the case of the hydroxyapatite implant, there may be an opening in the conjunctiva to accommodate a peg extending from the implant into the back of the prosthetic shell. This attachment can produce more normal motility of the prosthetic shell. Occasionally, the conjunctival surface may become irritated, for which ocular erythromycin may be helpful acutely with referral to the patient's primary ophthalmologist or orbital surgeon for timely evaluation.

Orbital bone fractures are frequently repaired with alloplastic materials such as silicone or, more frequently, *titanium plates* secured by screws. These can be seen on X-ray and computerized tomography imaging. Infrequently, these may erode through overlying tissues and become directly visible to the examiner. In cases of erosion of orbital plates through overlying tissues, referral to the surgeon or primary ophthalmologist is warranted.

Eye

Glaucoma may be treated by insertion of a silicone tube into the eye from the perilimbal area, which serves as a *shunt* for the drainage of aqueous from inside the eye, to a *silicone plate,* which is sutured to the eye and creates a large elevation under the conjunctiva known as a bleb. Sometimes, the conjunctiva may erode allowing direct visualization of the silicone plate attached to the outer wall of the eye typically in the superior temporal or superior nasal quadrants (Figures 16.2 and 16.3). Usually, this is found on pediatric evaluation in the emergency room as an incidental finding, rather than as the reason for evaluation. Evaluation of shunt function is beyond the scope of emergency room assessment. Consultation of the surgeon or ophthalmologist on-call should be considered in cases concerning inflammation to rule out ocular infection or endophthalmitis.

Figure 16.2 Direct visualization of a silicone plate.

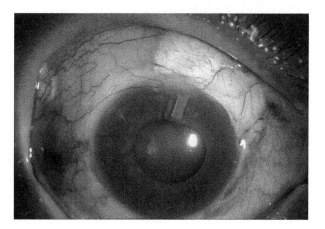

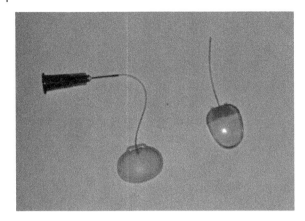

Figure 16.3   Glaucoma drainage devices.

Although infrequently used in recent times, silicone sponges and bands (Figure 16.4) may be used as part of surgical management of retinal detachment. These devices are sewn tightly to the exterior wall of the eye, causing the sclera to buckle (*scleral buckle*), thereby placing the retina and the nourishing choroid back into direct apposition and preserving the retinal function. These external silicone devices create unusual contours to the eye under the conjunctiva and, should the conjunctiva erode, can be directly visualized. In cases of significant inflammation of surrounding tissues, consultation of the on-call ophthalmologist or referral to the surgeon is warranted to rule out infection.

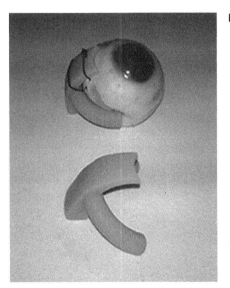

Figure 16.4   External silicone devices.

In summary, most of the ocular and orbital devices noted in children in the emergency room are found incidentally. Recognition of these devices is important in preventing unwanted injury to either the device function or the patient. In some cases, knowledge of these devices can assist the emergency room physician in determining potential need for urgent referral to the surgeon or consultation to the on-call ophthalmologist.

17

Breast Implants

R. Jason VonDerHaar[1,2] and Liza C. Wu[3,4]

[1]Department of Surgery, Indiana University Health, Indianapolis, IN, USA
[2]University of Indiana School of Medicine, Indianapolis, IN, USA
[3]Department of Surgery, Hospital of the University of Pennsylvania and the Children's Hospital of Philadelphia, Philadelphia, PA, USA
[4]Division of Plastic Surgery, Perelman School of Medicine at the University of Pennsylvania, Philadelphia, PA, USA

Introduction

Silicone breast implants were first introduced in 1964 and today are used frequently for both cosmetic and reconstructive purposes. Breast augmentation is the second most commonly performed cosmetic surgical procedure in the US, behind only liposuction. Implant-based breast reconstruction remains the most commonly performed type of reconstruction in the US, following mastectomy. The use of breast implants is generally considered very safe, but as with any surgical procedure, complications can occur.

Devices

Breast implants are designed with an outer shell of silicone, which is filled with either silicone gel or saline. Both types of implants are available in different sizes, shapes, and projections. The most common shape is the "round" implant, which is a symmetric disk. Shaped implants with more projection at the lower pole are also available and are commonly referred to as either "anatomic" or "tear drop" shaped implants. The outer silicone shell can be either smooth or textured (Figure 17.1).

While single-stage direct-to-implant reconstruction is possible in certain patients, most women undergoing implant-based reconstruction will first undergo placement of a tissue expander for the purpose of expanding to create a pocket for an eventual implant. The expander is composed of a silicone shell that can be filled with sterile saline through a port. The port can either be integrated into the shell or can be located at a remote location and connected to the expander by tubing.

Emergency Management of the Hi-Tech Patient in Acute and Critical Care, First Edition. Edited by Ioannis Koutroulis, Nicholas Tsarouhas, Richard J. Lin, Jill C. Posner, Michael Seneff, and Robert Shesser.
© 2021 John Wiley & Sons Ltd. Published 2021 by John Wiley & Sons Ltd.

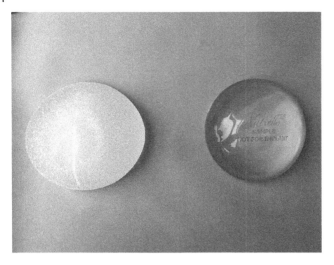

Figure 17.1 The implant on the left is a shaped textured silicone implant, while the implant on the right is a round smooth silicone implant.

Indications

Adults

- Mastectomy reconstruction
- Cosmetic breast augmentation

Pediatrics

- Poland's syndrome – breast hypoplasia or agenesis
- Severe developmental breast asymmetry
  - Adjustable saline implants can be placed to add volume as the contralateral breast grows

Management

Breast implants are placed surgically in an operating room. For breast reconstruction, the implant is usually placed into a submuscular pocket located just underneath the pectoralis major muscle. For cosmetic breast augmentation, the pocket can be located submuscular, subglandular, or a combination of the two, called *dual-plane*.

If the patient required a two-staged procedure in which a tissue expander is placed initially, the tissue expander is placed in either a prepectoral or a retropectoral plane and is gradually filled with saline over several weeks to create a pocket for the eventual implant prosthesis. For expanders with an integrated port, the port is located through the skin using a magnet. The overlying skin is then sterilized, and a needle is inserted through the skin into the port until the metal backing is hit. Saline can then be added or removed as desired. Remote ports are often able to be palpated under the skin and are then accessed in the same way.

Complications/Emergencies

As with any surgical procedure, implant placement can result in complications. Some complications such as infection, hematoma, and seroma are possible after any surgical procedure, while others are more specific to implants such as rupture, malposition, or capsular contracture.

Infection

Like all foreign bodies, breast implants are more likely to become infected compared to native tissue. This is one of the considerations that patients must take into account when choosing between implant-based and autologous reconstruction. The implant does not have a microcirculation, which limits the ability of the host immune system, as well as antibiotics to reach pathogens on the implant surface.

Following cosmetic breast augmentation, rates of infection have been reported around 1%. For implant-based breast reconstruction, the rate of infection is notably higher at 10.3%. This discrepancy may be caused by increased contamination of the surgical site by local flora during the mastectomy or may be related to the quality of the tissue in cancer patients, who may have undergone previous surgeries and/or received radiation to the area previously.

For acute and subacute implant infections, contamination with local flora at the time of implantation is thought to be a major cause. Breast skin as well as nipple ducts are colonized with bacteria that can be transferred to an implant during surgery. Most commonly, early-onset infections are caused by gram-positive organisms such as *Staphylococcus aureus*, *Staphylococcus epidermidis*, and streptococci. Infections with gram-negative organisms and anaerobes are also not uncommon. More rarely, nontuberculous mycobacterial and fungal infections can occur. Late-onset infections are hypothesized to be due to seeding from bacteremia.

Common signs and symptoms of implant infection include fever, erythema, pain, and purulent drainage at the incision and/or from the drains (Figure 17.2). Infection can also manifest as failure of the incision to heal or even exposure of the implant. The diagnosis is often made based on physical exam findings, although it can be difficult to differentiate a more superficial cellulitis compared to an actual deeper infection of the implant. Ultrasound imaging is used to look for a fluid collection around the implant. If one is present, the fluid can be aspirated and sent for culture and sensitivity to help guide future therapy. The fluid should be sent for Gram stain, aerobic and anaerobic cultures, and acid-fast and fungal cultures. Ultrasound guidance is recommended for the aspiration, as insertion of the needle too deep may inadvertently puncture the implant.

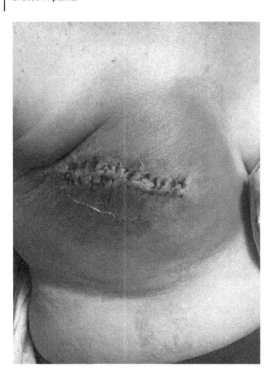

Figure 17.2 This implant-based breast reconstruction shows signs of swelling and erythema, consistent with infection.

Empiric treatment with antibiotics is the usual first step. In cases where the infection appears in its early stages, oral antibiotics may be appropriate. Coverage should include coagulase-negative *Staphylococcus* as well as methicillin-resistant *S. aureus* (MRSA), making trimethoprim-sulfamethoxazole or clindamycin good first choices. For patients with signs of systemic infection or sepsis, broad-spectrum, intravenous antibiotics such as vancomycin and piperacillin/tazobactam should be started. Once culture and sensitivity results are available, antibiotics should be tailored appropriately. Patients who are septic or do not improve with antibiotic therapy will need to have the implant removed. Fungal and mycobacterial infections are also notoriously difficult to treat effectively without removal of the implant.

While rare, there have been seven cases of toxic shock syndrome (TSS) reported in the literature following surgeries involving breast implants for both cosmetic and reconstructive purposes. Patients usually present with symptoms a few days after surgery (too early for a typical wound infection) and appear floridly septic without signs of a local wound infection. CDC criteria for TSS include fever, rash, desquamation, hypotension, and dysfunction in at least three organ systems. Despite a lack of signs of local wound infection, wound cultures will grow *S. aureus*. Treatment involves aggressive fluid resuscitation to treat the hypoperfusion and initiation of IV antibiotics targeted to *S. aureus*. In addition, the wound should be opened up and washed out to decrease the number of exotoxin-producing bacteria present. Other supportive measures will depend on the organ system dysfunctions that are present (i.e. dialysis for renal failure).

Given the potential for clinical decompensation and the possible need for removal of the implant, the patient's plastic surgeon should be notified of any concern for the presence of infection.

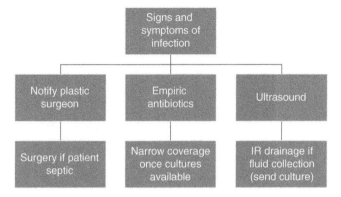

Exposure/Dehiscence

Implants or expanders can become exposed through either skin flap necrosis or incisional wound dehiscence (Figure 17.3). The presence of infection, poor wound healing due to systemic disease or history of radiation, or increasing expander volume too aggressively may all increase the risk of having an exposed implant. If the area of exposure is small and thought to be related to increased wound tension, surgical closure could be attempted if the wound tension can be decreased, such as through removing fluid from an expander or altering the implant pocket. For larger areas of exposure or those related to infection, the

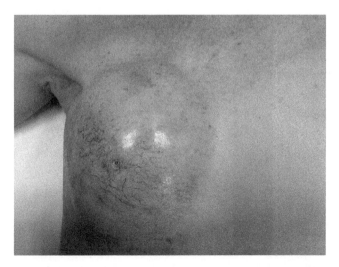

Figure 17.3 The center of this reconstructed breast mound has a small area of skin breakdown, resulting in exposure of the underlying implant. Even a small area of implant exposure necessitates an immediate call to the treating plastic surgeon in order to minimize the risk of implant loss or additional complications such as infection.

implant will usually need to be removed to allow the wound to heal. In either event, the patient will require surgical intervention and her plastic surgeon should be called for consultation.

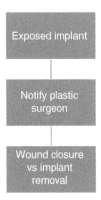

Hematoma

As with any operation, bleeding can occur following placement of a breast implant. Patients will present with a tender, swollen, and ecchymotic breast. Postoperative hematomas occur with an incidence around 1%. Most occur in the immediate postoperative period, but late hematomas can develop and may be related to coagulopathy, recent trauma, or overly strenuous activity.

Small hematomas can be observed, but evidence of expansion should prompt surgical exploration with washout of the hematoma and achievement of hemostasis. Frequently, the exact source of bleeding is unable to be identified at the time of surgery. The patient should also be evaluated for any underlying coagulopathy and have it corrected if possible. The treating plastic surgeon should be alerted to the development of a hematoma so they can determine whether operative intervention is required.

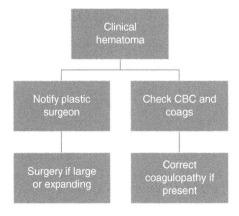

Skin Necrosis

Following a mastectomy, the remaining skin envelope is entirely dependent on its subdermal plexus for a vascular supply. If the blood supply to the flap is insufficient because the flap was made too thin, the dermal plexus received thermal injury during the operation, or pressure on the flap from an overfilled expander or external dressing is causing too much resistance, then portions of the skin may not be viable (Figure 17.4). After a mastectomy with immediate reconstruction, skin necrosis occurs in about 4% of patients. A nipple-sparing mastectomy may increase the risk even higher, with some reports indicating a rate of skin necrosis up to 16%.

If skin discoloration or other signs of poor perfusion are present in the early postoperative period, removing volume from the tissue expander will reduce pressure on the flap and may help improve perfusion. Topical nitroglycerin ointment has also been shown in studies to decrease the rate of mastectomy skin flap necrosis by about half compared to placebo (15.3 vs 33.8%). For this reason, some surgeons will routinely use topical nitroglycerin ointment postoperative in patients at increased risk for skin necrosis, such as those undergoing nipple-sparing mastectomies. Care must be taken when using topical nitroglycerin ointment, as it can be absorbed systemically leading to hypotension.

Depending on the size of necrosis, surgical debridement may be required. For small wounds, primary closure may be possible after debridement but should only be attempted if it can be done tension-free, which may require removing fluid from the expander. Otherwise, local wound care will be required. The patient's plastic surgeon should be immediately informed about any exposure of an implant so that they can determine the appropriate surgical treatment.

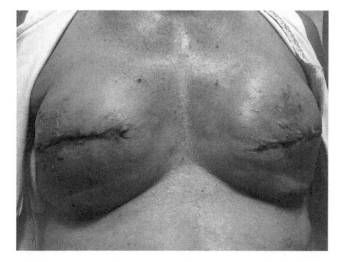

Figure 17.4   The dark skin discoloration, most prominent along the lateral aspect of the right breast incision, is consistent with ischemic changes and represents impending skin necrosis.

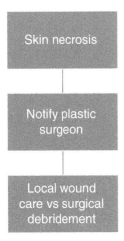

Seroma

Seromas can develop following both cosmetic augmentations and reconstructive implant procedures. Surgeon preference determines which patients will require a drain postoperatively, as well as how long the drains will stay in. In our practice, if a drain is placed, it is left in until the output is less than 30 ml per day for two consecutive days. Removing a drain too early may increase the risk of developing a seroma. The use of acellular dermal matrix may also increase the risk of seroma formation. Patients with a seroma can present with breast asymmetry, commonly enlargement of the affected breast, or may have breast discomfort. Seromas are also at risk for becoming infected.

Ultrasound is used to make the diagnosis, and treatment involves percutaneous drainage of the fluid collection, which again should be done under ultrasound guidance to minimize the risk of rupturing the implant with a needle. For larger collections, a drain is left in place until the output becomes low enough to remove it. If there is any concern for infection, the aspirated fluid is sent for culture.

Fluid collections occurring outside of the postoperative period are uncommon, but do occur and should prompt further workup. Differential diagnosis includes implant rupture, infection, malignancy, traumatic hematoma, implant-associated anaplastic large cell lymphoma (ALCL), or may simply be idiopathic. Imaging should include ultrasound and/or magnetic resonance imaging (MRI) based on clinical suspicion, and the fluid should be sent for cytology, cell counts, and culture. If the infectious and malignant workups come back negative, and the patient fails percutaneous drainage, the next step involves surgical exploration, capsulectomy, removal or replacement of the implant, and placement of drains. Some have theorized that late seromas can be caused by friction between the surface of a textured implant and the surrounding capsule, and, therefore, treatment involves exchanging the textured implant for a smooth one.

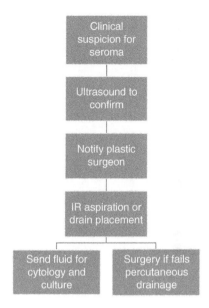

Rupture

Saline implant or tissue expander deflation will present as a decrease in breast size. Causes of deflation can be a defective valve, iatrogenic injury to the device during placement, inadvertent puncture during an expander fill, physical trauma, or from routine wear and tear over time. The diagnosis can be made clinically by the decrease in breast volume, and no further testing is required. The saline that leaks out is simply reabsorbed by the body and poses no threat to the patient. Patients should be referred back to their plastic surgeon to discuss removal or replacement of the deflated implant.

Silicone implant rupture, on the other hand, can be quite difficult to diagnose clinically. Intracapsular ruptures occur when the extruded silicone gel is completely contained within the surrounding implant capsule. Patients often will not notice any change in the implant, and the rupture may not be detectable on physical exam, only becoming identified when imaging is performed. MRI is the preferred modality for detecting an implant rupture, given its 96% sensitivity and 77% specificity. Extracapsular rupture means that the silicone gel has extended past the capsule and into the surrounding soft tissues. This may result in a palpable or tender mass on exam secondary to local inflammation (Figure 17.5). Because of the local inflammatory reaction to silicone gel, many would advocate for removal or replacement of known ruptured silicone breast implants. However, in patients who are asymptomatic, replacement is recommended but considered elective.

Because of the difficulty in detecting ruptured silicone implants, the Food and Drug Administration (FDA) has recommended that women with silicone-gel breast implants should undergo routine surveillance MRI starting three years after the implants are placed, followed by repeat imaging every two years.

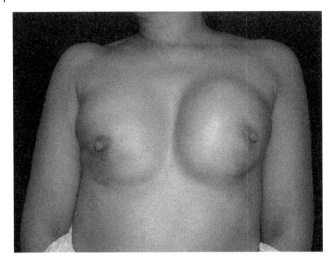

Figure 17.5 Bilateral capsular contracture causing significant visible distortion of the breast mounds (Baker IV). In addition, implant rupture has further altered the shape of the right breast mound.

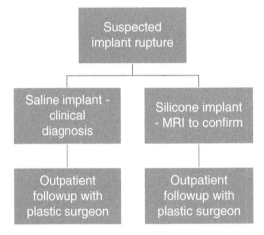

Rotation/Malposition

Round implants are symmetric and so rotation within the pocket will not be noticeable. However, anatomically shaped implants do have an orientation, and if they rotate, there can be significant disfigurement of the breast. Implants can also become malpositioned in a given direction due to an incorrectly dissected pocket at the time of surgery, repetitive forces exerted on the implant by overlying muscle, or by capsular contracture. While not dangerous to the patient, there can be substantial distress over the change in their appearance. Patients should be referred back to their plastic surgeon to discuss their options to reposition or replace the implant.

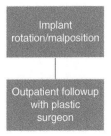

Capsular Contracture

When a breast implant is placed, the body recognizes it as a foreign object and walls it off with a fibrous capsule. A thin capsule is normal and usually asymptomatic, but, in some women, the capsule can become thickened, hard, and calcified, leading to discomfort and asymmetry (Figure 17.5). The severity of capsular contracture is commonly classified using the Baker system. Baker I appears normal and feels soft with no palpable capsule. Baker II still appears normal, but may feel a little firm with a palpable capsule. Baker III appears abnormal and feels firm with an easily palpable capsule. Baker IV appears significantly abnormal, feels hard, and is painful. In general, surgical treatment to either release (capsulotomy) or remove (capsulectomy) the capsule is offered to patients with Baker III or IV capsular contractures. Emergent treatment is not needed, and these patients can follow up with their plastic surgeon as an outpatient to arrange surgery if needed.

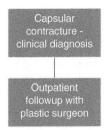

Lymphoma

Anaplastic large cell lymphoma (ALCL) is an uncommon peripheral T cell lymphoma that can develop around breast implants. The incidence is around one to three cases per million women with breast implants per year and can occur in patients receiving implants for both cosmetic and reconstructive reasons. Patients usually present with a fluid collection around the implant or less commonly a mass adjacent to the implant.

Ultrasound is used to visualize the fluid collection and any adjacent capsular masses. The fluid should be aspirated and any masses seen biopsied by fine needle aspiration (FNA). Any fluid collection occurring around an implant more than a year out from surgery without evidence of infection or trauma should raise suspicion for ALCL. Cytology on the aspirated fluid is used to confirm the diagnosis.

Complete surgical resection of the implant, capsule, and any involved mass is recommended for all patients with breast implant-associated ALCL.

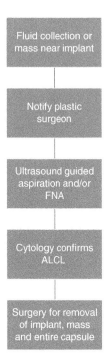

Mondor's Disease

Mondor's disease is a superficial thrombophlebitis of the breast. It can occur following either breast augmentation or reconstruction. The classic presentation is of a tender palpable cord on the breast that occurs three to six weeks after surgery. It is thought to be due to transection of superficial veins during surgery, which leads to venous stasis and then thrombosis, and is more common with transverse inframammary incisions. The disease itself is self-limited to about six to eight weeks, so treatment is focused on symptomatic relief with nonsteroidal anti-inflammatory drugs (NSAIDs) and warm compresses.

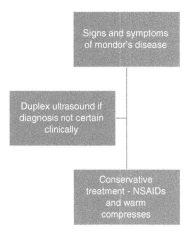

Consultation

A plastic surgeon should be involved in managing complications related to breast implants, whether they were placed for cosmetic or reconstructive indications. Complications such as infection, implant exposure, hematoma, and skin necrosis require urgent plastic surgery consultation. Many issues are able to be dealt with on an outpatient basis.

Further Reading

1 2015 Cosmetic Surgery National Data Bank Statistics. American Society for Aesthetic Plastic Surgery. http://www.surgery.org/sites/default/files/ASAPS-Stats2015.pdf (Accessed on February 17, 2017).

2 Kjoller, K., Holmich, L.R., Jacobsen, P.H. et al. (2002). Epidemiological investigation of local complications after cosmetic breast implant surgery in Denmark. *Ann. Plast. Surg.* 48: 229–237.

3 Olsen, M.A., Nickel, K.B., Fox, I.K. et al. (2015). Incidence of surgical site infection following mastectomy with and without immediate reconstruction using private insurer claims data. *Infect. Control Hosp. Epidemiol.* 36: 907–914.

4 Brand, K.G. (1993). Infection of mammary prostheses: a survey and the question of prevention. *Ann. Plast. Surg.* 30: 289–295.

5 Seng, P., Bayle, S., Alliez, A. et al. (2015). The microbial epidemiology of breast implant infections in a regional referral centre for plastic and reconstructive surgery in the south of France. *Int. J. Infect. Dis.* 35: 62–66.

6 Holm, C. and Muhlbauer, W. (1998). Toxic shock syndrome in plastic surgery patients: case report and review of the literature. *Aesthetic Plast. Surg.* 22: 180–184.

7 Collins, J.B. and Verheyden, C.N. (2012). Incidence of breast hematoma after placement of breast prostheses. *Plast. Reconstr. Surg.* 129: 413e–420e.

8 Antony, A.K., Mehrara, B.M., McCarthy, C.M. et al. (2009). Salvage of tissue expander in the setting of mastectomy flap necrosis: a 13-year experience using timed excision with continued expansion. *Plast. Reconstr. Surg.* 124: 356–363.

9 Rusby, J.E., Smith, B.L., and Gui, G.P. (2010). Nipple-sparing mastectomy. *Br. J. Surg.* 97: 305–316.

10 Gdalevitch, P., Van Laeken, N., Bahng, S. et al. (2015). Effects of nitroglycerin ointment on mastectomy flap necrosis in immediate breast reconstruction: a randomized controlled trial. *Plast. Reconstr. Surg.* 135: 1530–1539.

11 Sbitany, H. and Serletti, J.M. (2011). Acellular dermis-assisted prosthetic breast reconstruction: a systematic and critical review of efficacy and associated morbidity. *Plast. Reconstr. Surg.* 128: 1162–1169.

12 Bengtson, B., Brody, G.S., Brown, M.H. et al. (2011). Managing late periprosthetic fluid collections (seroma) in patients with breast implants: a consensus panel recommendation and review of the literature. *Plast. Reconstr. Surg.* 128: 1–7.

13 Hall-Findlay, E.J. (2011). Discussion: managing late periprosthetic fluid collections (seroma) in patients with breast implants: a consensus panel recommendation and review of the literature. *Plast. Reconstr. Surg.* 128: 10–12.

14 Vestito, A., Mangieri, F.F., Ancona, A. et al. (2012). Study of breast implant rupture: MRI versus surgical findings. *Radiol. Med.* 117: 1004–1018.

15 Holmich, L.R., Vejborg, I.M., Conrad, C. et al. (2004). Untreated silicone breast implant rupture. *Plast. Reconst. Surg.* 114: 204–214.

16 Austad, E.D. (2002). Breast implant-related silicone granulomas: the literature and the litigation. *Plast. Reconstr. Surg.* 109: 1724–1730.

17 Risks of Breast Implants. U.S. Food and Drug Administration. 2013 https://www.fda.gov/MedicalDevices/ProductsandMedicalProcedures/ImplantsandProsthetics/BreastImplants/ucm064106.htm (Accessed February 19, 2017)

18 de Jong, D., Vasmel, W.L., de Boer, J.P. et al. (2008). Anaplastic large-cell lymphoma in women with breast implants. *JAMA* 300: 2030–2035.

19 Brody, G.S., Deapen, D., Taylor, C.R. et al. (2015). Anaplastic large cell lymphoma occurring in women with breast implants: analysis of 173 cases. *Plast. Reconstr. Surg.* 135: 695–705.

20 Clemens, M.W., Medeiros, L.J., Butler, C.E. et al. (2016). Complete surgical excision is essential for the management of patients with breast implant-associated anaplastic large-cell lymphoma. *J. Clin. Oncol.* 34: 160–168.

21 Pignatti, M., Loschi, P., Pedrazzi, P., and Marietta, M. (2014). Mondor's disease after implant-based breast reconstruction. Report of three cases and review of the literature. *J. Plast. Reconstr. Aesthet. Surg.* 67: e275–e277.

18

Cutaneous Delivery Systems/Patches

Desiree M. Seeyave

Department of Emergency Medicine & Hospitalist Services, Children's Hospital of Georgia Emergency Department, Augusta, GA, USA

Introduction

Cutaneous delivery systems were first used in ancient China where medicated plasters were applied to the skin and left to dry. The transdermal route provides medication through the skin in a noninvasive manner. The medication is administered via a patch that is adhered to the patient's skin, and the medication is absorbed through the skin into the bloodstream. The patch can remain on the skin for as long as one week, if indicated.

The US Food and Drug Administration (FDA) classifies the transdermal patch as a combination product, which consists of a medical device (drug delivery system) combined with a drug. Safety and efficacy of any transdermal patch must be demonstrated for FDA approval and sales to proceed. The first transdermal patch approved by the FDA was in 1979; it was for scopolamine for motion sickness. Since then, numerous other drugs have been approved for use in the US.

Indications

Common uses of the transdermal patch:

- Nicotine patch – This is the highest selling transdermal patch in the US. It releases nicotine in small controlled doses to help with the cessation of tobacco smoking.
- Opioids, e.g. fentanyl and buprenorphine, are available in patch form for round-the-clock pain relief
- Hormones – Available as estrogen patches for treatment of menopausal symptoms, post-menopausal osteoporosis, in transgender women for hormonal replacement therapy. Contraceptive patches and testosterone patches are also available.

- Nitroglycerin patches – for angina treatment.
- Motion sickness – the scopolamine patch was the first that was commercially available.
- Hypertension – clonidine.
- Antidepressants – selegiline and 5-hydroxytryptophan are available in patch form.
- Attention deficit hyperactivity disorder (ADHD) – Daytrana is the first methylphenidate available in patch form.
- Alzheimer's treatment – rivastigmine.

Management

Equipment/Device

The transdermal patch consists of three basic layers:

- *Outer layer or backing*: It is water-resistant and provides protection from the environment, does not come into contact with the patient's skin.
- *Middle layer*: It contains medication and adhesive. Medication may be released from a reservoir through a porous membrane or via body heat melting the medication embedded in the adhesive.
- *Inner layer*: Clear release liner that is removed prior to patch application to skin.

Some transdermal patches have variations to the basic patch described above, with single or multiple layers of drug that allow for immediate and controlled release of drugs. Some patches contain reservoirs of medication in liquid or semisolid form that is released slowly from its compartment.

Vapor Patch

The adhesive layer is able to release vapor, such as essential oils for treatment of nasal congestion. Vapor patches are also used as sleep aids and smoking cessation.

Application of the Transdermal Patch

- Wash hands before and after application.
- Choose site of application, usually not the same site as the last patch application.
- Clean skin to remove dirt, lotions, powders, oils, or anything that may interfere with adherence.
- Remove packaging, make sure not to cut the patch with scissors.
- Remove protective inner liner.
- Apply patch firmly and press down around the edges.
- If patch starts to fall off before time for a new patch, try to press it back on or tape or cover with a sticky adhesive such as Tegaderm. A new patch may need to be placed if the old one does not stick back on.

Removal of the Transdermal Patch

- Peel patch away from skin
- Fold patch in half with adhesive sides touching and seal it shut
- Throw patch away securely or flush down the toilet – used patches may still contain medication and can be dangerous if ingested by children, adults, or pets

Advantages of the Cutaneous Route of Drug Administration Are

- Therapeutic effects are achieved at lower peak doses since first-pass hepatic metabolism is bypassed and there is no enzymatic degradation in the acidic gastrointestinal (GI) tract
- There is a more constant skin to bloodstream absorption, so peak and trough drug levels do not occur; hence, plasma drug levels remain constant
- Bypassing the GI tract leads to reduced risk of GI side effects
- Reduction in the need for frequent administration and improved patient compliance
- It is helpful for patients who have difficulty swallowing pills
- Not painful like intravenous or intramuscular injections
- With the removal of the patch, there is immediate cessation of drug administration

Disadvantages of Use

- Only medications with molecules that are small enough to be absorbed through the skin can be delivered this way
- Some patients may be concerned that the patch may be visible and less private than other methods of drug delivery, e.g. the contraceptive patch
- Skin hypersensitivity to any components of the transdermal patch system
- Patients with sensitive skin or exfoliative dermatitis may not be good candidates
- Potential for drug interactions or side effects of the particular drug contained in the patch
- If the patch falls off without the knowledge of the patient, there will be no medication administration

Complications/Emergencies

Drug overdose

Any drug used in transdermal patches can have adverse effects similar to effects from other routes of administration. Drug interactions with other medications can also occur.

Most notably, there have been multiple cases of death and serious opioid adverse effects from overdose of opioids from transdermal patches. There have also been case reports of ingestion and accidental skin application of fentanyl transdermal patches by pediatric patients causing serious adverse effects such as respiratory depression and toxic leukoencephalopathy.

Management

In cases of adverse events, drug overdoses, or toxicity, an advantage to the transdermal patch is that as soon as it is removed, drug delivery ceases. Treatment of the patient should proceed accordingly, e.g. opioid overdose reversal with naloxone, airway management.

Burns

- Magnetic resonance imaging (MRI)
  - Some transdermal patches contain metal in the backing or outer layer. The pieces of metal can overheat during an MRI scan and cause skin burns in the area of the patch in contact with the skin. In 2009, the FDA issued a public health advisory warning of the risk of burns and recommended that all patients wearing a patch should be reviewed before having an MRI. If it is unknown whether a transdermal patch contains metal or is not labeled, patches should be removed prior to an MRI and then replaced after. Burns that occur while wearing a patch during an MRI should be reported to the FDA through the MedWatch program by calling 1-800-FDA-1088 or via the Internet at http://www.fda.gov/Safety/MedWatch/HowToReport/default.htm
- Defibrillation
  - There have been reports of skin burns occurring when patients with transdermal patches containing metal in the backing receive shocks from external or internal defibrillators. If patients are known to have transdermal patches, these should be removed prior to defibrillation

Defective packaging

- The ADHD patch Daytrana was voluntarily recalled in 2007 by the manufacturer due to problems with removing the protective liner. There was no defect in the medication delivery system. Since then, there have been no further issues with the Daytrana patch

Skin complications

- Skin irritation or breakdown due to the transdermal patch should be treated by removal of the patch and replacing it with a new one in an area of unaffected healthy skin. Local wound care should then proceed as needed.

Further Reading

1 Nachum, Z., Shupak, A., and Gordon, C.R. (2006). *Transdermal scopolamine for prevention of motion sickness: clinical pharmacokinetics and therapeutic applications. Clinical Pharmacokinetics* 45 (6): 543–566.

2 *FDA Drug Safety Communication: FDA requiring color changes to Duragesic (fentanyl) pain patches to aid safety—emphasizing that accidental exposure to used patches can cause death.*

https://web.archive.org/web/20090307042455/http://www.fda.gov/cder/drug/advisory/transdermalpatch.htm. Archived from the original on January 18, 2017

3 Foy, L., Seeyave, D.M., and Bradin, S.A. (2011 Sept). *Toxic leukoencephalopathy due to transdermal fentanyl overdose. Pediatr Emergency Care* 27 (9): 854–856.

4 *FDA Public Health Advisory: Risk of burns during MRI scans from transdermal drug patches with metallic backing.* https://web.archive.org/web/20090307042455/http://www.fda.gov/cder/drug/advisory/transdermalpatch.htm. Archived from the original on January 18, 2017

5 Brown, M.R., Denman, R., and Platts, D. (2009 Nov). *Analgesic patches and defibrillators: a cautionary tale. Europace* 11 (11): 1552–1553.

19

Dental Emergencies Involving Oral Hardware

Chisom O.A. Agbim[1] and Ioannis Koutroulis[2]

[1] *Division of Emergency Medicine, Children's National Medical Center, Washington, DC, USA*
[2] *Department of Pediatric Emergency Medicine, Children's National Medical Center, Washington, DC, USA*

Introduction

Most oral emergencies involving dental hardware that present to the emergency department (ED) are not "true" emergencies and can be stabilized and referred for more permanent repair by a dental specialist at a later time. The purpose of this chapter is to review common orthodontic appliances for both pediatric and adult patients and describe a stepwise management of issues that may arise when they malfunction. Complications involving dental braces, fillings, crowns, bridges, and implants will be discussed below.

Dental Braces

Indications

Braces are perhaps one of the most common orthodontic devices. They are used to properly align and straighten the permanent teeth and correct issues including crowding, overbite/underbite, and misalignment of the teeth and jaw. Braces include three main components: brackets, bands, and archwires (Figure 19.1). Other components may include elastics (rubber bands and ligatures), springs, and power chains. Any of these individual components can malfunction. Most patients can troubleshoot small issues at home and follow up in an orthodontist clinic; however, complications may result in significant pain, bleeding, or potential for infection that require appropriate care in the ED.

Complications/Emergencies

Loose Bracket
Brackets are the small square component of braces that are cemented to the teeth. They are composed of metal or ceramic material. A bracket may become loose and completely separate from a tooth secondary to food, direct trauma, or manipulation. This is one of

Emergency Management of the Hi-Tech Patient in Acute and Critical Care, First Edition. Edited by
Ioannis Koutroulis, Nicholas Tsarouhas, Richard J. Lin, Jill C. Posner, Michael Seneff, and Robert Shesser.
© 2021 John Wiley & Sons Ltd. Published 2021 by John Wiley & Sons Ltd.

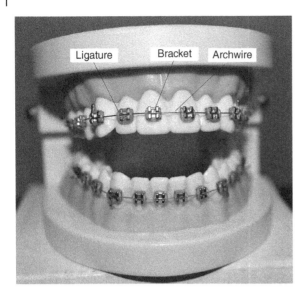

Figure 19.1 Components of orthodontic braces.

the most common complications regarding braces. If the bracket is still attached to the archwire, it should be left in place. Providers should use dental wax to cover the bracket and hold it in place until it can be recemented by an orthodontist. If the bracket has become completely loose, it should be removed from the mouth to prevent aspiration and saved if possible. Pain control should be top priority, and the patient should be advised to rinse his/her mouth regularly with salt water and transition to a soft food diet as tolerated.

Indications for Immediate Specialist Consultation

Loose or broken brackets do not meet criteria for immediate specialist consultation. A bracket that has become completely dislodged should be saved if possible. Patients should follow up with their orthodontist at the next available appointment.

Protruding/Broken Archwire

The orthodontic archwire is a guidewire that places force on the individual orthodontic brackets resulting in movement of teeth and correction of alignment. Occasionally, patients may experience pain and discomfort associated with a protruding archwire. Protruding archwires may also cause trauma and inflammation to the surrounding mucosa. If a wire becomes loose from its bracket, providers may use tweezers or forceps to place the wire back to its original position in the bracket. Often, the guidewire can be pushed back into position by sliding the wire toward the opposite end of the mouth. If a provider is unable to adjust the wire, a wire cutter can be used to clip the wire behind the last tooth where it is securely fastened. Special care should be taken to prevent the end that is clipped from becoming a loose foreign body. Using a piece of gauze to catch the loose fragment is strongly recommended as a secondary precaution measure. Dental wax can be placed over the newly cut end to help alleviate sharp corners. Immediate follow-up with the patient's orthodontist should be arranged.

Indications for Immediate Specialist Consultation

A protruding or broken archwire does not meet criteria for immediate specialist consultation. Patients should follow up with their orthodontist at the next available appointment.

Dental Implants

Implications

A dental implant is a metal post or frame that is surgically anchored in the mandible below the gumline and serves as a solid foundation for the placement of artificial teeth (crowns or bridges) as seen in Figure 19.2. Implants are made of titanium, which fuses with the bone over time through a process known as osseointegration. Because dental implants are fused to the bone, they offer a more stable base than fixed bridges or dentures.

Complications/Emergencies

Complications from dental implants usually include infection, local or referred pain, and failed osseointegration. Failed osseointegration occurs when the metal implant does not fuse correctly with the bone, which requires the expertise of a skilled provider. Infection of local tissue and nerve damage causing pain are the most common emergencies affecting

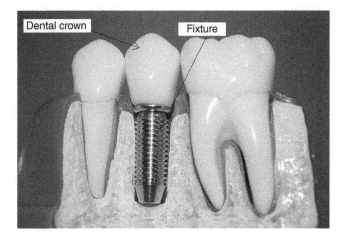

Figure 19.2 Components of an orthodontic crown.

patients with dental implants. For these patients, pain control with local anesthetics and a short course of systemic analgesics is a top priority. Signs of infection include gingival inflammation, localized pain, fever, bleeding, or purulent drainage at the implantation site. Patients with infection should be given a course of antibiotics and scheduled for urgent follow-up with a dental specialist or surgeon.

Occasionally, dental implant complications can warrant hospitalization. A recent study found that between 2008 and 2010, there were 1200 patients who visited the ED for implant failure with one-third of the visits related to osseointegration failures. Following the ED visit, 82.2% of these patients were discharged, while 13.3% were admitted to the hospital for further management. Although there are no clear criteria for hospital admission, providers should consider factors including medical comorbidities, the patient's ability to maintain hydration in an outpatient setting, the timing and availability of resources for repair, and medical stability when considering admission or discharge from the ED.

Indications for Immediate Specialist Consultation

Failed or infected dental implants require dental consultation to evaluate the extent of the complication and for management. Periodontal or periapical abscesses should be evacuated urgently by a dentist. In addition, implant complications due to failed osseointegration should be removed by a dentist using local anesthesia. Removal should not be attempted by emergency providers, as some failed dental implants may require further surgical management such as bone grafting.

Dental Crowns and Bridges

Implications

A dental crown is a covering or "cap" that is placed over a tooth to restore strength and shape as well as to protect the original tooth (Figure 19.2). Crowns can be made of a variety of materials including resin, ceramic, metal, and porcelain fused to metal. A dental bridge is a device that is used to approximate large gaps in the oral cavity caused by missing teeth. It consists of two or more anchoring (abutment) teeth on either side of the gap with a false tooth or teeth in between to fill the gap referred to as *pontics*.

Complications/Emergencies

Complications with dental crowns and bridges include chipping, loose crown, infection, discomfort, and sensitivity. A patient should be referred to a dentist for repair of chipped or loose crowns. In cases where the loose crown has completely detached from a tooth, providers should thoroughly clean the crown and replace it over the tooth using dental adhesive. If dental adhesive is not available in the ED, providers may use a small amount of petroleum jelly inside the crown and reinsert it on top of the original tooth. Sensitivity may be alleviated with the application of topical anesthetics such as benzocaine. Symptoms of infection include gingival swelling, sensitivity, pain, purulent drainage, foul odor, or, in some cases, lymphadenopathy. Infections require a short course of antibiotics and, in some cases, bedside drainage by a specialist in the ED.

Indications for Immediate Specialist Consultation

Patients experiencing complications from dental crowns or bridges should follow up with their dentist at the next available appointment. No immediate consultation is required in the ED.

Dental Fillings

Implications/Management

Dental fillings are used when a person presents with a dental caries or, in some cases, cracked tooth. In these instances, the decayed portion of the tooth is removed and "filled" with a synthetic material. Types of cavity fillings include amalgam, composite/filled resin (combination of glass or quartz filler), metals (gold or silver), ceramic, and glass ionomer (combination of acrylic or glass).

Complications/Emergencies

The two most common emergencies from dental fillings include sensitivity and infection. Tooth sensitivity can be managed with the application of topical anesthetic such as benzocaine. Occasionally, persons with fillings may present with periodontal infection or abscess. Signs of tooth abscess include swelling of the face or neck, sensitivity or pressure from chewing or biting, lymphadenopathy of the jaw or neck, fever, purulent drainage, or severe persistent throbbing of the affected tooth. Patients presenting with infection will require oral antibiotics and follow-up with a primary dentist. Depending on the extent of the infection, patients may require drainage by a skilled specialist, which may be performed on an outpatient basis if the patient is medically stable with no concern for sepsis.

Indications for Immediate Specialist Consultation

Complications involving dental devices present frequently to the ED. Providers should be familiar with common dental devices and be able to troubleshoot common complications associated with these devices in order to recognize issues and stabilize the patient in the ED for more permanent fixation by a dental specialist.

Patients who present with tooth or gingival abscesses from infected fillings require dental consultation in the ED for evacuation. Patients experiencing tooth sensitivity secondary to dental fillings should follow up with their dentist at the next available appointment.

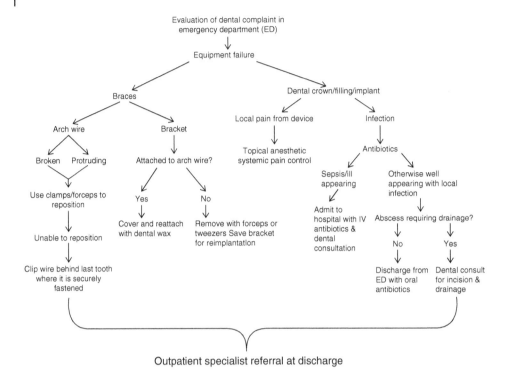

Outpatient specialist referral at discharge

Further Reading

1 Popat, H., Thomas, K., and Farnell, D.J.J. (2016). Management of orthodontic emergencies in primary care – self-reported confidence of general dental practitioners. *Br. Dent. J.* 221 (1): 21–24. http://proxygw.wrlc.org/login?url=https://search-proquest-com.proxygw.wrlc.org/docview/1802471700?accountid=11243. https://doi.org/10.1038/sj.bdj.2016.495.

2 Dowsing, P., Murray, A., and Sandler, J. (2015). Emergencies in orthodontics. Part 1: management of general orthodontic problems as well as common problems with fixed appliances. *Dent. Update* 42 (2) 4, 137. doi: https://doi.org/10.12968/denu.2015.42.2.131.

3 Buttaravoli, P. and Leffler, S. (2012). Chapter 55 – Orthodontic Complications. In: *Minor Emergencies*, 203–204. Elsevier Inc https://doi.org/10.1016/B978-0-323-07909-9.00055-6.

4 Camps-Font, O. (2015). Postoperative infections after dental implant placement: prevalence, clinical features, and treatment. *Implant Dent.* 24 (6): 713–719.

5 Elangovan, S. (2016). Estimates of hospital based emergency department visits due to dental implant failures in the United States. *J. Evid. Based Dent. Pract.* 16 (2): 81–85.

Section VI

Wound Management Devices

20

Emergency Management of Patients with Negative Pressure Wound Therapy Devices (NPWTD)

David Yamane[1] and Tenagne Haile-Mariam[2]

[1] *Department of Emergency Medicine and Department of Anesthesia and Critical Care Medicine, George Washington University Hospital, Washington, DC, USA*
[2] *Department of Emergency Medicine, George Washington University School of Medicine and Health Sciences, Washington, DC, USA*

Introduction

Negative pressure wound therapy treatment devices (NPWTDs) are used for both curative and palliative treatments of poorly healing wounds. They are most often prescribed for surgical or traumatic wounds intended to close by secondary or tertiary intention and to improve graft outcome. Although they are more likely to be prescribed by surgeons, they are utilized by other specialists and can be used to treat a wide range of wounds, including diabetic foot ulcers, pressure ulcers, thermal injuries, and closed but at-risk wounds. NPWTD therapy is often initiated in the hospital but can also be started at an outpatient clinic, a residential facility, or even a patient's home. Patients who initiate NPWTD treatment in the hospital are usually discharged to these other settings to complete their course of treatment. The duration of therapy is usually several weeks but can be extended for much longer periods in some patients, with dressing changes and wound evaluations occurring at least two to three times a week for most patients.

The use of NPWTD has increased greatly over the last two to three decades, and their increased use, coupled with the fact that they are used extensively in patients who are not hospitalized, meaning that patients will very likely present to an Emergency Department (ED) with device-related questions and complications. In addition, almost all deaths and many of the injuries associated with NPWTD occur in patients who are at home or in long-term care facilities. The ED practitioner must, therefore, be prepared to be the "first responder" for an emergent or even catastrophic device-related problem. Yet, addressing NPWTD-related problems can be a particularly vexing challenge to ED practitioners. NPWTDs are very rarely prescribed or placed in an ED and most emergency medicine practitioners have probably never observed an NPWTD dressing change. Most ED clinicians are unlikely to have received education or training on the care of patients with NPWTD during their residencies. Therefore, the primary goal of this chapter is to provide an ED practitioner with a framework for formulating a rational diagnostic and therapeutic plan for clinical and device-related problems that would lead a patient with an NPWTD to seek emergency care.

Mechanisms of Action

The mechanisms by which NPWTDs improve wound healing are not fully understood, but the application of negative pressure to damaged tissues appears to trigger structural and biochemical processes that accelerate and augment tissue repair. Negative pressure can induce micro- and macrodeformation of the wound bed, decrease local edema, and remove harmful exudates. The various wound dressings that are used with an NPWTD also improve wound healing by maintaining a warm and moist wound environment.

The net effect of negative pressure in a wound bed is difficult to quantitate, and although there is consensus that wounds improve, it is unclear how much of this improvement is attributable to mechanical forces. Macrodeformation of the wound by negative pressure can clearly result in approximation of wound edges, and some wounds will visibly shrink. This phenomenon is more noticeable in distensible tissues such as the anterior abdominal wall as opposed to less distensible tissues such as the scalp. Yet, there is evidence that such negative pressure might also hinder wound healing by increasing wound bed pressure and causing a decrease in local perfusion. This paradoxical effect is difficult to quantitate, is not fully understood, and can be clinically detrimental in some cases, especially in wounds in which tissue perfusion is tenuous.

Microdeformation of the wound bed can also trigger molecular processes, such as mechanotransduction, which are implicated in improved wound healing through structural and biochemical changes at the tissue and cellular level, which result in cellular migration, proliferation, and differentiation. Some authors state that since much of the published data on microdeformation in NPWTD reflect findings using specific types of foams, such data cannot be extrapolated across all NPWTD systems. Others have disagreed, stating that nonproprietary dressings, such as gauze, yield similar wound healing results in both experimental and clinical situations.

Lastly, the offloading of exudative fluid and accumulated wound debris from a wound bed is an established practice associated with improved healing and can be assumed to be a fundamental benefit of NPWTD. The added benefit of the NPWTD appears to be that biochemical changes are induced by the application of negative pressure that alter the balance of wound exudates in favor of restorative molecules. For example, wounds treated with NPWTD show a decrease in the relative concentration of caustic matrix metalloproteases to levels of tissue inhibitors of metalloproteases.

Equipment/Device

The Food and Drug Administration (FDA) approved the first NPWTD in 1997. Since then, new types of devices have been introduced and clinical indications for their use have increased. All NPWTDs share fundamental design features and key components necessary

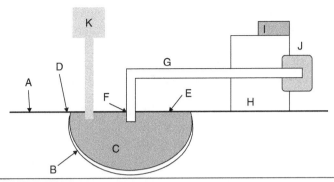

A)	Normal unaffected skin
B)	Contact layer (as needed, between wound and dressing)
C)	Gauze or foam wound dressing
D)	Protective interface between normal skin and wound dressing. It is essential to protect unaffected skin from suctioning, fluids, and cannot be covered with gauze.
E)	Occlusive dressing layer - must remain intact to maintain suction
F)	Connection between suction tubing and wound dressing. e.g. "Nipple"
G)	Suction tubing
H)	Vacuum source: can rely on continuous power supply or a spring loaded device (mechanical)
I)	Power supply: connected to wall unit with optional backup, rechargeable battery power
J)	Wound effluent collection unit (e.g. canister)
K)	In some units: instillation/infusion system for wounds that require vacuum-assisted drainage and controlled delivery of topical solutions

Figure 20.1   Schema of basic design and key components of an NPWTD.

for the production and maintenance of sub-atmospheric pressure within the treatment area (Figure 20.1). These include a power source that can generate negative pressure; a conduction system for delivering the pressure; a reliable seal to enclose the treatment area; an appropriate wound bed dressing to optimize wound healing; and, in most cases, a conduit for removing wound exudate. In most cases, power is supplied from a wall source and is backed up by a rechargeable or disposable battery. NPWTDs that rely on other power sources such as loaded springs or bellows to mechanically generate negative pressure can be used in small devices or in low resource settings. Most systems use continuous negative pressure, and the intensity can be controlled by the operator or cycled in a set pattern. Changes in the intensity or duration of negative pressure applied to a wound can be used to overcome device-related pain and/or minimize local tissue damage in friable or at-risk wounds while optimizing tissue moisture levels and local perfusion.

   The sub-atmospheric pressure is delivered to the wound through a sealable conduit, usually plastic tubing, that digitates with the wound through a foam or gauze dressing. Since such dressings can sometimes irritate the wound bed, it can be necessary to use a protective dressing, sometimes referred to as a "contact layer," directly onto the wound. To maintain negative pressure throughout the system, the treatment area is covered with a nonporous material such as adhesive film. If the wound produces an effluent, it is suctioned off the wound bed and is most often shunted into a sump to prevent back-drainage or blockage of the tubing. The sump is usually a portable canister, but units can also drain into a separate often larger receptacle, such as those commonly used with hospital wall suction devices.

Outside of these very basic design elements, there are numerous variations that apply to the many different types of NPWTDs available today. Units vary from reusable, complex, large, electrically powered durable medical devices with variable settings and permutations to small, spring-loaded, single-use devices with relatively few "bells and whistles." More recently, NPWTDs that allow for installation/dwell/removal cycles of a variety of topical wound solutions have been introduced and have proven especially useful in complex wounds. Topically placed wound solutions can flush the wound bed to better remove wound exudate and decrease bioburden while delivering antimicrobial or other restorative products to the wound. Such units are usually used in an inpatient setting.

As new designs and applications for NPWTDs emerge and as the patient population and the clinical conditions for which they are used broaden, we can expect to see different types and potentially more complications associated with NPWTD usage. Yet, the ED clinician who is familiar with components and features common to most devices still appreciates that there can be important differences between them, and will be able to formulate a logical and actionable approach in the evaluation and treatment of a patient with a variety of NPWTD-related complications.

Clinical Use

NPWTDs are prescribed for patients of all ages and for wounds of numerous etiologies. It is felt that they not only accelerate wound healing, shorten hospital stays, and decrease complications and expenditures but also improve patient and health care provider satisfaction. Indications for their use are growing, and new designs and associated products continue to be introduced.

Indications and Contraindications

The list of approved and/or widely accepted clinical uses and contraindications for NPWTDs would include the following clinical conditions.

Indications	Contraindications
1) Poorly healing soft tissue ulcers (diabetic, neuropathic, venous and/or pressure)	1) Untreated osteomyelitis
2) Traumatic wounds: acute, subacute, or chronic	2) Exposed internal organs
3) Surgical wounds: (closing by secondary intention), dehisced	3) Eschar or frankly necrotic tissue
	4) Exposed arteries, friable, or infected blood vessels
4) Wound bed preparation (e.g. in preparation for tertiary closure)	5) Exposed nerves, tendons, and ligaments
5) Over skin flaps or grafts	6) Exposed anastomotic sites (especially vascular anastomosis)
6) Partial-thickness burns	7) Nonenteric or unexplored fistulae
	8) Malignancy in wound bed (from increased cellular proliferation)

One would suspect that the accumulation of basic science and clinical research, therapeutic experience, increasing sophistication of NPWTD, improvement of dressings, and adjunct treatments will result in amendments to these lists. Even in clinical situations that fall within the above contraindications, evidence is being presented that NPWTDs can safely be used, although this usually requires closer follow-up and added precautions. Similarly, the FDA has not approved NWPTD use for infants and children, but NPWTDs are being used in children, including newborns, with good clinical outcomes.

What is also clear from the literature is that clinical reports of NPWTD success and increasingly broad usage have outpaced basic science research, comparative utility, and other important investigative efforts. For example, although there are numerous articles in the peer-reviewed literature on the clinical uses of NPWTD, randomized controlled trials are rare, and some authors have even questioned some of the available clinical and research data evidence as being unduly influenced by the NPWTD industry. In addition, the overall expenditures on NPWTD are growing in the US, (and globally) and there is a need to better understand the cost–benefit ratio of NPWTD use. In short, we should look for further clinical trials, improved clinical models, and an overall increase in our understanding of how to best use NPWTD.

Morbidity and Mortality

A comprehensive database of NPWTD-related morbidity and mortality does not exist but can be broadly attributed to hemorrhage, infection, and wound or peri-wound deterioration. The major cause of immediate mortality from NPWTD use is local, massive hemorrhage. For the period spanning 2007–2011, the FDA attributed 12 deaths and 174 injuries to NPWTD with bleeding as the major cause of death and a significant cause of morbidity. Bleeding can be caused by erosion of wound dressings or device structures into a highly vascular wound bed, organ, or blood vessel. Devices placed over arterial vascular repairs such as grafts or anastomosis, especially over large vessels, have the potential of inducing sudden and catastrophic hemorrhage. Yet, it is also important to remember that given the negative pressure that is delivered by an NPWTD, disruption of even low pressure (i.e. veins), components of the circulatory system can also lead to rapid exsanguination. As one would expect, bleeding complications are more likely to occur in patients who are anticoagulated or have an underlying coagulopathy. Retained or adherent dressings, especially foam dressings, have been implicated in causing bleeding not only by eroding into tissues but also by causing damage when they are being removed. Slower but sustained bleeding, especially if treatment is prolonged, can also lead to symptomatic blood loss.

Infection is the second highest cause of reported adverse outcome from NPWTD usage. Wounds that are encased within an NPWTD can develop worsening infection due to prolonged contact with wound exudate and the presence of foreign materials used to pack wounds. Surrounding skin, which can become macerated or denuded by prolonged contact with abrasive dressings, is more vulnerable to colonization and infection by contaminated wound exudate. In addition, patients with NPWTD are at greater risk of delayed diagnosis and, therefore, more advanced wound infections because they receive less frequent dressing changes. Therefore, special attention should be paid to the general state of the patient and any clues to early infection, such as increased pain. If infection of the wound bed is suspected, it is important that the dressing be taken down, and the wound thoroughly inspected. If an infection is noted, the removal of all wound bed dressings that could serve as a reservoir for infective agents is just as essential as the initiation of antibiotics and other treatments.

Patients often experience variable levels of pain with the use of an NPWTD. As pain is a frequent reason for a patient to come to the ED, it is essential to understand the potential causes for it in this patient population. Patients can experience variable levels of pain with wound dressing changes, but such pain can be increased with NPWTD dressing changes. The removal of the adhesive layer can cause pain, especially if the underlying skin has become irritated from a contact dermatitis, a local folliculitis, or even a fungal superinfection. Wound bed dressings can become adherent if they are not changed frequently enough or if a contact layer was omitted when indicated. The removal of adherent dressings from a wound bed can also cause significant pain and further traumatize the wound. Even components of the NPWTDs that are not in immediate contact with the wound and the surrounding tissues can result in pain and clinical deterioration. For example, direct and excessive pressure from device parts such as tubing or straps can induce pressure-related skin and soft tissue injuries, especially in patients who have poor sensation, cognition, or mobility.

Wounds with diminished or tenuous perfusion can become ischemic when sub-atmospheric pressure is applied to them, resulting in loss of tissue integrity and even frank necrosis. Although ischemia is expected to cause pain, if pain is not appreciated or reported by the patient, the only finding might be a worsening in the general clinical condition of the patient, a change in the amount or character of the wound effluent, or a deterioration of the wound. Penetration of the wound into surrounding tissue structures such as hollow viscous could also result from wound ischemia and might present in much the same ways. Thus, it is important that the clinician include the NPWTD as a potential source of any clinical deterioration in a patient.

Approach to the ED Patient with an NPWTD

General Considerations

The most common NPWTD-related complaints that patients present to the ED are pain, bleeding, fever (or other signs of infection), and mechanical problems including alarms that cannot be silenced or malfunctioning of a machine part. In some cases, it is very clear that the NPWTD and the associated wound are the cause of the patient's presenting complaint. In other cases though, the wound and the associated device/dressings are not readily recognizable as culprits or contributories to the patient's clinical condition. For example, a patient presenting with fever might have suppuration of the wound bed, possibly even caused by a retained wound sponge, without overt or local manifestations of a deep soft tissue infection. It, therefore, falls on the astute ED clinician to consider what role the NPWTD and the associated wound might play when evaluating and treating such patients. In general, the ED clinician who has a working knowledge of the basic components, mechanics, usages, and potential complications of NPWTD is most likely to make and communicate rational clinical decisions in all such cases.

After first evaluating the patient, if the ED clinician determines that the NPWTD should be removed and the wound bed examined, the next step is to determine how urgently this should occur. In a true emergency, such as when a patient is hemorrhaging into a canister or septic from a wound-related cellulitis, the immediate removal of the NPWTD and all associated dressings is required. This will allow for full exposure of the wound bed and initiation of standard investigations and therapies. If the NPWTD must be removed emergently, the ED clinician should not be deterred from doing so, especially if the reluctance stems from a lack of familiarity with NPWTD.

If the dressing does not have to be removed immediately, the treating physician should be contacted to discuss the patient's clinical situation. If the NPWTD must be removed, it is important to determine options for ensuing wound care. If NPWTD might need to be resumed in the ED, it should also be determined if adequate supplies and trained personnel are available to do so. If alternative dressings are to be used, it should likewise be determined what type of wound dressing would be indicated and what the wound care plan, including the follow-up care, would be.

Troubleshooting Alarms

One of the most common reasons for a patient with an NPWTD to seek ED care is for evaluation of an ongoing alarm. Most patients and caregivers will receive instruction on how to respond to common or critical alarms, and the ED practitioner should ask what, if any, measures the patient or caregiver has taken in response to the alarm. The ED clinician should then quickly determine if the alarm is due to a wound-related emergency, such as hemorrhage or infection that warrants immediate removal of the NPWTD and corrective measures. If the clinical condition is such that the ED practitioner does not have to immediately remove the NPWTD, a thorough inspection of the device and the associated dressings might reveal the cause of the alarm. Resources from the manufacturer, such as brochures or websites, are a great help in troubleshooting alarms.

In general, to be able to logically evaluate an NPWTD, the clinician should know several things, such as the level and mode of the negative pressure setting and the manner in which the device is powered. Suction is customarily set at a continuous 125 mmHg (but can vary from 20 to 150 mmHg) and may be intermittent or cycling. If negative pressure is interrupted for any reason, most machines are set to produce a "low pressure" alarm. Although the breach can occur anywhere in the system from the wound bed to the collecting canister, one should evaluate the most common, and most easily accessible and remediable, areas that could be causing the leak. A common cause for pressure loss is a loosening of the adhesive drape due to skin moisture or a distraction of the tubing from the porous dressing. Areas of increased stress on the tubing or the adhesive dressing such as tubing connection points or where adhesive dressing has been stretched over a skin fold should be examined as potential sites of pressure loss. If identified, such leaks can be closed with appropriately sized and applied occlusive skin dressing. Other wound-related problems, such as bleeding in the wound bed, can loosen the dressing and cause a "low pressure" alarm. Bleeding from the wound can be potentially catastrophic given the fact that negative pressure can lead to active removal of blood. In such cases, the NPWTD should be removed and associated wound beds examined with special attention given to potential sites of bleeding such as vascular anastomosis and retained sponges.

Loss of pressure within the system for any reason can result in retention of exudate on the wound bed, increase wound friability, cause dressings to become more adherent to the wound bed, and increase bioburden of wound and dressings. In general, if disruption of negative pressure has exceeded 2 or more hours (in systems that use foam dressings) or 24 hours (in systems that use gauze dressings), the wound should be exposed, cleansed, and the dressing should be changed. If wound dressings that are imbedded into the wound are not removed and negative pressure is reapplied, the chance of bleeding and/or infection of the wound bed is increased. Therefore, the resumption of negative pressure therapy to a wound bed without properly examining and cleansing the wound bed, and removing all retained dressings, can have serious consequences. If there is any question as to the potential contamination of the wound bed or if there is suspicion that negative pressure was disrupted for a prolonged period, it is best to fully remove the NPWTD and replace it with a "traditional" dressing (such as moist gauze) until therapy can be reinstated by the treating physician.

Low pressure alarms resulting from mechanical problems such as torn tubing or a cracked canister would require removal and replacement of parts that might not be available at the time of service. If immediate resumption of negative pressure is possible and is tolerated by the patient, safe discharge should be possible after a short observation period to make sure that the alarm does not restart. When restarting an NPWTD, it is important to know what kind of wound filler (type of sponge or gauze) is being used and how many pieces were placed in the wound during the last dressing change, both to make sure that all are removed and to better understand how to best dress the wound. The ED practitioner should, therefore, review clinical notes, interview the patient and caregivers, and review the manufacturer's information and recommendations when trying to elucidate the cause of an alarm and preparing the patient for discharge. An algorithmic approach to troubleshooting a low-pressure alarm is presented in Figure 20.2.

In most NPWTDs, an alarm will also sound if the power source is disrupted and/or if the backup power source is depleted. Most NPWTDs are electrically powered and have a backup battery that is used when the patient is ambulatory or if electrical power is disconnected. It is important to know how long the battery can be used without recharging since the vacuum delivered to the wound bed should not be interrupted for a prolonged period. In a patient who is to be discharged from the ED, it is just as important to ensure that the unit has enough power to sustain negative suction after discharge.

In all cases of an NPWTD alarm that cannot be easily elucidated or fixed, it is important to seek the advice of the treating physician. By obtaining the relevant history from the patient, understanding the potential causes for an alarm, and consulting with the treating physician, the ED practitioner should be able to successfully troubleshoot a device and properly address the problem triggering the alarm. Variations to this practice should be made on individual patients only in consultation with the treating physician.

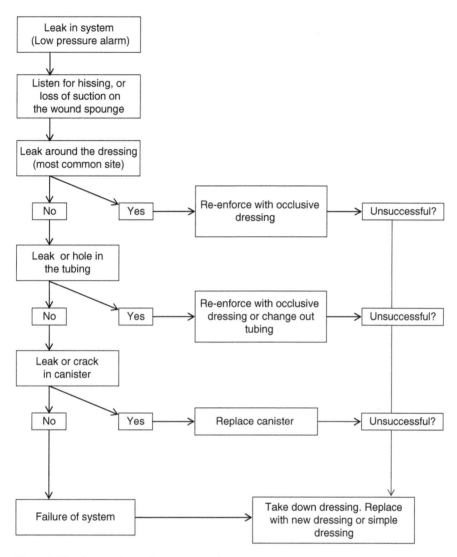

Figure 20.2 Approach to a low pressure alarm.

Pain

Pain is a common complaint among patients seeking emergent care. Application of negative pressure to a wound bed can cause pain from direct irritation of denuded tissue or cause local hypoperfusion, which will also induce pain. Often, this is detected when the NPWTD is first applied, allowing for adjustments, such as decreasing the level of suction or changing from continuous to cyclical mode, until the patient is able to comfortably tolerate treatment. Yet, patients can present at any time after the initial application with the consequences of hypoperfusion, with or without resultant pain. Breakdown of peri-wound skin occurs from accumulation of moisture or exudate under occlusive dressings or from prolonged contact with abrasive dressings. Pressure from tightly applied dressings, tubing, or other machine parts that are not elevated away from soft tissues can result in pressure-related skin and soft tissue injuries with resultant pain. Therefore, it is important to thoroughly examine the wound and surrounding tissues for signs of infection, hypoperfusion, or pressure-related injury that could be the cause of the patient's pain.

In patients who are unable to perceive or report pain, the level of tissue injury from hypoperfusion, abrasion, or pressure could be severe before it is discovered and treated. Such patients can present with seemingly unrelated symptoms such as diaphoresis, agitation, and nausea, and the evidence that the NPWTD and/or the wound are/is a cause of the patient's pain or distress might not be very clear. This is especially true in patients in whom the treatment has been used without complication for some time. In such patients, an increase in wound odor or alteration in the quantity or character of wound drainage can be an overlooked and unreported clue to wound deterioration. It is, therefore, especially important that the ED clinician elicit pertinent history from caregivers and conduct a thorough examination of patients with a diminished level of consciousness or decreased ability to feel or report pain when they come to the ED for seemingly unrelated problems. For example, although it is contraindicated, a dressing might have slipped and/or been inappropriately applied over the whole circumference of an anatomic site, resulting in strangulation and hypoperfusion of the area. An algorithmic approach to pain in NPWTD patients who present to the ED is presented in Figure 20.3.

Bleeding

Bleeding, a possible complication of any wound, can be a devastating complication in the setting of negative pressure. Catastrophic hemorrhage from perforation of an underlying vascular structure is the most common cause of NPWTD-related mortality, and it is essential for the ED practitioner to recognize and treat it. Significant bleeding in the wound should be manifested by rapid filling of the collection vessel with blood. In this event, it is essential for the NPWTD to be discontinued and the wound bed to be accessed to ascertain what the cause of bleeding is and to institute all measures to stem the loss of blood. Accelerated bleeding can also be the result of a coagulopathy, and a review of associated diseases, such as liver disease, and the use of anticoagulant medications is crucial if proper treatment is to be instituted.

Wound-related blood loss in most patients is less dramatic but can result from continuous low-grade bleeding in the wound bed in association with the variety of anemias that result from malnutrition and chronic disease. Such patients might present with the expected constitutional symptoms of slow blood loss such as malaise and fatigue, and it is important that the ED practitioner consider this when evaluating and planning for patient disposition.

Infection

NPWTDs are not indicated for use in actively infected wounds, but infection may develop after placement and during use and can range from superficial soft tissue infections to systemic, life-threatening ones. If the wound or surrounding tissues show signs of

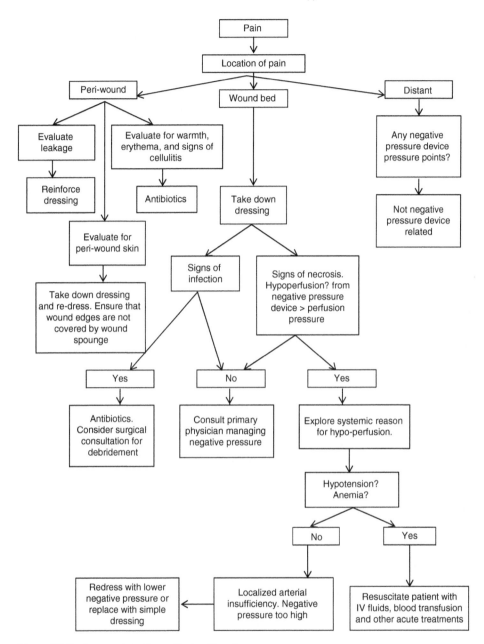

Figure 20.3 Approach to the patient with pain.

inflammation or infection, the NPWTDs must be discontinued and the wound bed thoroughly cleansed and investigated. If the wound bed is clean, but there is a surrounding cellulitis not associated with any devitalized tissue or retained foreign bodies, it is likely that the use of appropriate antibiotics and withholding of the NPWTD until the infection improves will result in a good outcome. In such cases, empiric antibiotics would be directed at organisms associated with more common, albeit healthcare-related, organisms that cause skin and soft tissue infections such as Methicillin-resistant *Staphylococcus aureus.* On the other hand, if the wound infection is associated with the necrotic tissue or a foreign body such as an imbedded/retained piece of sponge, treatment would have to include debridement of tissue and/or removal of colonized foreign material. In some cases, the characteristics of the wound or the surrounding tissue (such as a foul odor of the wound or proximity to a colostomy site) warrant broader antibiotic coverage.

For many patients, it will be clear to the ED physician that the wound is the nidus of the infection. In others, overt signs or symptoms associating the wound with the patient's symptom complex will not be found. Therefore, in all patients in whom the cause of infection is not clear, especially in those who are ill, it is important that the wound be considered and actively investigated as a cause for the patient's clinical state. As was mentioned above, if the ED clinician feels that the wound must be examined, it is best to engage the treating physician in shared decision-making. If the patient is too ill or such a consultation cannot occur, it is important that the ED clinician remove the dressing, inspect the wound, and replace the NPWTD with an appropriate dressing. It is also very important to document one's decision-making process and communicate the options as well as the treatment plan to the patient. In general, more harm can be done by leaving an infected dressing and NPWTD in place than would ever result from removing them. For example, if an NPWTD needed to be removed from a postsurgical wound to evaluate it for potential infection, it would be reasonable to bridge restarting the negative pressure treatment with regular moist to dry gauze dressing changes until definitive therapy could be reinstituted.

Although NPWTDs are not indicated in grossly infected wounds, they can be used with close attention in patients who are being treated with systemic antibiotics. In addition, the introduction of instill/dwell/suction NPWTDs that apply antibiotics and antimicrobials to the wound, with cyclic cleansing and removal of debris from the wound bed, has allowed for their use in deep, infected wounds. Development or worsening of infection in all patients using NPWTD should lead to a thorough evaluation with close attention to local causes of infection, removal of all foreign bodies that might be a nidus of infection, and institution of antibiotics as indicated by the clinical scenario. Always involve the treating physician in the care of the patient if it is at all possible.

Special Considerations

As the usage of NPWTD increases and indications for treatment are expanded, the ED practitioner should be prepared to factor in the continued use of the device in relation to other diagnostic or therapeutic interventions. If, for instance, a patient requires a magnetic resonance imaging (MRI), hyperbaric therapy, thrombolytic therapy, or must undergo a prolonged procedure with the potential of losing power to the device, the ED practitioner must be able ask the questions that would allow one to best manage the patient.

In general, NPWTDs must be discontinued if a person is to undergo an MRI or enter a hyperbaric chamber although wound dressings do not usually have to be removed in these situations. If suction is interrupted for a prolonged period, some dressings (such as foam) must be removed, as they cannot be left in the wound without continued negative pressure. Other treatments, such as thrombolysis, can be undertaken in patients who have an

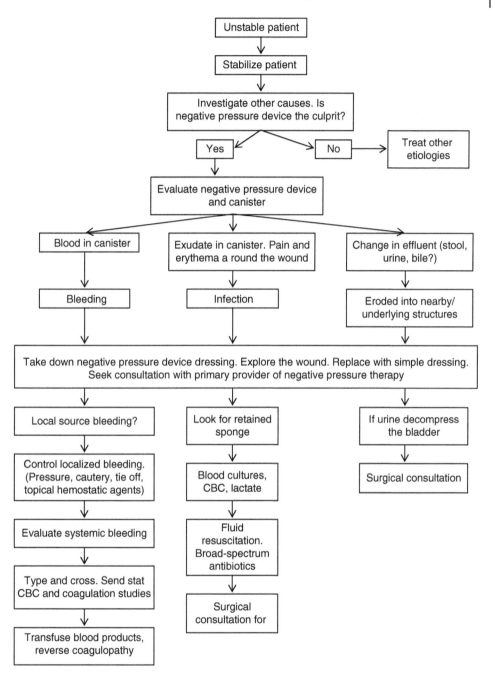

Figure 20.4   Evaluating the patient with NPWTD.

NPWTD in place, but attention should be given to potential complications, such as accelerated bleeding from the wound bed. If there is any doubt about the safety of continuing negative pressure during a procedure or treatment, it is best to consult the manufacturer or the treating physician to insure the safety of the patient.

In conclusion, by having a basic understanding of the risks and benefits associated with NPWTD, the ED clinician can work with other members of the patient's health care team to successfully diagnose and safely treat patients who present with NPWTD-related clinical problems. "Just-in-time" literature reviews will often yield useful guidelines and information on how to troubleshoot a device and avoid therapeutic and diagnostic pitfalls. An example of such a guide is one published by WoundSource, a site that provides wound information on wound care companies and products. Figure 20.4 offers a unified initial approach for the ED care of patients with the most common NPWTD-related problems.

Further Reading

1 Anghel, E.L. and Kim, P.J. (September 2016). Negative-pressure wound therapy: a comprehensive review of the evidence. *Plastic & Reconstructive Surgery* 138 (3S) Current Concepts in Wound Healing: Update 2016: 129S–137S.

2 Krug E, Berg L, Lee C, Hudson D, Birke-Sorensen H, Depoorter M, Dunn R, Jeffery S, Duteille F, Bruhin A, Caravaggi C, Chariker M, Dowsett C, Ferreira F, Martinez JM, Grudzien G, Ichioka S, Ingemansson R, Malmsjo M, Rome P, Vig S, Runkel N, Martin R, Smith J. Evidence-based recommendations for the use of negative pressure wound therapy in traumatic wounds and reconstructive surgery: steps towards an international consensus International Expert Panel on Negative Pressure Wound Therapy [NPWT-EP]. *Injury* 2011;42(Suppl 1):S1–12. DOI: https://doi.org/10.1016/S0020-1383(11)00041-6.

3 Dumville JC, Hinchliffe RJ, Cullum N, Game F, Stubbs N, Sweeting M, Peinemann F. Negative pressure wound therapy for treating foot wounds in people with diabetes mellitus. *Cochrane Database of Systematic Reviews* 2013, Issue 10. Art. No.: CD010318. DOI: https://doi.org/10.1002/14651858.CD010318.pub2

4 Lavery, L.A., Davis, K.E., Berriman, S.J. et al. (January/February 2016). WHS guidelines update: diabetic foot ulcer treatment guidelines. *Wound Repair & Regeneration* 24 (1): 112–126.

5 Sandoz, H. (April 7, 2015). Negative pressure wound therapy: clinical utility. *Chronic Wound Care Management and Research* 2: 71–79.

6 Rhee SM, Valle MF, Wilson LM, Lazarus G, Zenilman J, Robinson KA. Negative pressure wound therapy technologies for chronic wound care in the home setting. Rockville (MD): Agency for Healthcare Research and Quality (US); 2014 Sep 15. Available from: https://www.ncbi.nlm.nih.gov/books/NBK285361/

7 Desai, K.K., Hahn, E., Pulikkottil, B., and Lee, E. (2012). Negative pressure wound therapy: an algorithm. *Clinics in Plastic Surgery* 39 (3): 311–324.

8 US food and drug administration: FDA safety communication: Update on serious complications associated with negative pressure wound therapy systems Silver Spring, MD, US Food and Drug Administration February 24, 2011, Available at: http://www.fda.gov/MedicalDevices/Safety/AlertsandNotices/ucm244211.htm [Accessed: 15 May 2017].

9 Huang, C., Leavitt, T., Bayer, L.R., and Orgill, D.P. (2014). Effect of negative pressure wound therapy on wound healing. *Current Problems in Surgery* 51 (7): 301–331.

10 Orgill, D.P., Manders, E.K., Sumpio, B.E. et al. (2009). The mechanisms of action of vacuum assisted closure: more to learn. *Surgery* 146 (1): 40–51.

11 Kairinos, N., Voogd, A.M., Botha, P.H. et al. (February 2009). Negative-pressure wound therapy II: negative-pressure wound therapy and increased perfusion. Just an illusion? *Plastic & Reconstructive Surgery* 123 (2): 601–612.

12 Birke-Sorenson, H., Malmsjo, M., Rome, P. et al. (2011). Evidence-based recommendations for negative pressure wound therapy: treatment variables (pressure levels, wound filler and contact layer) – steps towards an international consensus. *Journal of Plastic, Reconstructive and Aesthetic Surgery* 64: S1–S16.

13 Wiegand, C. and White, R. (Nov/Dec 2013). Microdeformation in wound healing. *Wound Repair and Regeneration* 21 (6): 793–799.

14 Borgquist, O., Gustafsson, L., Ingemansson, R., and Malmsjo, M. (June 2010). Micro- and macromechanical effects on the wound bed of negative pressure wound therapy using gauze and foam. *Annals of Plastic Surgery* 64 (6): 789–793.

15 Dorafshar, A.H., Franczyk, M., Gottlieb, L.J. et al. (July 2012). A prospective randomized trial comparing subatmospheric wound therapy with a sealed gauze dressing and the standard vacuum-assisted closure device. *Annals of Plastic Surgery* 69 (1): 79–84.

16 Nguyen, T., Franczyk, M., Lee, J. et al. (March/April 2015). Prospective randomized controlled trial comparing two methods of securing skin grafts using negative pressure wound therapy: vacuum-assisted closure and gauze suction. *Journal of Burn Care & Research* 36 (2): 324–328.

17 Glass, G.E., Murphy, G.F., Esmaeili, A. et al. (December 2014). Systematic review of molecular mechanism of action of negative-pressure wound therapy. *British Journal of Surgery* 101 (13): 1627–1636.

18 Moues, C., van Toorenenbergen, A., Heule, F. et al. (July/August 2008). The role of topical negative pressure in wound repair: expression of biochemical markers in wound fluid during wound healing. *Wound Repair & Regeneration* 16 (4): 488–494.

19 Anghel, E. and Kim, P.J. (September 2016). Negative-pressure wound therapy: a comprehensive review of the evidence. *Plastic & Reconstructive Surgery* 138 (3S) Current Concepts in Wound Healing: Update 2016: 129S–137S.

20 Zurovick, D.R., Mody, G., Riviello, R., and Slocum, A. (October 2015). Simplified negative pressure wound therapy device for application in low-resource settings. *Journal of Orthopaedic Trauma* 29 (Supplement 10): S33–S36.

21 Serena, T., Buan, J.S., and Anghel, A. (April 2016). The use of a novel canister-free negative-pressure device in chronic wounds: a retrospective analysis. *Advances in Skin & Wound Care.* 29 (4): 165–168.

22 Anghel, E.L., Kim, P.J., and Attinger, C.E. (2016). A solution for complex wounds: the evidence for negative pressure wound therapy with instillation. *International Wound Journal* 13 (suppl.S3): 19–24.

23 Suissa, D., Danino, A., and Nikolis, A. (November 2011). Negative-pressure therapy versus standard wound care: a meta-analysis of randomized trials. *Plastic & Reconstructive Surgery* 128 (5): 498e–503e.

24 Childs, D.R. and Murthy, A. (2017). Overview of wound healing and management. *The Surgical Clinics of North America* 97: 189–207.

25 Aldridge, B., Ladd, A.P., Kepple, J. et al. (2016 Mar.). Negative pressure wound therapy for initial management of giant omphalocele. *American Journal of Surgery* 211 (3): 605–609.

26 Kairinos, N., Pillay, K., Solomons, M. et al. (2014 May). The influence manufacturers have on negative-pressure wound therapy research. *Plastic & Reconstructive Surgery* 133 (5): 1178–1183.

27 Li, Z. and Yu, A. (2014 Jul-Aug). Complications of negative pressure wound therapy: a mini review. *Wound Repair & Regeneration.* 22 (4): 457–461.

28 Strategies for the Effective Management of Challenges Associated with Negative Pressure Wound Therapy. White Paper online publication: WoundSource. Beth Hawkins Bradley author. Downloaded on 5/15/2019 from http://www.woundsource.com/white-papers.

21

Emergency Management of Patients with Wound Infections

David Yamane[1] and Tenagne Haile-Mariam[2]

[1] *Department of Emergency Medicine and Department of Anesthesia and Critical Care Medicine, George Washington University Hospital, Washington, DC, USA*
[2] *Department of Emergency Medicine, George Washington University School of Medicine and Health Sciences, Washington, DC, USA*

General Considerations

Wound infections can be subtle. It is important to differentiate between a surgical site that is progressing through the inflammatory stages necessary for healing and an infected site that is undergoing the disordered inflammation that can lead to wound dehiscence and surgical site failure. Most health care workers can identify an obviously infected wound from a pristine well-healing wound. In order to provide timely diagnosis and early intervention for a surgical site that is undergoing a disorder in healing, a physician must rely on thorough review of the patient's premorbid conditions, the events leading up to the surgical intervention, and those that occurred during surgery and perform a focused but comprehensive physical exam.

The medical literature provides us with many examples of subtle manifestations that if missed will result in significant morbidity and even mortality. The postsurgical state is in itself a state of great stress that resembles an immunocompromised state. The classic signs and symptoms of inflammation may not always be present. But the physician must always be cognizant that this period is one in which heightened surveillance is imperative. For example, foreign bodies are purposely introduced to the body to obtain wound management (i.e. sutures, staples, and drains). These can be niduses for systemic inflammatory reactions such as toxic shock syndrome.

The following is an algorithm for the management of wounds.

Emergency Management of the Hi-Tech Patient in Acute and Critical Care, First Edition. Edited by Ioannis Koutroulis, Nicholas Tsarouhas, Richard J. Lin, Jill C. Posner, Michael Seneff, and Robert Shesser.
© 2021 John Wiley & Sons Ltd. Published 2021 by John Wiley & Sons Ltd.

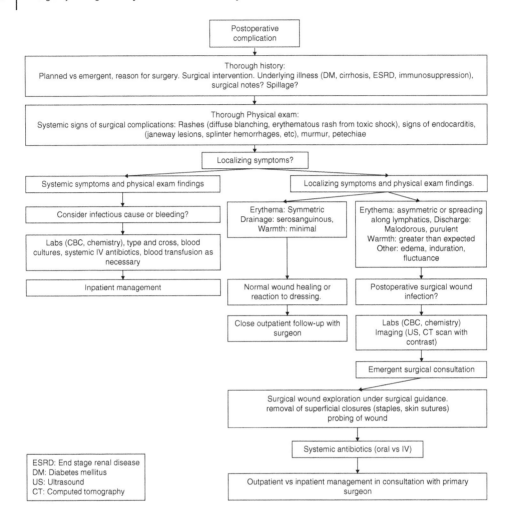

Further Reading

1 Prevaldi, C., Paolillo, C., Locatelli, C. et al. (2016). Management of traumatic wounds in the Emergency Department: position paper from the Academy of Emergency Medicine and Care (AcEMC) and the World Society of Emergency Surgery (WSES). *World J. Emerg. Surg.* 11: 30.

2 Edlich, R.F., Rodeheaver, G.T., Morgan, R.F. et al. (1988). Principles of emergency wound management. *Ann. Emerg. Med.* 17 (12): 1284–1302.

Section VII

GU Devices

22

Emergency Management of Patients with Genitourinary Prostheses

Katie Wagner[1], Michael Phillips[1], and Kelly Chiles[2]

[1] *George Washington University School of Medicine and Health Sciences, Washington, DC, USA*
[2] *Urology, Private Practice, Washington, DC, USA*

Introduction

In the 1980s, the introduction of the prostate-specific antigen, first as a tumor marker, and then as a screening tool for prostate cancer, resulted in a significant increase in the number of men diagnosed with prostate cancer. This in turn led to an increase in individuals receiving treatment for their disease, including radical prostatectomy and/or pelvic radiation therapy. Common and much feared side effects of these treatments include erectile dysfunction (ED) and urinary incontinence (UI). These side effects, however, are not limited to the treatment of prostate cancer; any pelvic surgery or radiation can also result in similar outcomes. Furthermore, common medical comorbidities such as diabetes and hypertension are also strongly linked to the development of ED. The growing prevalence of ED necessitated the development of novel treatment modalities.

Recent estimates place the prevalence of ED among men younger than 50 at 1–10%, 20–40% for men in their 60s, and as high as >50% for men older than 70. In 1998, the Food and Drug Administration (FDA) approved oral phosphodiesterase-5 inhibitors (Sildenafil) for the treatment of ED. This event led to not only more men seeking remedy for their ED, but also to greater dialog about quality-of-life issues for the aging male. Up to 35% of ED patients will fail oral therapy, and many men have turned to the use of implanted prosthetic devices to address the problem.

At some point in time, many of these individuals will present to the emergency room (ER) for nonurologic health issues. It is incumbent upon the staff to recognize that the patient has undergone urologic prosthetic surgery so that measures may be taken to insure that complications associated with mishandling of the device do not occur in the course of dealing with the problem that brought the patient to the facility in the first place. Alternatively, patients may also present with malfunction or complications of the

Emergency Management of the Hi-Tech Patient in Acute and Critical Care, First Edition. Edited by Ioannis Koutroulis, Nicholas Tsarouhas, Richard J. Lin, Jill C. Posner, Michael Seneff, and Robert Shesser.

prosthetic devices, which is reported to occur in as many as 15% after 10 years. Prosthetic dysfunction or complications should always be referred to a urologist, but the ED physician should be familiar with the various devices and how to initially troubleshoot issues with them.

The presence of these devices is also not limited to older men. Males and females born with developmental abnormalities such as spina bifida may have had corrective treatment involving prosthetic implants. Transgender patients, primarily female to male, should also be questioned as to the presence of a prosthetic implant, prior to any manipulation involving the urinary tract. Furthermore, individuals of both sexes may have undergone placement of an InterStim™ in the course of treating urinary or fecal incontinence, urinary urgency, frequency, or rarely urinary retention. This device, which is not universally effective and undergoes a testing period before permanent implantation, neuromodulates the sacral plexus to improve urinary and fecal control. The knowledge that this implant is present may dictate diagnostic studies ordered by ER personnel; for example, this device is not magnetic resonance imaging (MRI) compatible.

Artificial Urinary Sphincter

The artificial urinary sphincter or AUS is an increasingly common surgical solution for stress UI, primarily in men with incontinence after prostatectomy. The device has three components: an inflatable cuff placed around the proximal urethra, a pump placed in the scrotum or labium, and a balloon, which acts as a fluid reservoir that is placed in the patient's abdomen (Figure 22.1). The pump in the scrotum or labium is connected to both the cuff and the balloon reservoir by fluid-filled tubing. When in use, the urethral cuff stays inflated to compress the urethra and support continence. When the patient is ready to void,

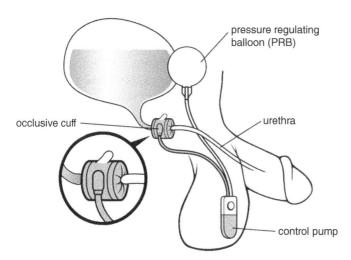

Figure 22.1 AUS components. (*Source:* https://www.bostonscientific.com/content/dam/bostonscientific/uro-wh/general/ams/Resources/1001248_AMS_800_Patient_Instruction_Card_EN.pdf).

he or she depresses the pump in the scrotum or labium, which diverts fluid from the cuff to the intra-abdominal balloon, opening the urethra to allow urine to flow. Fluid then refills the cuff over the next few minutes to recompress the urethra. In the first few weeks after implantation, the pump is generally locked in place with the urethral cuff decompressed to allow for healing before the patient begins using the device. The device is locked with a button located just above the pump.

Penile Prostheses

Inflatable penile prostheses (IPPs) are a definitive option for ED that is not adequately treated by nonsurgical methods. There are multiple types of penile implants for ED, including the three-piece IPP, which is the most common, the two-piece IPP, and the malleable penile prosthesis (Figure 22.2). Similar to the AUS, the three-piece IPP consists of three components: a fluid reservoir in the abdomen, a pump placed in the scrotum, and two cylinders which are implanted within each corpora cavernosa. The two-piece option consists of a combined pump and reservoir in the scrotum without an abdominal fluid reservoir. With either inflatable models, the patient presses the scrotal pump several times causing fluid to move into the cylinders to achieve erection. The cylinders are decompressed by pressing the release button on top of the scrotal pump to divert fluid back into the reservoir. Another option for men with ED is the malleable penile prosthesis, which involves a malleable rod implanted in each corpora. The malleable implants are not inflatable and are instead bent into position when the patient desires an erection.

InterStim

This device, manufactured by Medtronic, comprises two components (Figure 22.3): the lead and the intermittent pulse generator (IPG). The lead is usually placed into the S3 foramen percutaneously. The IPG is placed through a small incision, under the fat pad, at the superior aspect of the patient's gluteal muscle. The device is operated with an external controller, which can be used to alter the amplitude of the stimulation, as well as the program.

Physical Exam Findings in Patients with Genitourinary Implants

Physical exam can aid to identify genitourinary implants in a patient who cannot provide a clear history and can also determine if the device is nonfunctional, eroding, or infected. Both the AUS and IPP devices have a pump component located in the scrotum or labium. The AUS pump component is smooth and flat, with a depressible pump on the distal aspect and a firmer proximal component housing a small button used to lock the fluid in place (Figure 22.1). The IPP pump component is rounder and has ridges; it also contains a

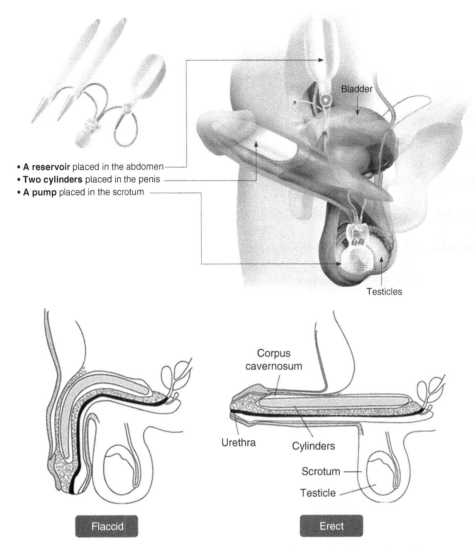

- **A reservoir** placed in the abdomen
- **Two cylinders** placed in the penis
- **A pump** placed in the scrotum

Bladder

Testicles

Corpus cavernosum

Urethra

Cylinders

Scrotum

Testicle

Flaccid

Erect

Figure 22.2 Penile prostheses. (*Source:* https://www.coloplastmenshealth.com/erectile-dysfunction/penile-implants/)

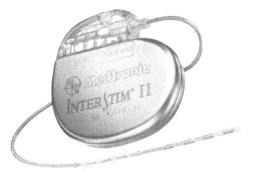

Figure 22.3 InterStim device. (*Source:* https://www.medtronic.com/us-en/healthcare-professionals/products/urology/sacral-neuromodulation-systems/interstim-ii.html)

proximal portion housing the locking button (Figure 22.2). The malleable penile prosthesis unit consists only of the two rigid cylinders placed in the corpora.

The scrotal and labial pumps should be easily palpated and freely mobile outside of the immediate postoperative period. If they feel adherent to the surrounding tissue or are not easily identified on palpation, infection is likely, especially if there are other signs or symptoms of infection including erythema, induration, fluctuance, localized pain, fever, or elevated white blood cell count. Alternatively, a patient with a genitourinary implant who has signs or symptoms of systemic infection but a completely normal genitourinary exam with the device in place, supple and nontender scrotum or labium, and no issues voiding likely has another source of infection.

Management of Genitourinary Prosthesis Complications

Infections

The complications associated with AUS and IPP are similar: both run the risk of infection, although infection rates have decreased with improved surgical technique. Both are also complicated by a relatively frequent need for revision surgery due to infection, device migration, or erosion into surrounding structures.

Most infections occur in the postoperative period as extension of a surgical site infection, but hematogenous seeding of the device is also possible, and thus, device infection does not always exist with obvious wound infection. Infections can also present in a delayed fashion weeks to months after the initial surgery. Any infection associated with a genitourinary prosthesis will always require urgent urologic consultation. In cases of purulent drainage, especially when there are systemic symptoms of infection, blood, urine, and wound cultures should be sent and broad-spectrum antibiotics initiated promptly. The causative organism can sometimes be predicted by other patient factors, but the initial choice of antibiotics should cover typical enteric gram-negative and gram-positive organisms, including methicillin-resistant *Staphylococcus aureus*. The addition of an antifungal agent can be considered, particularly if there is evidence of concomitant fungal satellite lesions or if the patient is immunocompromised.

Patients with an InterStim device may possibly present to the ER with an infection of either the IPG site or the lead. In these instances, cultures should be obtained, and antibiotics should be initiated with broad-spectrum coverage. The patient should be seen by a urologist to arrange explantation. In the absence of infection, it is possible that a patient may present with pain due to stimulation at high amplitudes. If the patient has the remote device with him/her, it can be used to turn off the device altogether. The individual may then contact his/her physician or the patient helpline at Medtronic at an elective time.

Erosion

Erosion of genitourinary prostheses into surrounding structures or through the skin itself is often not an emergent complication despite its alarming appearance. Erosion is frequently seen in patients with longstanding penile prostheses, where the cylinders can erode through the corpora or glans. In addition, over time, AUS and IPP pumps can erode through the skin of the scrotum or labium. This is especially common in patients who have decreased or absent sensation of the genitalia, including those with spinal cord injuries or poorly controlled diabetes. Unless there are also signs of infection such as erythema, induration, purulent drainage, pain, or signs of systemic infection including any systemic inflammatory response syndrome (SIRS) criteria or altered mental status, the patient can follow up with his/her urologist in the outpatient setting the following day.

Erosion with possible infection mandates that cultures should be sent from any purulent material or from the exposed device; broad-spectrum intravenous antibiotics started; blood, urine, and wound cultures sent; and urgent consultation with the patient's urologist or the urologist on call for prompt device removal.

There are rare reports of device erosion into viscera, including AUS cuff erosion into the bladder or abdominal reservoir erosion into the colon, but these are exceedingly rare and, of course, would require an urgent surgical consultation.

Mechanical Malfunction

A patient with an AUS may experience acute urinary retention if the device is accidentally locked with the urethral cuff inflated. The locking mechanism is a button located just above the pump in the scrotum or labium. Once unlocked, the pump should be depressed to deflate the cuff and allow urine to flow. If this maneuver does not result in voiding, a urology consult is required to determine the cause of the device malfunction and to decompress the bladder. Urinary retention secondary to AUS which does not allow voiding is an emergency requiring urologic consultation. *A transurethral catheter must never be placed in a patient with an activated AUS device.*

If a urologist is not available for a patient with urinary retention with an AUS, the emergency physician or general surgeon should decompress the bladder by suprapubic aspiration, preferably under image guidance with ultrasound. *Only a urologist should attempt to deactivate the device and place a urethral catheter in any patient with an AUS.*

A patient with an inflatable penile prosthesis may experience malfunction associated with an inability to inflate or deflate the penile cylinders. This malfunction is not urgent and, therefore, does not require urgent urologic consultation. Failure to inflate can be addressed by the patient's surgeon at a routine office visit if there are no other issues or complaints. In the case of inability to deflate an IPP, also known as autoinflation, the patient can follow up in the outpatient setting with his urologist as long as he is still able to void and there is no local pain or discomfort. Unlike in patients with an AUS, *a foley catheter may safely be placed in a patient with an IPP or malleable penile prosthesis*; the need for a urethral catheter in a patient with a penile prosthesis does not require a urology consultation.

Imaging in Patients with Urologic Implants

In most instances, presentation to an emergency facility by a patient with a urologic implant will not be implant related. Many of these visits will require imaging of some type. Both the penile implants and the AUS are largely silicone and are not expected to cause issues with ultrasound, computerized tomography, or MRI. If at all possible, MRI should be

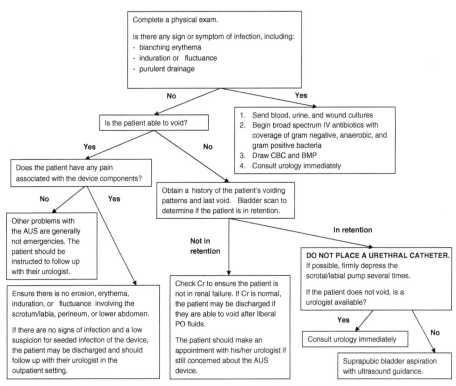

*AUS: Artificial urinary system; Cr: Creatinine; CBC: Complete blood count; BMP: Basic metabolic profile

Figure 22.4   Algorithm for emergency patient presenting with InterStim device.

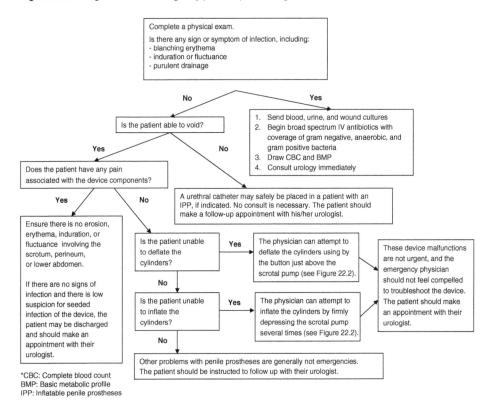

*CBC: Complete blood count
BMP: Basic metabolic profile
IPP: Inflatable penile prostheses

Figure 22.5   Algorithm for emergency patient presenting with a penile prosthesis.

avoided in patients with an InterStim. If this is not possible, the device should be turned off, and if available, the patient should be imaged in a 1.5 Tesla magnet. Given the pelvic location of the device, MRI of the brain is acceptable.

Figures 22.4 and 22.5 summarize a troubleshooting approach to the emergency department (ED) patient presenting with a urologic prosthesis. This algorithm is not meant to cover all possible situations, and in general, if an ED physician is unsure about whether a urological device is contributing to a patient's illness, a urologist should be consulted.

Further Reading

1 Shauloul, R. and Ghanem, H. (2013). Erectile dysfunction. *Lancet* 381: 153–165.
2 Goldstein, I., Lue, T.F., Padma-Nathan, H. et al. (1998). Oral sildenafil in the treatment of erectile dysfunction. *N. Engl. J. Med.* 338: 1397–1409.
3 Carson, C.C. (2004). Efficacy of antibiotic impregnation of inflatable penile prostheses in decreasing infection in original implants. *J. Urol.* 171: 1611–1614.
4 Carson, C.C. and Robertson, C.N. (1988). Late hematogenous infection of penile prostheses. *J. Urol.* 139: 50–52.
5 Linder, B.J., Piotrowski, J.T., Ziegelmann, M.J. et al. (2015). Perioperative complications following artificial urinary sphincter placement. *J. Urol.* 194: 716–720.
6 Mulcahy, J.J. (2010). Current approach to the treatment of penile implant infections. *Ther. Adv. Urol.* 2: 69–75.
7 Ravier, E., Fassi-Fehri, H., Crouzet, S. et al. (2015). Complications after artificial urinary sphincter implantation in patients with or without prior radiotherapy. *BJU Int.* 115: 300–307.
8 Schoepen, Y. and Staerman, F. (2002). Penile prostheses and infection. *Prog. Urol.* 12: 377–383.

Section VIII

Cardiac Devices

23

Management of Prosthetic Valve Complications

Massoud Kazzi[1,2] and Guenevere V. Burke[1]

[1] *Department of Emergency Medicine, George Washington University School of Medicine and Health Sciences, Washington, DC, USA*
[2] *Critical Care Medicine, Washington Adventist Hospital, Takoma Park, MD, USA*

Introduction

For some patients with valvular heart disease, there is the possibility of valve replacement. While prosthetic valves can significantly improve the patient's clinical condition, it is said that the patient exchanges the risks and complications of native valve disease for that of the prosthetic valve.

While there are different models, designs, and manufacturers, prosthetic valves come in two basic types: mechanical and bioprosthetic. Each valve is associated with its own potential advantages and disadvantages. The type of valve used is ultimately determined by the patient's characteristics, underlying clinical condition, and shared decision between the patient and surgeon as to what best fits the patient's needs. The indication for long-term anticoagulation depends on both the type of valve placed and certain patient characteristics. In addition, the introduction of a nonnative device into the patient's body poses a risk of infection and device failure with hematologic and hemodynamic sequela. Clinically, such complications often mimic acute heart failure; a thorough history and physical exam combined with imaging (usually echocardiography) will help in the diagnosis. Acute care providers caring for such patients need to coordinate with the patient's cardiologist and cardiac surgeon. This chapter will review prosthetic valves and their complications.

Patient Populations

Since valvular heart disease can be congenital and/or acquired, the emergency physician may encounter sequelae of valvular disease in diverse patient populations. Prosthetic valves are most frequently encountered in older adult patients as a result of age-related degeneration and calcification. The frequency of repair and replacement procedures is anticipated to increase with population aging and the proliferation of minimally invasive techniques. However, prosthetic valve emergencies may also be encountered in young

Emergency Management of the Hi-Tech Patient in Acute and Critical Care, First Edition. Edited by Ioannis Koutroulis, Nicholas Tsarouhas, Richard J. Lin, Jill C. Posner, Michael Seneff, and Robert Shesser.
© 2021 John Wiley & Sons Ltd. Published 2021 by John Wiley & Sons Ltd.

adults, notably pregnant women. Pregnancy in the setting of mechanical or bioprosthetic valve is associated with significant maternal and fetal morbidity and mortality. Thrombosis induced by the hypercoagulable state is the greatest concern, and anticoagulation profiles place one or the other, expectant mother or baby, at risk.

In pediatric populations, valve disease is fortunately rare. The overall incidence of congenital heart disease is approximately 8 per 1000 live births, with isolated ventricular septal defects most common. Valvular disease and procedures are still less frequently encountered. When required, valve repair is generally favored over replacement.

Equipment/Device

Prosthetic heart valves are generally divided into mechanical valves and bioprosthetic heart valves. Mechanical valves are made from synthetic materials (metals, polymers, etc.) and are modeled in three basic types: bileaflet, monoleaflet, and caged ball valves, the last of which are no longer routinely implanted due to unfavorable hemodynamic qualities and increased thrombogenicity. An example of a mechanical valve is depicted in Figure 23.1. Bioprosthetic valves are made from biologic tissue and are commonly bovine or porcine in origin and can be stented or stentless (see Figure 23.2).

Mechanical valves are more durable but have higher thrombogenicity, thus requiring lifelong anticoagulation to prevent thrombotic complications. Bioprosthetic valves, on the other hand, do not usually require lifelong anticoagulation but are known to have less durability. When deciding which type of valve to implant, the medical team may consider a patient's age and preference. Generally speaking, a mechanical valve is recommended for patients under the age of 50 years with no contraindications to anticoagulation or who are already on anticoagulants for another indication. Meanwhile, a bioprosthesis is recommended for patients in whom there are contraindications to anticoagulation or difficulties managing anticoagulation therapy or if the patient has a strong preference for not taking

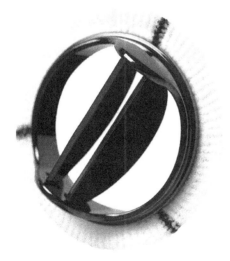

Figure 23.1 SJM Regent™ mechanical heart valve. SJM Regent and St. Jude Medical are trademarks of St. Jude Medical, LLC or its related companies.(*Source:* Reproduced with permission of St. Jude Medical ©2017. All rights reserved.)

Figure 23.2 Medtronic Mosaic™
bioprosthetic valve. (*Source:* Photograph
courtesy of Medtronic. Reproduced with
permission of Medtronic ©2017. All rights
reserved.)

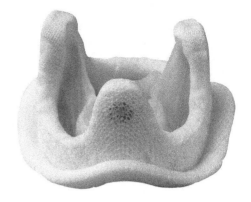

anticoagulation. Additionally, the most recent focused 2017 update of the 2014 American College of Cardiology and American Heart Association (ACC/AHA) guidelines on valvular heart disease state that it is "reasonable" to use bioprosthetic valves in patients over the age of 70 years. For patients between the age of 50 and 70 years, an individualized approach is recommended.

Even with identical valve subtypes, long-term complications and mortality rates after valve replacement vary widely. Rigorous device testing appears to have been effective in limiting variation in device performance characteristics, such that patient age and comorbid conditions (e.g. heart failure and coronary artery disease) are more important predictors of morbidity and mortality than the type of prosthetic valve *within* each of the two major categories. From the standpoint of the emergency or acute care provider, the most important variables to learn from the patient are the type of prosthetic valve, location, and whether the patient is on anticoagulation.

As previously noted, in the pediatric patient population, treatment options are limited by the available device sizes. Mechanical heart valves have not yet been successfully constructed for younger patient populations such as neonates, infants, and toddlers. This size restriction generally means that, in these patient populations, valvular disease may be treated with valve repair, valvuloplasty, or more advanced surgical techniques depending on the underlying condition. An in-depth review of treatment for such patients is beyond the scope of this chapter.

Indications

Patients with a diseased valve causing symptoms may be considered for operative management. Valvular disease generally entails infection (e.g. endocarditis), and primary or secondary stenosis or regurgitation. A multidisciplinary team including the patient's primary physician, cardiologist, and cardiothoracic surgeon, among others, will generally be involved in the decision-making. The decision of whether to perform surgery for valvular heart disease is generally case-based and may include factors such as valve anatomy, valve hemodynamics, patient age, symptom severity, and other complicating comorbidities.

A risk calculator developed by the Society of Thoracic Surgeons is available online and can help determine the operative risk for the patient. Should the decision be made to pursue surgery, there is the option of valve repair instead of valve replacement. This decision-making process is so sufficiently nuanced and detailed that it is out of the scope of this chapter.

The ACC/AHA guidelines on valvular heart disease lay out a number of decision-making algorithms that can be useful in deciding in which patients to pursue surgery. In practice, valve replacement is most frequently encountered in patients with a history of severe, symptomatic left-sided valvular disease, including aortic stenosis, aortic regurgitation, mitral stenosis, and mitral regurgitation. Symptoms are typical of heart failure, including exertional dyspnea, decreased exercise tolerance, and exertional angina.

Management

Routine postoperative follow-up after valve surgery involves management of anticoagulation, imaging of the valve by echocardiography, and physical examination, screening for new signs of heart failure. The frequency for such evaluations is determined by the patient's cardiologist and cardiothoracic team. The most active management issue pertaining to the valve is generally the management of anticoagulation therapy.

Anticoagulation and Antiplatelet Therapy

Patients with mechanical valves and high-risk patients with bioprosthetic valves require lifelong anticoagulation. Vitamin K antagonists (warfarin) and heparin (generally for bridging) are the only anticoagulants approved for use in this patient population. Direct thrombin inhibitors such as dabigatran are contraindicated due to excessive bleeding and thromboembolic risk as compared with warfarin. Direct factor Xa inhibitors such as apixaban and rivaroxaban are not approved for anticoagulation in patients with prosthetic heart valves. Of note, both the European Society of Cardiology and the American College of Chest Physicians have guidelines which pertain to antithrombotic therapy in this patient population. Additionally, each individual institution may have its own institution-specific guidelines or protocols. Thus, it is of utmost importance to coordinate care in the acute setting with the patient's consistent providers. Figure 23.3 demonstrates the 2014 ACC/AHA Valvular Heart Disease report's algorithmic approach to anticoagulation in prosthetic valve patients.

Complications/Emergencies

Complications of valves fall generally into three broad categories: infectious, hematologic, and functional failure, although there is overlap between the three.

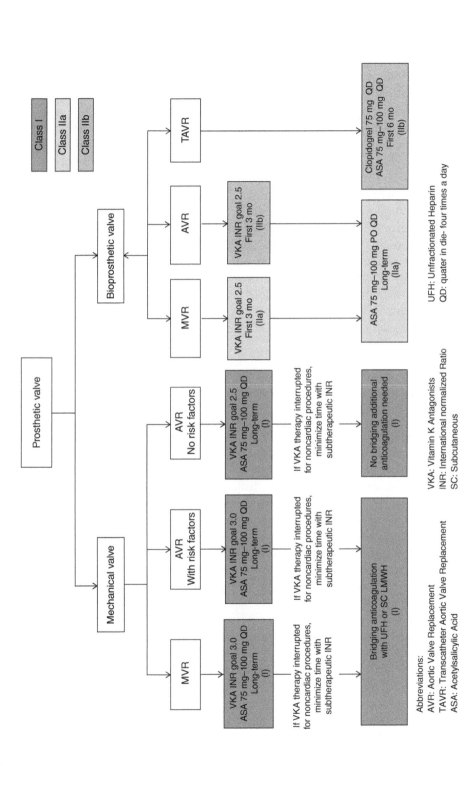

Figure 23.3 Anticoagulation of prosthetic valves. *Source:* Nishimura et al. © 2014, Elsevier. Risk factors include AF, previous thromboembolism, left ventricle (LV) dysfunction, hypercoagulable condition, and older generation mechanical AVR. Reprinted with permission Circulation. **2014;** CIR0000000000000029©**2014** American Heart Association**, Inc.**

Infective Endocarditis

Nonnative tissue introduced into an environment of abnormal flow is susceptible to seeding of bacteria and other organisms. Patients at risk of native valve endocarditis due to underlying medical condition (intravenous drug use (IVDU), diabetes, etc.) have a predisposition for infection of the prosthetic heart valve. The clinical presentation of infective endocarditis (IE) may be diverse and includes, among other manifestations, fever, new or worsened murmur, skin manifestations, sepsis, unexplained heart failure, stroke, abscesses, or infarcts of solid organs. Any febrile patient with multiple sites of infection should immediately raise suspicion for IE. Moreover, any prolonged fever without an obvious source should also raise the index of suspicion for valvular infection. The Modified Duke Criteria is a useful scoring system for establishing a diagnosis of IE. The cornerstones of diagnosis, however, are blood cultures and echocardiography. The Infectious Diseases Society of America (IDSA) recommends three sets of blood cultures from different venipuncture sites and transthoracic echocardiogram (TTE) as the initial diagnostic modality of choice. However, because prosthetic valve patients are at high risk for complications, a transesophageal echocardiography (TEE) should be performed to help determine valve function, hemodynamics, and vegetation size in order to inform decision-making regarding necessity of surgical intervention. In the emergency setting, early intravenous (IV) antibiotic administration and consultation with cardiothoracic surgery are essential steps in management.

Supratherapeutic International Normalized Ratio and Anticoagulation Reversal

The second category of complications is hematologic. Patients who are on anticoagulation for valve replacement will be on a vitamin K antagonist (warfarin) as the novel oral anticoagulants are not approved nor indicated for mechanical heart valves, and are generally only used in the first three to six months of bioprosthetic heart valves placement, if at all. Bleeding is thus a higher risk in mechanical valves than in bioprosthetic.

The long list of drug interactions and possible individual difficulty in maintaining a therapeutic international normalized ratio (INR) pose a risk to the patient of developing supratherapeutic anticoagulation. Anticoagulation reversal in the setting of prosthetic valves involves an individualized evaluation of risks and benefits with high-risk bleeding necessitating more aggressive reversal. Generally speaking, if not faced with a major life-threatening bleed, then optimal management decisions require a multidisciplinary approach. It is always prudent to refer to institutional protocols where relevant.

One approach, in patients who have a supratherapeutic INR > 4.5 without bleeding, is to consider the administration of small doses of vitamin K (1–2 mg orally) or just allow the INR to fall gradually. If the INR > 10, then higher doses of oral vitamin K (e.g. 5 mg) may be required.

Immediate reversal of anticoagulation would be necessary if the patient has a major bleed (intracranial or extracranial) or the patient requires an emergency surgery with significant bleeding risk. In these scenarios, four-factor prothrombin complex concentrate are generally more effective at reversal than fresh frozen plasma. However, the 2017 AHA guidelines state that either is reasonable for reversal prior to an urgent procedure. Generally, in major bleeding, IV vitamin K would be recommended as well. Recombinant Factor VIIa should not be used in this patient population due to higher thrombotic risks. The decision of when to initiate anticoagulation after a major bleed would depend on a number of factors, including site of bleeding, whether an intervention was performed, and the risk of rebleeding. However, in most patients, anticoagulation can be reinitiated after 7–14 days.

Hemolytic Anemia

Hemolytic anemia is a rare complication occurring in <1% of patients with newer prosthetic valves. An echocardiogram is indicated to rule out paravalvular leak. If the leak is due to either IE or severe symptoms such as causing a patient to have multiple blood transfusions, then operative management is recommended. If there is no IE and a patient is not a surgical candidate or does not desire repeat surgery, then medical management may include erythropoietin, iron supplementation, and beta-blockade.

Prosthetic Valve Thrombosis, Thromboembolism, and Valve Obstruction

Prosthetic valve thrombosis (PVT) and thromboembolism are two complications which can be part of the same spectrum of disease. PVT involves the formation of an in-situ thrombus that may interfere with blood flow across the valve and thromboembolism entails embolic phenomena. Prosthetic valves are the primary culprits in PVT and thromboembolism; both complications can occur in patients with bioprosthetic valves, but the incidence is much lower in comparison to mechanical valves. Thrombosis may be associated with valve obstruction. However, pannus growth and stenosis can also lead to the same end pathway.

PVT is rare in bioprosthetic valves but occurs in up to 1.3% patient years of mechanical valve patients. Thromboembolic events are also more common in mechanical valve patients, occurring in 0.6–7% patient years. A significant portion of patients will have had inadequate anticoagulation as a contributing cause. A patient can present asymptomatically or with symptoms of obstruction such as dyspnea, fatigue, decreased exercise tolerance, or, more seriously, heart failure and shock. Therefore, a patient with subtherapeutic INR who has any symptoms of emboli or heart failure should be suspected of having PVT.

When PVT is suspected, the AHA, in its most recent guidelines, suggests multimodal imaging including echocardiography (TTE and/or TEE), fluoroscopy, and/or computerized tomography (CT) scanning of the chest. Echocardiography will evaluate the velocity and flow across the valve, estimate the valve orifice, and possibly visualize a thrombus. If no thrombus is seen and there are elevated transvalvular gradients suggesting obstruction, then pannus growth may be suspected.

The two basic treatment modalities are surgery (valve replacement) and medical therapy, which includes anticoagulation and fibrinolysis. The 2017 AHA guidelines highlight an expanded role for fibrinolysis, but ultimately the decision will come down to a series of factors, including patient's choice, surgical risk, thrombus size, institutional experience with each approach, and surgeon recommendations.

If a thrombotic or thromboembolic event occurs, then it is incumbent upon the team to assess the adequacy of anticoagulation. If it is subtherapeutic, then evaluating the patient's dosage, dietary compliance, and possible institution of more frequent INR checks may be necessary.

If the patient has a therapeutic INR when the thrombotic event occurs, then generally one of the two interventions is selected: either a higher INR is targeted or the addition of an antiplatelet agent to the current regimen is considered. Again, in this scenario, the primary cardiology or cardiac surgery team will be involved in making such decisions.

Consultation

Infectious Disease

Consider consultation in the occasion of infectious complications. Empiric therapy is likely to reflect the IDSA guidelines. But input regarding dosing, double empiric coverage, or certain organisms based on local antibiograms and resistance patterns may be warranted.

Cardiothoracic Surgery

Early consultation with the patient's cardiothoracic surgeon is essential to help guide management. Each institution or provider may have certain protocols in place based on their local experience, thus early input to establish a course of action would be ideal.

Cardiology

An essential step in the decision tree is the performance and interpretation of the echocardiogram. Thus, accelerated diagnostic interpretation of the echocardiogram can determine acuity of the patient's condition, the urgency of initiating treatment, and the necessary initial steps (antibiotics, anticoagulation, urgent surgical intervention, etc.)

Hematology

Consultation may provide help in decision-making with regard to anticoagulation reversal, bridging therapy, or in deciding the timing for reinitiation of anticoagulation therapy.

Further Reading

1 Vahanian, A., Alfieri, O., Andreotti, F. et al. (2012). Guidelines on the management of valvular heart disease (version 2012). *Eur. Heart J.* 33 (19): 2451–2496.
2 Lawley, C.M., Lain, S.J., Algert, C.S. et al. (2015). Prosthetic heart valves in pregnancy, outcomes for women and their babies: a systematic review and meta-analysis. *BJOG* 122 (11): 1446–1455.

3 Alshawabkeh, L., Economy, K.E., and Valente, A.M. (2016). Anticoagulation during pregnancy: evolving strategies with a focus on mechanical valves. *J. Am. Coll. Cardiol.* 68 (16): 1804–1813.

4 Bhagra, C.J., D'Souza, R., and Silversides, C.K. (2017). Valvular heart disease and pregnancy part II: management of prosthetic valves. *Heart* 103 (3): 244–252.

5 Henaine, R., Roubertie, F., Vergnat, M., and Ninet, J. (2012). Valve replacement in children: a challenge for a whole life. *Arch. Cardiovasc. Dis.* 105 (10): 517–528.

6 Singhal, P., Luk, A., and Butany, J. (2013). Bioprosthetic heart valves: impact of implantation on biomaterials. *ISRN Biomater.* 2013: 728791. https://doi.org/10.5402/2013/728791.

7 Hammermeister, K., Sethi, G.K., Henderson, W.G. et al. (2000). Outcomes 15 years after valve replacement with a mechanical versus a bioprosthetic valve: final report of the veterans affairs randomized trial. *J. Am. Coll. Cardiol.* 36 (4): 1152.

8 Pibarot, P. and Dumesnil, J.G. (2009). Prosthetic heart valves: selection of the optimal prosthesis and long-term management. *Circulation* 119 (7): 1034–1048.

9 Nishimura, R.A., Otto, C.M., Bonow, R.O. et al. (2017). 2017 AHA/ACC focused update of the 2014 AHA/ACC guideline for the management of patients with valvular heart disease: a report of the American College of Cardiology/American Heart Association Task Force on Clinical Practice Guidelines. *Circulation* 135 (25): e1159–e1195.

10 Nishimura, R.A., Otto, C.M., Bonow, R.O. et al. (2014). 2014 AHA/ACC guideline for the management of patient with valvular heart disease: a report of the American College of Cardiology/American Heart Association task force on practice guidelines. *J. Am. Coll. Cardiol.* 63 (22): e57–e185.

11 Rahimtoola, S.H. (2003). Choice of prosthetic heart valve for adult patients. *J. Am. Coll. Cardiol.* 41 (6): 893–904. https://doi.org/10.1016/S0735-1097(02)02965-0.

12 Alsoufi, B. (2011). Aortic and mitral valve replacement in children: current options and outcomes. *Expert Rev. Cardiovasc. Ther.* 9 (7): 805–809.

13 Society of Thoracic Surgeons [internet]. Chicago c2017 [cited 2017 Apr 15]. Available from https://www.sts.org/quality-research-patient-safety/quality/risk-calculator-and-models/risk-calculator

14 Eikelboom, J.W., Connolly, S.J., Brueckmann, M. et al. (2013). Dabigatran versus warfarin in patients with mechanical heart valves. *N. Engl. J. Med.* 369 (13): 1206. Epub 31 August 2013.

15 Whitlock, R.P., Sun, J.C., Fremes, S.E. et al. (2012). Antithrombotic and thrombolytic therapy for valvular disease: antithrombotic therapy and prevention of thrombosis, 9th ed.: American College of Chest Physicians Evidence-Based Clinical Practice. *Chest* 141 (2 suppl): e576S–e600S.

16 Hoen, B. and Duval, X. (2013). Clinical practice. Infective endocarditis. *N. Engl. J. Med.* 368 (15): 1425–1433.

17 Li, J.S., Sexton, D.J., Mick, N. et al. (2000). Proposed modifications to the Duke criteria for the diagnosis of infective endocarditis. *Clin. Infect. Dis.* 30: 633–638.

18 Baddour, L.M., Wilson, W.R., Bayer, A.S. et al. (2015). Infective endocarditis in adults: diagnosis, antimicrobial therapy, and management of complications: a scientific statement for healthcare professionals from the American Heart Association. *Circulation* 132 (15): 1435–1486.

19 Brennan, J.M., Edwards, F.H., Zhao, Y. et al. (2013). Long-term safety and effectiveness of mechanical versus biologic aortic valve prostheses in older patients: results from the Society of Thoracic Surgeons Adult Cardiac Surgery National Database. *Circulation* 127 (16): 1647.

20 Goldstein, J.N., Refaai, M.A., Milling, T.J. Jr. et al. (2015). Four-factor prothrombin complex concentrate versus plasma for rapid vitamin K antagonist reversal in patients needing urgent surgical or invasive interventions: a phase 3b, open-label, non-inferiority, randomised trial. *Lancet* 385 (9982): 2077. Epub. 27 February 2015.

21 Panduranga, P., Al-Mukhaini, M., Al-Muslahi, M. et al. (2012). Management dilemmas in patients with mechanical heart valves and warfarin-induced major bleeding. *World J. Cardiol.* 4 (3): 54–59.

22 Shapira, Y., Vaturi, M., and Sagie, A. (2009). Hemolysis associated with prosthetic heart valves: a review. *Cardiol. Rev.* 17: 121.

23 Roudaut, R., Serri, K., and Lafitte, S. (2007). Thrombosis of prosthetic heart valves: diagnosis and therapeutic considerations. *Heart* 93 (1): 137–142.

24 Deviri, E., Sareli, P., Wisenbaugh, T., and Cronje, S.L. (1991). Obstruction of mechanical heart valve prostheses: clinical aspects and surgical management. *J. Am. Coll. Cardiol.* 17 (3): 646.

24

Emergency Management of Patients with Vascular Occlusion Devices, Stents, or Filters

Amy Caggiula

Department of Emergency Medicine, George Washington University School of Medicine and Health Sciences, Washington, DC, USA

Introduction

This chapter focuses on emergency management and diagnosis of complications from vascular occlusion and filtration devices. While symptoms can be nonspecific or indolent, an overriding theme of this chapter is the need for urgent consultation with specialty services. Due to the high-risk nature of many of these devices, surgical and/or endovascular consultation is often immediately indicated for retrieval, repositioning, or recanalization. Expeditious treatment can greatly reduce the risk of long-term complications. Emergency physicians should also have a high index of suspicion for device malfunction or complication, particularly in the immediate postprocedural period.

Congenital Heart Defect Management and Occlusion Devices

Congenital heart defect occlusion devices include devices for the repair of atrial and ventricular septal defects and patent foramen ovales. While treatment of these congenital heart defects has traditionally been surgical, endovascular repair is becoming more common as a mainstay of therapy.

Complications for septal occlusion devices are relatively uncommon. When a patient does present to the emergency department (ED) with issues related to his or her device, treatment is often surgical or endovascular removal or repositioning. As such, the role of the ED physician is really one of diagnosis rather than management, and treatment usually involves calling the appropriate service (surgery, cardiology, or interventional radiology) for definitive management. This chapter will discuss some of the serious complications and their presentations, but we stress the importance of early consultation in all cases.

Emergency Management of the Hi-Tech Patient in Acute and Critical Care, First Edition. Edited by Ioannis Koutroulis, Nicholas Tsarouhas, Richard J. Lin, Jill C. Posner, Michael Seneff, and Robert Shesser.

Atrial Septal Defect Occlusion Devices

Atrial septal defects are a relatively common type of congenital heart defect affecting approximately 1 out of every 770 live births. Most defects are small and require only observation and frequent monitoring, but large defects often mandate surgical or endovascular repair to prevent serious complications from the defect, such as right-sided heart failure and pulmonary hypertension.

Devices

Amplatzer® Septal Occluder
Gore Cardioform® Septal Occluder
Risk factors for complications: Older age at repair, large defect, preexisting complications (pulmonary hypertension and right-sided heart failure)

Types of Complications
- Atrial and ventricular arrhythmias
  - Symptoms – Palpitations, chest pain, and syncope.
  - Treatment – If stable, admit to monitored bed with cardiology consultation. Usually self resolves and is most common in the immediate and subacute preprocedural periods.
- Device embolization – Most commonly occurs in the immediate postprocedural period, and the device usually embolizes to the pulmonary vasculature. Left-sided migration is very rare.
  - Risk factors – Very large Atrial Septal Defect and thin atrial rim.
  - Treatment – Immediate endovascular retrieval.
- Endocarditis
  - Symptoms – Fever, septicemia and shock, and symptoms related to septic embolic.
  - Treatment – Broad-spectrum antibiotics and device removal.
- Cardiac erosion
  - Symptoms – Shock, undifferentiated hypotension, and shortness of breath.
  - Findings – Hemopericardium and/or cardiac tamponade.
  - Treatment – Immediate CT surgery consultation.

Ventricular Septal Defect (VSD) Occlusion Devices

Ventricular septal defect is the most common type of congenital heart defect, affecting 1 in every 240 live births in the US. Decision to repair a ventricular septal defect depends on many factors, including age at diagnosis, size of the defect, symptoms, and presence of complications such as arrhythmias, left to right shunt, pulmonary hypertension, or heart failure. Small VSDs may close on their own, but large defects often necessitate surgical or endovascular repair. For the purposes of this chapter, we will focus only on congenital heart defects rather than VSDs secondary to cardiac lesions such as MI or iatrogenic defects after cardiac surgery such as septal myomectomy.

Of note, open repair of moderate and large VSDs is still the modality of choice, with endovascular repair with devices considered a second option. As such, literature is lacking with regard to the long-term sequelae and complications of these relatively uncommon devices. The complications that have been described in the literature are similar or analogous to ASD repair devices with the exception of heart block, which will be discussed here.

Devices

Amplatzer Occluder Device for VSD
CardioSEAL® Septal Occlusion System

Types of Complications
- Heart block
  - Risk factors – Age at repair (older age associated with higher rates of heart block), anatomy and size of the defect, and etiology of the defect (congenital versus secondary).
    - Signs and symptoms – Hypotension, bradycardia, palpitations, and shock.
  - Diagnosis – EKG and echocardiogram.
  - Management – Consultation and immediate removal of device if recently implanted. If heart block is present as a late outcome of VSD repair, pacemaker implantation is indicated.
- Device embolization and/or migration
  - Signs and symptoms – Presents similarly to ASD, and management, consultation, and monitoring are analogous.
  - Management – Immediate consultation with CT surgery and interventional radiology is indicated

Patent Ductus Arteriosus (PDA) Occlusion Devices

The ductus arteriosus, a passage through which aortic blood can pass into the pulmonary vascular system, usually closes within a couple of days of birth. It affects approximately 8 in 1000 live births. A patent ductus arteriosus is a ductus that remains open, and is often small and asymptomatic into adulthood (silent PDA). Patients with audible PDAs on exam or who present with symptoms are at serious risk for complications such as pulmonary hypertension and heart failure. Almost all patients, with the exception of those with silent PDAs, should be repaired by either embolization or a PDA occlusion device.

Devices

Amplatzer Duct Occluder

Complications
- Migration and/or embolization of the device – Infrequently described in the literature and usually occurs in the immediate postprocedural period.
  - Signs and symptoms – Varies depending on the site of migration but can present as aortic stenosis or obstruction with exertional fatigue, syncope, and chest pain.

- Diagnosis – echocardiogram, CTA, or angiography.
- Management – surgical or endovascular removal.
- Left pulmonary artery stenosis or obstruction
  This complication has only been described in case reports, so evidence for its workup is extremely limited.
  - Signs and symptoms – Presents only in children due to the size of the pulmonary vasculature in adults. Can present with tachypnea, fatigue, tachycardia, and edema.
  - Diagnosis – CTA and echocardiogram.
  - Management – CT surgery and endovascular consultation. Stent angioplasty may be indicated to relieve obstruction.
- Infective endocarditis
  - Symptoms – Fever, septicemia and shock, and symptoms related to septic embolism.
  - Treatment – Broad-spectrum antibiotics and consultation with CT surgery and/or IR for device removal.

Arterial Stents

Far and away, the most commonly encountered complication of any stent is in-stent thrombosis or stenosis leading to ischemia of the organ or structure distal to the stent. Signs and symptoms are consistent hypoperfusion and are diagnosed with angiography, CT/CTA, MRA, ultrasound, or direct visualization through endovascular intervention. Serum markers such as troponin and creatinine can be helpful in certain cases.

Device Examples

Protégé Rx® Carotid Stent
Resolute Onyx® Drug-Eluting Stent
Resolute Integrity® Drug-Eluting Stent
Integrity Bare Metal Stent
Itrix® Rapamycin Eluting Coronary Stent
Everflex® Self-Expanding Peripheral Stent
Protégé GPS® Self-Expanding Peripheral Stent
FACILE® Self-Expanding Peripheral Stent
Supera® Peripheral Stent System
Thalis® Balloon Expandable Stent
Neurolink® Stent System
Wingspan® Stent System
Cheatham® Platinum Stent

Stent Thrombosis or Stenosis
- Coronary arteries
  - Signs and symptoms – Acute MI, chest pain, elevated cardiac enzymes, and EKG changes.
  - Evaluation and management – Interventional cardiology consultation, catheterization, and recanalization. Serum troponin can be helpful in the absence of acute EKG changes.

- Renal arteries
  - Signs and symptoms – flank pain, acute or subacute renal failure, and hypertension
  - Evaluation – CTA, angiography, ultrasound, and MRA
- Carotid arteries
  - Signs and symptoms – Acute CVA or TIA manifesting as unilateral muscle weakness, facial droop, and aphasia.
  - Evaluation – CTA or MRA of the head and neck.
- Intracranial arteries
  - Signs and symptoms of thrombosis/stenosis – Acute CVA or TIA in the corresponding vascular distribution.
  - Evaluation – CT/CTA of the brain.
  - Management – Neurology and endovascular consultation
- Femoral or iliac arteries
  - Signs and symptoms of thrombosis/stenosis – Acute, subacute, or gradual limb ischemia; leg or foot pain; and pallor.
  - Evaluation – Angiography or CTA.
  - Management – Vascular surgery consultation and anticoagulation.

Coarctation of the Aorta Stenting

Coarctation of the aorta is a congenital narrowing of the aorta affecting approximately 1 in 2500 live births in the US. It is repaired surgically or with balloon angioplasty and stenting to restore normal blood flow through the aorta. While this disease entity is relatively uncommon, restenosis of these stents is a frequent complication.

Devices

Cheatham Platinum Stent

Complications
- Stent stenosis
  - Signs and symptoms – Elevated blood pressure, fatigue, syncope, shortness of breath, chest pain, and heart failure. Symptoms are usually subacute, and mild stenosis is usually detected on routine follow-up imaging.
  - Evaluation – ECHO and angiography.
  - Management – Consultation and endovascular intervention of recanalization of the stenosed stent.
- Aortic aneurysm:
  - Signs and symptoms – There have been no cases in the literature of symptomatic aneurysm following coarctation stenting.
  - Evaluation – Usually detected incidentally on imaging studies for unrelated symptoms such as echo or chest CT. Aneurysms are most commonly discovered on routine post-procedure follow-up echocardiograms.
  - Management – Consultation with CT surgery, especially for large aneurysms.

Inferior Vena Cava (IVC) Filters

Inferior vena cava filters are common devices used for the prevention of dangerous pulmonary emboli in patients for whom anticoagulation is contraindicated or ineffective.

Indications

- Known acute VTE and a contraindication to anticoagulation
- Hemodynamically unstable PE
- Anticoagulant failure
- Prophylaxis in massive trauma or spinal cord injury*
- Adjunct to PE with thrombolysis*
- Mobile thrombus*
- Ileocaval thrombus*

*Not recognized by all societies as a true indication

Complications

Broadly defined as periprocedural or delayed. For the purposes of this text, this chapter focuses on delayed complications.

- Filter thrombosis (approximately 2–20%)
  - Symptoms – Depend on the location of the filter. Bilateral lower extremity swelling is common. If the stent is proximal to the renal vasculature, acute kidney failure can be the presenting symptom.
  - Diagnosis – CT scan in the venous phase or venography.
  - Management – Endovascular consult for thrombectomy, stent, and balloon angioplasty.
- Migration – Very challenging to diagnose
  - Symptoms – Often nonspecific or systemic. Symptoms also depend entirely on the site of migration and can include back pain, sepsis, and chest or abdominal pain. The most serious is intracardiac migration, which can lead to ventricular tachycardias, cardiac rupture, and death.
  - Diagnosis – CT scan.
  - Treatment – Surgical or endovascular extraction of filter.
- Penetration of the caval wall and subsequent injury to surrounding organs
  - Symptoms – If the IVC filter penetrates into an adjacent organ, patients can present with severe abdominal pain, acute abdomen, hemodynamic instability and shock, fever, and other symptoms related to the damaged organ. Potential sites include the aorta, liver parenchyma, portal vein, retroperitoneum, and bowel. Duodenal perforation has been described in the literature. While exceedingly uncommon, duodenal perforation can present with abdominal pain, peritoneal symptoms, hematemesis and melena, obstructive symptoms, and back pain.
  - Diagnosis – Often found incidentally on imaging studies for unrelated symptoms. Perforations most often occur slowly and are asymptomatic upon diagnosis. In patients with IVC filters, providers must have a high index of suspicion when patients present with nonspecific or systemic symptoms. Diagnosis is usually made with CT scan.

- Management: Immediate surgical consultation and operative exploration and repair of damaged organs and vasculature. If symptoms are subacute and perforation appears chronic, IR consultation for removal is indicated.

Left Atrial Appendage Devices

One of the most common and morbid complications of long-standing atrial fibrillation is the formation and embolization of blood clots leading to acute cerebrovascular accident. However, due to medical comorbidities, allergies, and fall risks, many patients are not candidates for prophylactic anticoagulation. The left atrial appendage (LAA) is a common site of clot formation in patients with atrial fibrillation. Closure or occlusion of the LAA helps mitigate stroke risk in these patients for whom anticoagulation is contraindicated or fails.

Devices

WATCHMAN® device
Amplatzer Plug Device

Complications
- Pericardial effusion secondary to LAA perforation
  - Symptoms – Shortness of breath, chest pain, hypotension, shock.
  - Diagnosis – Echocardiogram.
  - Management – Pericardiocentesis for unstable patients and immediate CT surgery consultation.
- Device-associated thrombosis (DAT) – Relatively uncommon and usually asymptomatic. Often detected incidentally on ECHO during postprocedure monitoring.
  - Risk factors – poor EF at the time of insertion and a high CHA_2DS_2-VASc score.
  - Symptoms – Extremely rare but can present with neurological manifestations consistent with TIA or stroke. Have a low index of suspicion for DAT if patient is within one year of device implantation. Risk factors for DAT include poor EF at the time of insertion and a high CHA_2DS_2-VASc score.
  - Diagnosis – usually diagnosed incidentally on echocardiogram. Physicians should have a high index of suspicion for patients with a known LAA occlusion device at high risk for DAT.
  - Management – Neurology and cardiology consultations indicated, and treatment consists of anticoagulation and close monitoring.

Further Reading

1 Behjati-Ardakani, M., Rafiei, M., Behjati-Ardakani, M. et al. (2015). Long-term results of transcatheter closure of patent ductus arteriosus in adolescents and adults with Amplatzer Duct Occluder. *North American Journal of Medical Sciences* 7 (5): 208–211.
2 Bélénotti, P., Sarlon-Bartoli, G., Bartoli, M. et al. (2011). Vena cava filter migration: an unappreciated complication. About four cases and review of the literature. *Annals of Vascular Surgery* 25 (8): 1141.e9–1141.e14.

3 Caplin, D., Nikolic, B., Kalva, S. et al. (2011). Quality improvement guidelines for the performance of inferior vena cava filter placement for the prevention of pulmonary embolism. *Journal of Vascular and Interventional Radiology* 22 (11): 1499–1506. https://doi.org/10.1016/j.jvir.2011.07.012.

4 Feltes, F., Bacha, H., Beekman, P. et al. (2011). Indications for cardiac catheterization and intervention in pediatric cardiac disease: a scientific statement from the American Heart Association. *Circulation* 123 (22): 2607–2652. https://doi.org/10.1161/CIR.0b013e31821b1f10.

5 Fox, M. and Kahn, S. (2008). Postthrombotic syndrome in relation to vena cava filter placement: a systematic review. *Journal of Vascular and Interventional Radiology* 19 (7): 981–985.e3.

6 Gabriels, C., De Backer, J., Pasquet, A. et al. (2017). Long-term outcome of patients with perimembranous ventricular septal defect: results from the Belgian registry on adult congenital heart disease. *Cardiology* 136 (3): 147–155.

7 Ghosh, S., Sridhar, A., and Sivaprakasam, M. (2018). Complete heart block following transcatheter closure of perimembranous VSD using amplatzer duct occluder II. *Catheterization and Cardiovascular Interventions* 92 (5): 921–924.

8 Ivanovic, V., Mckusick, M., Johnson, C. et al. (2003). Renal artery stent placement: complications at a single tertiary care center. *Journal of Vascular and Interventional Radiology* 14 (2): 217–225.

9 Jazayeri, M., Vuddanda, V., Turagam, M. et al. (2018). Safety profiles of percutaneous left atrial appendage closure devices: an analysis of the Food and Drug Administration Manufacturer and User Facility Device Experience (MAUDE) database from 2009 to 2016. *Journal of Cardiovascular Electrophysiology* 29 (1): 5–13. https://doi.org/10.1111/jce.13362.

10 Lempereur, M., Aminian, A., Freixa, X. et al. (2017). Device-associated thrombus formation after left atrial appendage occlusion: a systematic review of events reported with the Watchman, the Amplatzer Cardiac Plug and the Amulet. *Catheterization and Cardiovascular Interventions* 90 (5): E111–E121. https://doi.org/10.1002/ccd.26903.

11 Liem, N., Tung, C., Van Linh, N. et al. (2014). Outcomes of thoracoscopic clipping versus transcatheter occlusion of patent ductus arteriosus: randomized clinical trial. *Journal of Pediatric Surgery* 49 (2): 363–366.

12 Mahmud, E. (2005). Renal artery stenting. *Journal of the American College of Cardiology* 46 (5): 784–786.

13 Malgor, R. and Labropoulos, N. (2012). A systematic review of symptomatic duodenal perforation by inferior vena cava filters. *Journal of Vascular Surgery* 55 (3): 856–861.e3.

14 Martínez-Quintana, E. and Rodríguez-González, F. (2016). Risks factors for atrial Septal defect occlusion device migration. *The International Journal of Angiology* 25 (5): e63–e65.

15 Mcelhinney, B., Quartermain, D., Kenny, D. et al. (2016). Relative risk factors for cardiac erosion following transcatheter closure of atrial septal defects: a case–control study. *Circulation* 133 (18): 1738–1746.

16 Meadows, B., Minahan, B., Mcelhinney, B. et al. (2015). Intermediate outcomes in the prospective, multicenter coarctation of the aorta stent trial (COAST). *Circulation* 131 (19): 1656–1664.

17 Reller, M., Strickland, M., Riehle-Colarusso, T. et al. (2008). Prevalence of congenital heart defects in Metropolitan Atlanta, 1998–2005. *The Journal of Pediatrics* 153 (6): 807–813.

18 Riaz, I., Husnain, M., Riaz, H. et al. (2014). Meta-analysis of revascularization versus medical therapy for atherosclerotic renal artery stenosis. *The American Journal of Cardiology* 114 (7): 1116–1123.

19 Sarosiek, S., Crowther, M., and Sloan, J. (2013). Indications, complications, and management of inferior vena cava filters: the experience in 952 patients at an academic hospital with a level I trauma center. *JAMA Internal Medicine* 173 (7): 1–5. https://doi.org/10.1001/jamainternmed.2013.343.

25

The Emergency Department Approach to the Patient with an Implantable Mechanical Circulatory Support Device

Robert Shesser

Department of Emergency Medicine, George Washington University School of Medicine and Health Sciences, Washington, DC, USA

The advent of aggressive treatment for coronary artery occlusive disease and better understanding and treatment of heart failure of all types with the long-term use of beta blockers and angiotensin converting enzyme (ACE) and angiotensin receptor blockage (ARB) inhibitors has increased the prevalence of end-stage heart disease in our population. Despite these advances, the one year mortality rate is 7.2% and about 1/3 of patients with heart failure are hospitalized each year. over. The inexorable advance of technology in mechanical circulatory support (MCS) is being applied to extend the lifespan and improve the quality of life of heart failure patients in a variety of clinical scenarios. Many emergency physicians are familiar with in hospital circulatory support devices such as an intra-aortic balloon pump and ECMO, each of which is being used more frequently in the emergency department (ED). This chapter, however, will focus on the ED presentation of outpatients with implantable MCS devices. The types and configurations of devices will be described, and the most frequent complications associated with these devices will be reviewed.

The lifetime risk of heart failure in the US is about 20%, and the incidence rises with age, but the overall incidence has remained stable for several decades. There are about equal numbers of heart failure patients with preserved and reduced ejection fraction. Patients presenting to the ED with MCS devices will be those with reduced ejection fractions whose symptoms have not been controlled by medical and device management. The majority (53%) will have nonischemic cardiomyopathies and 38% will have ischemic cardiomyopathies. This group will have a 50% 1–2 year mortality rate.

The gold standard for the treatment of end-stage heart disease is still heart transplantation. Currently, there are about 2300 transplants per year performed in the US. The scoring systems for advanced heart failure include a combination of the New York Heart Association and American College of Cardiology Foundation/American Heart Association classification where there is a combination of a patient's functional status

Emergency Management of the Hi-Tech Patient in Acute and Critical Care, First Edition. Edited by Ioannis Koutroulis, Nicholas Tsarouhas, Richard J. Lin, Jill C. Posner, Michael Seneff, and Robert Shesser.
© 2021 John Wiley & Sons Ltd. Published 2021 by John Wiley & Sons Ltd.

(classes I–IV for functional status) and objective disease severity (classes A–D). A patient with class IV D disease, for example, would be unable to carry out any physical activities without heart failure (HF) symptoms, have these symptoms at rest, and have objective evidence of severe heart disease. The Interagency Registry for Mechanical Assisted Circulatory Support (INTERMACS) has a seven-category (1–7) classification system that describes the timeframe for intervention where category 1 is the most severe where a patient is in critical cardiogenic shock, is persistently hypotensive despite escalating inotropic support and needs an intervention within hours.

The annual rate of patients receiving MCS has been increasing each year since 2007. The INTERMACS is the North American registry for all patients who have received an implantable MCS device. It was established in 2005 through a collaboration between the National Heart, Lung and Blood Institute (NHLBI), the Food and Drug Administration (FDA), the Centers for Medicare and Medicaid Services, and industry representatives and is located at the University of Alabama in Birmingham. All US MCS programs participate in INTERMACS, and participation is mandated by Joint Commission on the Accreditation of Healthcare Organizations (JCAHO) standards for these programs.

INTERMACS collects clinical data relevant to mechanical circulatory support devices (MCSDs) from index hospitalization through follow-up evaluations. Post implant follow-up data are collected at one week, one month, three months, six months and every six months thereafter. Major outcomes after implant, e.g. death, explant, rehospitalization and adverse events, are entered within 30 days of occurrence and also as part of the defined follow-up scheduled intervals. A separate database, Pediatric Registry for Mechanical Assisted Circulatory Support (PEDIMACS), maintains the data for pediatric MCS patients.

A review of adult data from September 2016 shows that 168 centers provided data on 18 385 patients. There are about 2500 new implants per year in the data base and there has been 10–15% growth in the number of new implants each year for the past several years. There are about 300 North American children with implants followed in PEDIMACS with about 40–50 new devices per year implanted.

There are several well accepted indications for MCS.

- *Bridge to transplant* (BTT) – Prior to the refinement of the MCS devices, BTT was the primary indication for implantation, as patients with end-stage congestive heart failure (CHF) were at high risk for mortality while awaiting their transplant. The problem has been that there are too few hearts available for transplant relative to the need. Approximately 2300 HT are performed per year in North America, and it is estimated that 10% of 6.6 million North American patients with heart failure are stage D (ACC/AHA system) and, therefore, eligible for transplantation.

As the initial clinical trials of patients awaiting transplant demonstrate about double the survival rate in patients receiving MCS compared with those treated with medical therapy, it was then surmised that these devices could improve survival and quality of life in any patient with end-stage heart failure whether they were a transplant candidate or not.

- *Destination therapy* (DT) – This is when the patient receives an MCS device as a long-term, permanent treatment and is not considered a transplant candidate at the time of device implantation. It is generally offered to patients with ejection fractions <25% at high one-year risk for death from HF and are without other life-limiting organ dysfunction and are failing optimal medical therapies.

- *Bridge to recovery (BTR)* – This is generally an indication for short-term MCS with devices such as a balloon pump; however, a proportion of BTT or DT patients do have improvement in left ventricular (LV) function during device implantation. Changes have been noted in patients who received an left ventricular assist device (LVAD) as BTT or DT in their myocyte structure and function, with normalization of LV shape that has been termed "reverse remodeling." At the moment, there are no universally agreed-upon protocols for VAD weaning for explantation, but many groups have reported sufficient LV functional improvement to permit this in individual cases.

The devices themselves have gone through a rapid evolutionary process. There is variation in the ventricles supported (left, right, or biventricular), the type of flow (continuous or pulsatile), and the way blood is moved (axial versus centripetal), and there are also a series of devices termed total artificial hearts which, as the name suggests, totally replace the patient's native organ.

The two systems in most frequent use in the US are the St. Jude's Medical HeartMate system and the Medtronic HeartWare HVAD. In the HeartMate system, a pump is itself is surgically implanted into a "pump pocket" below the diaphragm. In the HeartMate II, a rotary pump, the blood enters the device at one end of a rotor affixed with helical blades and is impelled along the length of the rotor to the pump's outflow. In the newer, HeartMate 3, a centrifugal control pump, the blood enters at the central axis of the rotor and is driven outward centrifugally to the pump outflow. The rotor is "magnetically levitated," meaning that it has no mechanical bearings that eliminates friction among the device's components. In the HeartWare system, the pump, similar to the Heartmate 3, is a continuous-flow frictionless design and is implanted into the pericardial space. In both cases, the pump is then connected to the LV apex via a short inflow cannula and to the ascending aorta via an end-to-side anastomosis. There is a percutaneous drive line that connects the pump to an external controller that the patient wears on a belt. The controller is connected to external batteries when the patient is mobile, but can be plugged into an alternating current power source when the patient is sedentary (Figure 25.1).

The controller is the main interface between the LVAD and the outside world; it has a number of functions including controlling motor power and speed, providing redundant system operation, performing diagnostic monitoring, providing hazard and advisory alarms, recording and storing events in memory, and transferring system performance data to the system. The LVAD generally operates in a "fixed speed mode" where a designated number of revolutions per minute are set at the time of implantation using a sonographic ramp test. This speed cannot be altered by the controller, but the controller can automatically vary the speed if a number of conditions occur. For example, if a "suction event" (see below) occurs, the controller will automatically decrease the pump's speed to a preset "low speed limit," then gradually increase the speed back to its preset value as the cardiac performance returns to its prior levels.

(a)

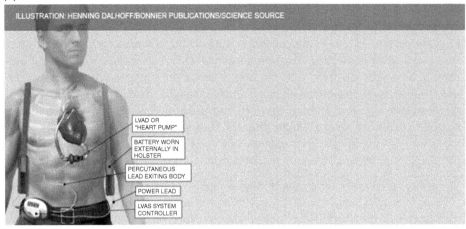

(b)

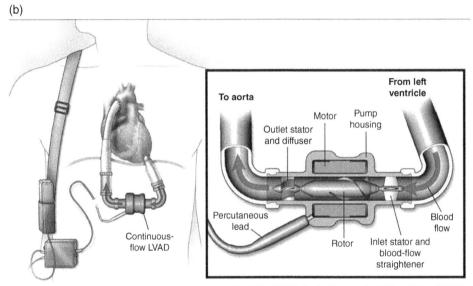

Figure 25.1 (a) Left ventricular assist device components. (b) Left ventricular assist device (continuous flow). *Source:* Perez, YP, McGovern TM. How to Manage Emergency Department Patients with Left Ventricular Assist Devices, ACEP Now, American College of Emergency Physicians, August 2017.

The frequency of complications between these two types of devices is generally similar, but one study suggested that pumps running at lower RPMs might have a lower frequency of complications due to the maintenance of pulsatile flow. Such lower speeds were more difficult with the HVAD compared with the HM pump.

Regardless of the device's mechanical properties, LVADs continually unload the left ventricle and pump blood into the aorta. Their hemodynamic effects are illustrated by the use of ventricular flow-volume loops that compare the normal heart to the failing heart and the failing heart after implantation of an LVAD. (Figure 25.2). This figure demonstrates reductions in LV end diastolic volume, reductions in peak LV systolic pressure and a decrease in aortic pressures. Thus, as the pump speed increases, the aortic valve remains closed throughout the cardiac cycle, and although the heart pumps, the total cardiac output is going through the LVAD.

The clinical evaluation of the patient with an assist device challenges normal clinical paradigms for a variety of reasons. The clinician should become familiar with the controller settings and warning monitors. When these devices are implanted, the patient is on cardio-pulmonary bypass. There are a variety of considerations in optimizing the initial pump settings, but the speed is set in a range (usually 8600–9800 rpm for the HeartMate and 2200–2800 rpm for the HeartWare) to provide a sufficient cardiac output. A number of valvular pathologies that would have been deleterious to the patient after LVAD implantation may have been partially or completely corrected at implantation. As the speed of the pump increases, diastolic pressure tends to rise while systolic pressure remains constant. The mean blood pressure is generally set between 70 and 80 mmHg with a pulse pressure of 10–20 mmHg and the aortic valve opening once every three beats. Such low pulse pressures often lead to the absence of a palpable pulse. Similarly, pulse oximetry may not be accurate in LVAD patients.

Symptomatic LVAD patients presenting to an ED should be placed on a cardiac monitor and receive the standard 12 lead electrocardiogram. Observed arrhythmias should be treated in a similar manner as would occur in a non-LVAD patient. There is some concern about the danger of external chest compressions disrupting an LVAD, but the emergency physician really has no choice but to initiate external chest compressions in a patient with complete circulatory collapse. Neither external cardioversion nor defibrillation is contraindicated in an LVAD patient, but a mean blood pressure can be obtained by attaching a

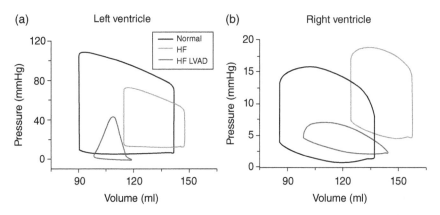

Figure 25.2 Pressure–volume loops of a. left ventricle and b. right ventricle. There is a decrease in LV end-diastolic volume, peak LV systolic pressure, and aortic pressures. *Source:* Park JIK, Heikhmakhtiar AK, Kim, CH et al. The effect of heart failure and left ventricular assist device treatment on right ventricular mechanics: a computational study, Biomed Eng Online 2018, 17: 62

manual blood pressure cuff, inflating it to about 120 mmHg and listening with a Doppler; the mean pressure is when flow is audible with the Doppler. Automated blood pressure cuffs will not be reliable in LVAD patients.

Look at the controller and take note of the pump speed (rpm), flow (l/min), power (watts), pulsatility index (1–10), and battery life. The pulsatility index (PI) reflects how much of the patient's cardiac output is supplied by the pump and how much represents native heart activity. Higher PI's indicate that a greater degree of cardiac output is supplied by the patient's heart and a lower PI reflects greater pump activity. It should also be remembered that the flow displayed on the controller is a value calculated from the speed and power and may be inaccurate during pathophysiologic perturbations. A change from the patient's normal parameters might provide a clue as to the cause of a problem.

Additionally, each type of LVAD has a series of alarms of graded severity that could provide the clinician with a starting place to intervene. These include hazard and advisory alarms. Generally, the hazard alarms are related to pump power issues that might need an electrical intervention, while the advisory alarms relate to a perturbation of pump function from the interaction of the pump and the patient's physiology. The types and exact meaning of these alarms are somewhat complicated and confusing. Physicians should remember that the LVAD operating manuals are all available online and easily retrieved with an Internet search. It would be highly advisable to approach a patient with this manual, particularly if there is a delay in speaking with the patient's LVAD center.

The ability to perform a bedside cardiac echo evaluation is a crucial skill for the emergency physician in the evaluation of an LVAD patient with hemodynamic instability and will provide crucial information to guide therapy. Increasingly, most EPs will have this skill and will be able to make a decent bedside assessment of LV and RV (right ventricular) size and the presence of a pericardial effusion.

Returning to the patient, we can present several basic scenarios and discuss the approach. As noted above, the patient should be assessed for adequate peripheral perfusion in the usual clinical fashion and by taking the mean blood pressure with the Doppler. A bedside echo should be performed to assess LV size, RV size, shift of the interventricular septum, and the presence of a pericardial effusion.

A) Hypotension, no pulmonary congestion
- *Reduced preload with small LV and small RV* – The most frequent and easily treated problem is reduced preload from hypovolemia. LVAD function is very volume sensitive, and the patient could be hypovolemic from any relatively minor cause such as overdiuresis, or a vomiting–diarrhea syndrome. More serious causes of hypovolemia such as gastrointestinal (GI) bleeding or septic shock (see below) should be excluded using the normal approach for these conditions. A nonvolume-related cause of reduced preload is when there is mechanical kinking of the inflow cannula that is positioned in the LV. This situation, termed a "suction" event, can occur either de novo (as a result of mechanical obstruction of the inflow channel) or secondarily as a result of anything causing hypovolemia. When this occurs, the LVAD will react automatically decreasing the pump speed down to a preset "low speed limit," which is the lowest speed thought to be able

to maintain hemodynamic stability. The pump will maintain this speed until the event is over at which time it will automatically, gradually increase back to its original speed. A bedside cardiac echo should demonstrate a small LV and a small RV.

- *Reduced preload with small LV and large RV* – The possibility of right heart failure as a precipitant of LV dysfunction and systemic hypotension. Although as many as 25% of LVAD patients have RV dysfunction at some point, this most frequently occurs soon after LVAD implantation. Any acute pulmonary insult such as a pulmonary embolus or RV infarct should be sought. Fluids should be given gingerly while conditions producing a cause is sought. RV failure is generally treated with inotropic therapy and RV afterload reduction.

B) Hypertension with or without pulmonary congestion

Hypertension must be closely monitored in an LVAD patient where the mean arterial pressure (MAP) should be 70–80 mmHg. Patients with MAPs > 90 mmHg are at risk for cerebral ischemia or hemorrhage, and pressures should be promptly lowered with systemically acting after-load reducers. Both LV and RV volumes may be increased in this situation.

C) Normotension or hypotension with pulmonary congestion, large biventricular chamber sizes

Pump thrombosis is a major complication of an LVAD, seen in 1–2% of patients during the first two years after implantation. This is why, LVAD patients are maintained on both antithrombin and antiplatelet agents. Regardless of where in the pump mechanism a thrombosis occurs, the clinical picture can be quite variable and may include pulmonary congestion, large biventricular chamber sizes, a decrease in the patient's baseline pulsatility index, and increases in the pump speed and power. No data are available on ED presentations of pump thrombosis, but presumably patients would have some degree of hemodynamic compromise. However, pump thrombosis should be suspected in patients with an isolated complaint of hematuria or jaundice. If thrombosis is suspected, the clinician should search for objective measures of hemolysis that would include lactic dehydrogenase (LDH) elevation > 2.5 times the upper limit of normal, haptoglobin decreases, hemoglobinuria, and anemia with red cell morphologic evidence of hemolysis. Intravenous heparin can be started upon reasonable suspicion of thrombosis, and thrombolytic therapy can be considered if the patient is unstable, particularly in patients with the HeartWare VAD where medical therapy has been more effective than in the HeartMate II. But most of these patients are not unstable, and a subspecialty consultation can be obtained for helping to plot further diagnostic and treatment strategies.

Bleeding – As noted above, LVAD patients require continuous antithrombin and antiplatelet agents to avoid device-related thrombosis. Up to 22% of these patients may be admitted to the hospital with a GI bleed. In addition to the therapeutic anticoagulation, LVAD patients are at additional bleeding risk from a form of acquired Von Willebrand's (VWF) disease, as VWF reductions occur from high sheer stresses as blood moves through the LVAD. Additionally, the continuous, non (or low) pulsatile blood flow associated with LVAD patients seems to promote the development of angiodysplasia at a variety of GI tract locations from the stomach to colon, but most frequently in the upper GI tract.

Stroke – The annual rate of stroke in LVAD patients is between 4 and 10% with a slightly higher stroke rate for both thrombotic and hemorrhagic strokes reported for LVADs with axial rather than centrifugal flow pumps. The major risk factors for strokes in LVAD patients were nonadherence with anticoagulation treatment, elevated MAP, and a concomitant infection. Patients with LVADs who sustain an acute thrombotic stroke with a high NIH study section (NIHSS) should be considered for endovascular treatment rather than tissue plasminogen activator (tPA) if available.

Infection – Given the presence of indwelling, percutaneous lines, it is not surprising that infection is an ongoing risk for LVAD patients. Risk factors for infection are high BMI, diabetes, malnutrition, and a low lymphocyte count. Infections in this population have been characterized as LVAD-specific, LVAD-related, and non-LVAD. In LVAD-specific infection, although any portion of the system can be infected, the driveline is most frequently involved, usually as a result of local trauma to the line. Of driveline infections, 80% occurs >30 days after implantation, and the average infection presents six months after implant. VAD-related infections, such as endocarditis or mediastinitis, can occur in non-VAD patients but will be seen with greater frequency in the LVAD population. VAD-specific infections may be subtle, and patients may lack characteristic systemic signs of infection. Coagulase-negative Staphylococci, *Staphylococcus aureus*, and Pseudomonas are three of the most frequent organisms causing blood stream infections in LVAD patients.

Further Reading

1 Alraies, M.C. and Eckman, P. (2014). Adult heart transplant: indications and outcomes. *J. Thorac. Dis.* 6: 1120–1128.

2 https://www.uab.edu/medicine/intermacs/about-us. March 21, 2017.

3 Enciso, J.S. (2016). Mechanical circulatory support: current strategies and future directions. *Prog. Cardiovasc. Dis.* 58: 444–454.

4 Selzman, C.H., Madden, J.L., Healy, A.H. et al. (2015). Bridge to removal: a paradigm shift for left ventricular assist device therapy. *Ann. Thorac. Surg.* 99: 360–367.

5 Hetzer, R. and Delmo Walter, E.M. (2017). Mechanical circulatory support devices – in progress. *N. Engl. J. Med.* 376: 487–489.

6 Kirkpatrick, J.N., Wieselthaler, G., Strueber, M. et al. (2015). Ventricular assist devices for treatment of acute heart failure and chronic heart failure. *Heart* 101: 1091–1096.

7 Lalonde, S.D., Alba, A.C., Rigobon, A. et al. (2013). Clinical differences between continuous flow ventricular assist devices: a comparison between HeartMate II and HeartWare HVAD. *J. Card. Surg.* 28: 604–610.

8 Slaughter, M.S., Pagani, F.D., Rogers, J.G. et al. (2010). Clinical management of continuous-flow left ventricular assist devices. *J. Heart Lung Transplant.* 29: S1–S39.

9 Robertson, J., Long, B., and Koyfman, A. (2016). The emergency management of ventricular assist devices. *Am. J. Emerg. Med.* 34: 1294–1301.

10 Partyka, C. and Taylor, B. (2014). Review article: ventricular assist devices in the emergency department. *Emerg. Med. Australas.* 26: 104–112.

11 Nguyen, A.B., Uriel, N., and Adatya, S. (2016). New challenges in the treatment of patients with left ventricular support: LVAD thrombosis. *Curr. Heart Fail. Rep.* 13: 302–309.

26

Emergency Management of the Patient with an Implantable Pacemaker or Defibrillator

Michael J. O'Neal

Department of Emergency Medicine, University of San Francisco, San Francisco, CA, USA

Introduction

Cardiovascular implantable electronic devices (CIEDs) include permanent pacemakers (PM), implantable cardioverter-defibrillators (ICD), cardiac resynchronization therapy (CRT) devices, and devices capable of a combination of therapies. CIEDs are used to re-approximate physiologic electrical rhythm generation, restore conduction and the timing of chamber contraction, and abort lethal arrhythmias in susceptible patients. The mean age of pacemaker placement in the US is now 75, and the incidence of cardiac device implantation continues to rise, as indications for implantation have expanded.

In 2010, approximately 370 000 pacemakers and 97 000 implantable cardiac defibrillators were placed in the US. Since the introduction of the first single-chamber pacemaker in 1958, implantable cardiac devices have become increasingly more complex. Newer devices pace multiple chambers, improve atrioventricular (AV) synchrony, and are rate adaptive as the rate of pacing can adjust to physiologic changes, including activity and minute ventilation. Currently, 40% of implanted devices in the US are CRT-D (cardiac resynchronization therapy and defibrillation); they employ one atrial and two ventricular leads to improve cardiac synchrony and are increasingly used in patients with heart failure. Estimates of devices complications vary widely, with lead, electrode, or generator-related problems, affecting approximately 1.8–14% of patients. Permanent cardiac devices are employed in pediatric patients, especially those prone to ventricular dysrhythmias from congenital heart disease or cardiomyopathy; however, the incidence of implantation and device failure in pediatric patients is not well known. As the use of cardiac devices continues to rise, understanding the functions, potential malfunctions, and management of device complications will be increasingly important for the emergency clinician.

Emergency Management of the Hi-Tech Patient in Acute and Critical Care, First Edition. Edited by Ioannis Koutroulis, Nicholas Tsarouhas, Richard J. Lin, Jill C. Posner, Michael Seneff, and Robert Shesser.

The Structure and Functions of Implanted Cardiac Devices (ICD's)

The two essential parts of an implantable pacemaker or defibrillator are the pulse generator and the lead(s). The pulse generator includes hardware capable of sensing intrinsic cardiac activity and delivering electrical impulses, programmable software, RAM memory storage, and a battery (with a typical life span of 5–10 years) and is often enclosed in a titanium case. The lead consists of a conductor to conduct the electrical impulse, an electrode to contact the myocardium, a fixation mechanism, known as a terminal connector pin that connects the lead to the pulse generator, and insulation. Defibrillators can be distinguished by the addition of a shock coil, which is seen as a thick radiopaque stripe on chest x-ray (see Figure 26.1).

ICDs are typically placed in the left infraclavicular area, while pacemakers are usually implanted under the nondominant clavicle. Endocardial leads are floated via the subclavian vein to their desired location in the heart. Atrial leads are typically placed in the right atrial appendage. Right ventricular (RV) leads are placed in the RV apex (this is the location of most defibrillator leads), the RV outflow tract, or occasionally in the intraventricular septum. Left ventricular (LV) leads are delivered through the coronary sinus into a tributary vein of the LV.

Pacemakers are classified by their lead location and function and are assigned a five-letter code according to the North American Society of Pacing and Electrophysiology and British Pacing and Electrophysiology Group. The first three letters describe the basic functionality of the pacemaker, with the fourth and fifth letters expressing its programmability, rate modulation, and multisite pacing. *The first letter designates the chamber*

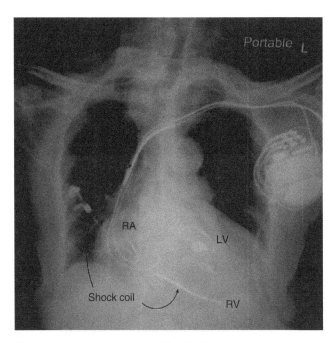

Figure 26.1 Demonstration of Shock coil.

Table 26.1 The North American society for pacing and electrophysiology/British pacing and electrophysiology group generic pacemaker code.

I	II	III	IV	V
Chamber(s) paced	Chamber(s) sensed	Response to sensing	Programmability, rate modulation	Multisite pacing
A = Atrium V = Ventricle D = Dual (A+V) O = None	A = Atrium V = Ventricle D = Dual (A+V) O = None	T = Triggered I = Inhibited D = Dual (triggered + inhibited) O = None	P = Simple programmable M = Multiprogrammable C = Communicating R = Rate modulation O = None	A = Atrium V = Ventricle D = Dual (A+V) O = None

being paced, the second letter states what chamber is being sensed, and the third letter describes the pacemaker's response to a sensed impulse (see Table 26.1). Pacemakers capable of rate modulation are assigned R for their fourth letter. As an example, a patient with symptomatic sinus bradycardia (with preserved AV conduction) may have an AAI pacemaker placed. The pacemaker is set to a desired rate, e.g. 60 bpm (or one impulse every five seconds). If an atrial impulse is sensed within five seconds of the preceding atrial impulse, the pulse generator is inhibited; if not, the pacemaker will deliver an atrial stimulus. The majority of pacemakers in the US are DDD/DDD-R, with AAIR and VVIR also frequently placed.

The functions of a defibrillator, or ICD, include sensing (recognition of atrial and ventricular signals), rhythm determination (based on the rate, location of electrical stimuli, and wave morphology), and programmable therapy for ventricular tachycardia (VT) and ventricular fibrillation (VF). If high-energy defibrillation is needed, a shock of 1–40 J is delivered between the coil electrode and the ICD casing or another electrode. In the setting of VT, antitachycardia pacing (ATP) or overdrive pacing is employed: 6–10 ventricular impulses are generated at a rate faster than the VT. If ATP fails to convert the rhythm from VT, the ICD delivers shocks. Most ICDs also have pacemaker capabilities which are triggered if bradycardia is detected.

All patients with a PM or ICD are given an identification card with manufacturer and model information and are enrolled in a patient registry. Device manufacturers include Medtronic, Boston Scientific/Guidant, St. Jude, Biotronik, and Sorin/ELA, with the first three companies accounting for >90% of the devices placed in the US. In cases where the manufacturer cannot be identified from personal history or the electronic medical record, manufacturer-specific alphanumeric codes can be visible on chest x-ray. Unfortunately, correct device identification using alphanumeric codes has been found to be successful in less than 20% of cases. In 2011, Jacob et al. published an algorithm to determine the manufacturer using battery and device shape (see Figure 26.2).

Placing a magnet over a pacemaker will turn off the sensing function of the device, placing it in asynchronous mode. The pacemaker will emit a manufacturer-specific set rate, which is dependent on the device's battery life. This can be the easiest way to test the battery life.

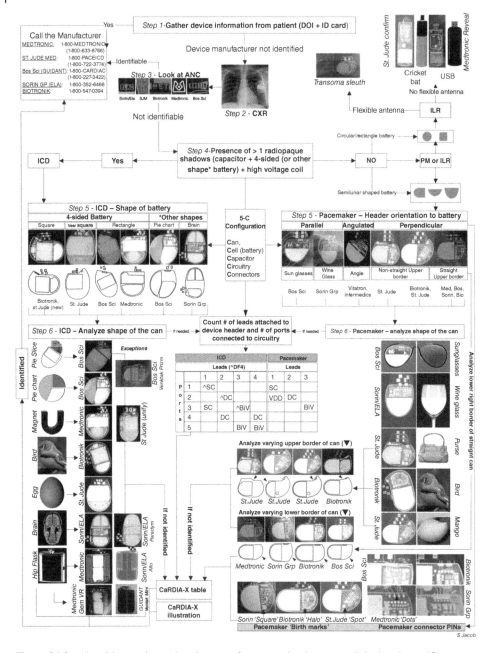

Figure 26.2 Algorithm to determine the manufacturer using battery and device shape. (*Source:* Jacob et al. © 2011, Elsevier.)

Indications for Placement of Pacemakers and Defibrillators

Permanent pacemakers are indicated in the setting of symptomatic inappropriate bradycardia from sinus node dysfunction or atrio-ventricular (AV) block. Symptoms may include dizziness, fatigue, exertional symptoms, or syncope. Long-term (Holter) monitoring may be necessary to correlate symptoms with the presence of a brady-dysrhythmia. Asymptomatic sinus node dysfunction does not require a pacemaker. The indication for pacemaker placement in the setting of asymptomatic Type I and II AV blocks is dependent on the risk of progression of the conduction abnormality to a ventricular escape rhythm. Reversible causes (drug toxicity or Lyme disease) carry a lower risk of progression than structural cardiac causes. *Patients with asymptomatic AV blocks and coexisting left bundle branch block (LBBB) or bifascicular blocks, pulse rates less than 40, or asystolic pauses greater than three seconds while awake should be evaluated for pacemaker placement.*

Traditionally, dual chamber (RA/RV) pacemakers were implanted in patients with AV blocks to restore AV synchrony. However, studies have shown an increased progression of heart failure in patients with LV dysfunction that are RV paced, likely as a result of dyssynchronous ventricular contraction from the widened QRS. To combat ventricular dyssynchrony, biventricular pacemakers capable of CRT have been used more and more over the past two decades. Recent studies have demonstrated a significant reduction in both hospitalization and all-cause mortality in patients with ejection fraction (EF) < 30% and QRS duration > 150 ms that received a CRT pacemaker compared to medical management. Therefore, *current indications for CRT placement include patients with LBBB and QRS > 150 ms; New York Heart Association (NYHA) functional class II, III, or IV; and an LVEF of 35% or less on guideline-directed medical therapy (GDMT).*

ICDs should be considered in the primary prevention of sudden cardiac death (SCD) from lethal ventricular arrhythmias. High-risk cardiac diseases in which ICD placement is indicated include:

- LVEF less than 35% on guideline directed medical therapy (GDMT) with NYHA class II or III HF
- LVEF less than 30% on GDMT, NYHA class I HF, and a history of myocardial infarction
- Hypertrophic cardiomyopathy, Brugada, or long QT syndrome

ICDs should be employed in the secondary prevention of SCD in patients with a history of life-threatening sustained VT or VF, or those who have survived a cardiac arrest caused by VT/ VF that was not from a reversible cause.

The benefits of CRT-D devices in preventing heart failure admissions and death have resulted in expanded use as well as expanded indications for their placement, and clinicians in all settings should expect to increasingly encounter these devices.

Routine Management of Implanted Cardiac Devices

PMs and ICDs are placed by electrophysiologists (EPs), typically as part of a short inpatient stay. Routine monitoring in EP clinic is needed with device interrogation every one to six months to ensure desired device performance and adequate battery life, as well as patient symptomatology. Some devices emit an audible tone when battery life is exhausting.

During interrogation, manufacturer-specific computers wirelessly communicate with devices to obtain information and modify device settings. Information gathered with interrogation includes the underlying cardiac rhythm, the percent time paced, tachycardiac events, battery voltage, lead impedance, sensing threshold, pacing output, and ICD charge time. Emergency physicians are increasingly interrogating cardiovascular implantable electronic devices (CIEDs), gaining useful device information that can be used in concert with a cardiologist to make management decisions.

Complications and Emergencies of Patients with Implanted Cardiac Devices

Emergency Department Evaluation

History acquisition should include the date and indication for device placement, device type and model, and a detailed past medical and past cardiac history. Any known device complications, recent EP clinic visits, or programming changes should be sought. Patients should be questioned for symptoms of decreased perfusion or heart failure (fatigue, dizziness or syncope, or exertional dyspnea), palpitations, chest pain, and muscle twitching. Possible device exposures should be elucidated, including trauma, environmental extremes, or electromagnetic interference, which can include cellphone use or medical causes such as magnetic resonance imaging, electrocautery, or radiation therapy. In addition to standard cardiopulmonary exam, the implantation site should be examined for signs of infection or swelling, and the neck and upper extremities should be inspected for edema.

Electrocardiogram (ECG) evaluation of a patient's underlying rhythm and search for pacer artifacts is critical in the evaluation of device functioning. Atrial-paced devices produce a pacer spike followed by a p wave. Bipolar leads produce smaller pacer spikes that can be barely perceptible in some leads. Pacemaker leads in the RV produce a pacer spike followed by a widened QRS with LBBB morphology and discordant ST segments. Biventricular-paced devices typically produce a wide QRS with a dominant R wave in V1–V2. Comparison with a previous ECG is helpful, especially to evaluate for lead migration or displacement. Change from LBBB morphology to RBBB in an RV-paced patient can indicate lead malposition or lead perforation through the intraventricular septum.

PA/lateral chest radiographs are not required for all patients, but can help verify the location and integrity of each lead, correct positioning of the connector pins in the header of the pulse generator, as well as evaluate for possible implant-related complications. RA leads have a J-shape, curving anteriorly and medially into the right atrial appendage. RV leads slope anteriorly and caudally toward the cardiac apex (see Figure 26.1). A common site for lead fracture occurs in the subclavian vein between the first rib and the clavicle, termed subclavian crush syndrome.

CIED Emergencies

Implantable cardiac device emergencies can be due to implantation-related problems, pacing or defibrillation malfunctions, and various medical emergencies in patients with cardiac devices. Most complications related to device implantation are seen early in the postoperative period Immediate postprocedure complications include pneumothorax and hemothorax, diagnosed by chest x-ray. Hematoma formation around the pulse generator, termed a pocket hematoma, occurs in 2–2.5% of patients (patients on anticoagulants and antiplatelet agents are especially prone) and generally managed expectantly. Large, tense pocket hematomas may require evacuation or discontinuation of anticoagulant therapy and are associated with an increased risk of device infection.

Cardiac device-related infections, which include pocket infection, endocarditis, and bacteremia (without signs of device infection), are grave diagnoses with high morbidity and mortality. Cardiac device infective endocarditis (CDIE) has an incidence of approximately 0.4%. Without device removal, CDIE carries a mortality rate of 66%, which lowers to 13–22% with explantation and long-term antibiotics. Implantation site erythema or purulence, dehiscence, or erosion, as well as systemic signs of infection, should be carefully sought in all patients with recent device placement. If signs of infection are present, admission with blood cultures and trans-esophageal echocardiogram is indicated. Superficial or incisional infections can be treated with a short course of antibiotics targeting skin flora; however, infections tracking to the implanted device are most often refractory to antibiotics. All device-related infections, confirmed with local inspection, positive blood cultures, or TEE, generally require removal of the device (and its leads) and prolonged antibiotics aimed at gram-positive organisms, as *Staphylococcus aureus* and *Staphylococcus epidermidis* cause the majority of infections.

The incidence of thrombosis and occlusion of veins containing device leads varies widely (2–32%), likely related to the high rate of asymptomatic venous occlusions found years after implantation. Patients with ipsilateral arm swelling or pain should be evaluated for acute venous thrombosis with Doppler ultrasound. In patients with facial or neck swelling, superior vena cava syndrome should be considered. Sonography may be diagnostic, but if negative, contrast venography or CT venogram can be used to rule out a central venous thrombosis.

Lead dislodgement occurs in approximately 1.5–2.4% of cases, typically occurs in the initial weeks after placement and can result in a lack of sensing or lack of capture of the device. Patients may have recurrence of their preimplantation symptoms, or device malfunctioning may be discovered on ECG or telemetry. Large distortions may be picked up on chest x-ray; however, device interrogation and echocardiogram are often required for diagnosis. Leads may migrate across the intraventricular septum, altering QRS morphology. They can travel near the phrenic nerve or diaphragm causing hiccups or irregular breathing. Leads may also pierce the myocardium, resulting in pericardial effusion, and possible tamponade. In a patient with recent device placement and hypotension, early recognition via bedside echocardiogram and pericardiocentesis can be lifesaving.

RV leads may cause interference, thrombosis, or scarring of the tricuspid leaflets and result in tricuspid regurgitation (TR). The prevalence of TR in patients with CIEDs may be as high as 29%; however, the majority of the patients are asymptomatic. Patients with signs or symptoms of right-sided heart failure should receive an echocardiogram and may require lead extraction, with or without valve repair or replacement.

Twiddler syndrome is an uncommon entity characterized by compulsive manipulation of a patient's pulse generator, resulting in coiling and dislodgement of the leads. Coiled leads around a pulse generator may be seen on chest x-ray. Pulse generators can be placed inside a pouch or in a subpectoral location to remedy this problem.

Complication	Management
Pneumothorax or hemothorax	Thoracostomy or thoracentesis
Pocket hematoma	Conservative (rarely evacuation)
Pocket infection	Explantation and antibiotics
Endocarditis	Explantation and antibiotics
Venous thrombosis	Anticoagulation, angioplasty, or surgery
Lead dislodgement	Lead repositioning or replacement
Cardiac perforation	Pericardiocentesis, lead repositioning
Tricuspid regurgitation	Lead extraction +/− annuloplasty/valve replacement

Pacing malfunctions can be grouped into three categories: *failure to pace, failure to capture, and failure to sense* and are generally caused by *generator failure, lead failure, interference, or functional failure*. Generator failure is rare (an annual incidence of 4.6 per 1000 for PMs and 20.7 per 1000 for ICDs), and battery depletion is the most common cause. The most common cause of lead failure is an insulation break; this can be diagnosed with device interrogation showing low impedance.

In failure to pace, no stimulus is delivered, often due to *oversensing*, in which a stimulus is inappropriately identified as a cardiac depolarization. Oversensing can result in pulse rate below the lower limit of the device. Crosstalk is a term that describes when a paced atrial stimulus is registered as a ventricular depolarization and a ventricular stimulus is withheld. *Failure to capture occurs when a pacing stimulus is delivered but does not result in depolarization,* appearing as a pacing artifact without a subsequent P wave or QRS. This pacing malfunction can be functional, when a stimulus is delivered to a refractory myocardium, or results from problems with the lead, the electrode-myocardium interface (often from scarring), or the status of the myocardium. *Failure to sense results from undersensing of intrinsic depolarizations.* Pacemakers have programmed blanking and refractory periods after a sensed depolarization; long programmed periods can miss intrinsic signals, causing functional undersensing.

Hyperkalemia is of particular importance in evaluating a pacing malfunction, as it can delay conduction and increase the pacing threshold, causing increased latency, loss of capture, or loss of sensing. Severe hyperkalemia widens the QRS and can result in a sine wave.

Pacing Malfunction	Common causes
Failure to pace	Battery depletion; lead failure; oversensing of P waves, T waves or skeletal myopotentials; crosstalk; trauma; external electromagnetic interference
Failure to capture	Lead fractures or insulation defects; cardiac scarring; ischemia; electrolyte changes (hyperkalemia); medications (class IC antiarrhythmics); infiltrative diseases
Failure to sense	Lead failure; electrolyte changes (hyperkalemia); medications (class IC antiarrhythmics); high sensing threshold or blanking period; scarring

Pacemaker syndrome is an intolerance to ventricular pacing due to AV dyssynchrony. Ventriculoatrial conduction leads to increased atrial pressures, high vagal tone, and symptoms of heart failure or low cardiac output (dyspnea or dizziness). Treatment includes replacing a ventricular-paced pacemaker with a dual chamber device, or device reprogramming.

Pacemaker-mediated tachycardia (PMT) is a re-entrant dysrhythmia that can occur in patients with dual-chamber devices. A sensed atrial complex induces the pacemaker to generate *a ventricular stimulus that travels retrograde through the AV node*. This atrial stimulus is again sensed by the atrial lead, completing the loop and delivering a ventricular stimulus. The ECG shows a regular wide-complex tachycardia with a pacer spike preceding each QRS and is rate limited by the maximum programmed rate. PMT appears identical to ventricular-paced sinus tachycardia; differentiation can be done by treating the PMT with a magnet or interrogation. If a magnet is not available, AV nodal blockers (e.g. adenosine) can be used to increase the refractory period of the AV node and terminate PMT.

Placing a magnet over a pacemaker turns off sensing, initiates a device-specific set rate, and may initiate recording. Magnets can remedy PMT. They can also be helpful in the case of oversensing (and underpacing) by restoring a physiologic rate. Magnet placement over an ICD will turn off antitachycardia functions, which is helpful for the patient receiving inappropriate shocks, while preserving backup bradycardia pacing. If there is no pacemaker response to a magnet, the magnet may not be sensed, the battery may be depleted, or the device may be placed in magnet-off mode.

ECG evaluation for acute myocardial infarction (AMI) in ventricular-paced patients presents a diagnostic challenge. In RV-paced patients with a baseline LBBB pattern, the Sgarbossa criteria has shown excellent specificity in the diagnosis of AMI. To improve the sensitivity and specificity of AMI diagnosis in LBBB, the use of modified Sgarbossa criteria have been proposed (see table below). Patients with biventricular pacemakers typically have a prominent R wave in V1–V2. Thus, ST elevation in the anterior leads is a concordant ST change and consistent with AMI in a patient with concerning symptoms.

Modified Sgarbossa Rule (Positive if 1 Criterion is Present):
- ≥ 1 lead with ≥1 mm of *Concordant ST Elevation*
- ≥ 1 lead of V1-V3 with ≥1 mm of *Concordant ST Depression*
- ≥ 1 lead anywhere with ≥1 mm ST Elevation and *Excessively Discordant ST Deviation*, as defined by ≥25% of the depth of the preceding S-wave

A patient with a reported shock of their ICD may have a received appropriate therapy, inappropriate therapy, or a phantom shock (no therapy). Appropriate therapy after recognition of VT or VF occurs in over 30% of patients within the first two years of device placement. After a shock, determination of a patient's underlying rhythm and excluding ischemia and metabolic derangements are key steps. In a patient who experiences a single shock with no complaints prior to or after the shock, the AHA recommends no further workup and outpatient cardiology evaluation. Inappropriate therapy is usually caused by misclassification of supraventricular tachycardia (SVT) or of electrical noise as a ventricular dysrhythmia. Repeated inappropriate shocks from an SVT may require magnet placement to inactivate antitachycardia therapy. Any patient with a disabled ICD should be placed on a monitor and have pacer pads applied. As defibrillation can cause elevation in cardiac biomarkers, measuring their levels should be reserved for patients with symptoms or ECG changes concerning for cardiac ischemia.

Electrical storm is a morbid event, defined as three or more shocks from VT/VF in a 24-hour period. While assessing for ischemia or metabolic abnormalities, amiodarone should be initiated, as well as consideration for beta-blockade. A magnet should not be used in treating a patient with repeated appropriate shocks; however, sedation or general anesthesia may be necessary.

In the hemodynamically unstable patient, advanced cardiac life support (ACLS) should proceed in a similar manner as patients without cardiac devices. Atropine and transcutaneous pacing may be used in unstable bradycardia or AV block, and cardioversion may be employed. Transcutaneous pads should be applied in an anterior–posterior orientation, ideally 8 cm away from the pacemaker. Veins containing device leads should be assumed to be thrombosed and avoided when selecting a site for central venous access. Depending on the clinical scenario, placement of a magnet may be helpful in preventing unwanted pacing or shocks during resuscitation.

Consultation

Patients with symptoms of potential pacemaker dysfunction (palpitations, dyspnea, weakness, etc.) or ECG evidence of malfunction require device interrogation in the emergency department (ED). Patient symptoms, vital signs, rhythm abnormalities, and ability to obtain close EP follow-up will determine whether inpatient or outpatient management is most appropriate for these patients.

See above for ED management and consultation of ICDs. Asymptomatic patients with a single shock can be reassured; all other patients should be evaluated for ischemia or metabolic derangements, undergo interrogation, and monitored for subsequent dysrhythmias.

Further Reading

1 Go, A.S., Mozaffarian, D., Roger, V.L. et al. (2014). Heart disease and stroke statistics 2014 update. A report from the American Heart Association. *Circulation* 129 (3): e28–e292.

2 Kurtz, S.M., Ochoa, J.A., Lau, E. et al. (2010). Implantation trends and patient profiles for pacemakers and implantable cardioverter defibrillators in the United States: 1993–2006. *Pacing Clin. Electrophysiol. Actions* 33 (6): 705–711.

3 Colquitt, J.L., Mendes, D., Clegg, A.J. et al. (2014). Implantable cardioverter defibrillators for the treatment of arrhythmias and cardiac resynchronisation therapy for the treatment of heart failure: systematic review and economic evaluation. *Health Technol. Assess.* 18 (56): 1–560.

4 Martindale, J. and deSouza, I.S. (2014). Managing pacemaker-related complications and malfunctions in the emergency department. *Emerg. Med. Pract.* 16 (9): 1–21.

5 Stevenson, W.G., Chaitman, B.R., Ellenbogen, K.A. et al. (2004). Clinical assessment and management of patients with implanted cardioverter-defibrillators presenting to nonelectrophysiologists. *Circulation* 110 (25): 3866–3869.

6 Samii, S.M. (2015). Indications for pacemakers, implantable cardioverter-defibrillator and cardiac resynchronization devices. *Med. Clin. North Am.* 99 (4): 795–804.

7 Essebag, V., Verma, A., Healey, J.S. et al. (2016). Clinically significant pocket hematoma increases long-term risk of device infection: BRUISE CONTROL INFECTION study. *J. Am. Coll. Cardiol.* 67 (11): 1300–1308.

8 Rodriguez, Y., Garisto, J., and Carrillo, R.G. (2013). Management of cardiac device-related infections: a review of protocol-driven care. *Int. J. Cardiol.* 166 (1): 55–60.

9 Rozmus, G., Daubert, J.P., Huang, D.T. et al. (2005). Venous thrombosis and stenosis after implantation of pacemakers and defibrillators. *J. Interv. Card. Electrophysiol.* 13 (1): 9–19.

10 Ghani, A., Delnoy, P.P.H.M., Ramdat Misier, A.R. et al. (2014). Incidence of lead dislodgement, malfunction and perforation during the first year following device implantation. *Neth. Heart J.* 22 (6): 286–291.

11 van Rees, J.B., de Bie, M.K., Thijssen, J. et al. (2011). Implantation-related complications of implantable cardioverter-defibrillators and cardiac resynchronization therapy devices. A systematic review of randomized clinical trials. *J. Am. Coll. Cardiol.* 58 (10): 995–1000.

12 Al-Bawardy, R., Krishnaswamy, A., Bhargava, M. et al. (2013). Tricuspid regurgitation in patients with pacemakers and implantable cardiac defibrillators: a comprehensive review. *Clin. Cardiol.* 36 (5): 249–254.

13 Maloy, K.R., Bhat, R., Davis, J. et al. (2010). Sgarbossa criteria are highly specific for acute myocardial infarction with pacemakers. *West J. Emerg. Med.* 11 (4): 354–357.

14 Smith, S.W., Dodd, K.W., Henry, T.D. et al. (2012). Diagnosis of ST-elevation myocardial infarction in the presence of left bundle branch block with the ST-elevation to S-wave ratio in a modified Sgarbossa rule. *Ann. Emerg. Med.* 60 (6): 766–776.

15 Jacob, S., Shahzad, M.A., Maheshwari, R. et al. (2011). Cardiac rhythm device identification algorithm using X-rays: CaRDIA-X. *Heart Rhythm* 8 (6): 915–922.

Section IX

Pulmonary Devices

27

Invasive Ventilation

A Discussion of Equipment and Troubleshooting

Pelton A. Phinizy[1,2], Joseph J. Bolton[3], and John F. Tamasitis[4]

[1] *Division of Pulmonary and Sleep Medicine, Children's Hospital of Philadelphia, Philadelphia, PA, USA*
[2] *Department of Pediatrics, Perelman School of Medicine at the University of Pennsylvania, Philadelphia, PA, USA*
[3] *Department of Respiratory Care Services, Children's Hospital of Philadelphia, Philadelphia, PA, USA*
[4] *Children's Hospital Home Care, Children's Hospital of Philadelphia, King of Prussia, PA, USA*

Introduction

Invasive mechanical ventilation is a routine therapy for many critically ill or chronically critically ill children and adults. The primary goal of mechanical ventilation is to normalize and/or stabilize the patient's gas exchange by augmenting ventilation and oxygenation in patients with respiratory failure. Mechanical ventilation may be used acutely, subacutely, or chronically depending on the need of the patient. Most patients will need mechanical ventilation all through the day and night, while some may only need mechanical ventilation while sleeping. Whatever the need for mechanical ventilation, invasive mechanical ventilation involves a wide range of complex equipment. This chapter will review that life-sustaining equipment, its purpose in mechanical ventilation, and pay particular attention to identifying and correcting many issues common to invasive mechanical ventilation. This chapter will focus on invasive ventilation: respiratory support provided by endotracheal tube or tracheostomy tube. A discussion of noninvasive mechanical ventilation will be covered in another chapter. This chapter is not meant to be exhaustive, but rather to provide a reasonable discussion of and management plan for typical problems with the goal of correcting the issue or stabilizing the patient while waiting for the evaluation of an expert.

Background Components of the Patient Ventilator System and Their Uses

Positive pressure ventilators support a patient's breathing by assisting or replacing the work of the muscles of respiration. In general, the ventilator does this by delivering a gas mixture rapidly through a humidifier and tubing circuitry into the patient's lungs via an artificial airway. The patient then passively exhales, and the gas travels through the

Emergency Management of the Hi-Tech Patient in Acute and Critical Care, First Edition. Edited by
Ioannis Koutroulis, Nicholas Tsarouhas, Richard J. Lin, Jill C. Posner, Michael Seneff, and Robert Shesser.
© 2021 John Wiley & Sons Ltd. Published 2021 by John Wiley & Sons Ltd.

artificial airway and out an exhalation valve in the ventilator circuit. There are a number of options for the various parts in the patient-ventilator system that may differ depending on region, vendors, and provider preferences. It is important to have a general understanding of the various components of the patient-ventilator system and their roles, as this can make troubleshooting easier.

The Ventilator

There are a wide variety of hospital and portable ventilators available for use with newer models being developed, which often expand upon the functionality of older models. Nonetheless, ventilators typically have four main components: a power supply, controls, monitors, and safety systems. Power supplies differ ventilator to ventilator – the three main categories are:

• Ventilators that use pressurized gas to drive the inspiratory flow and control the valves and switches.
• Ventilators that use pressurized gas to drive the inspiratory flow but use electricity to power the controls and monitors.
• Ventilators that rely entirely on electricity for the controls and monitors but also use a power source to drive a turbine to supply the inspiratory flow of gas.

The first two groups rely on a consistent delivery of pressurized gas. Because of this, they are very energy efficient but generally need to remain in a hospital setting where they can be hooked up to a source of pressurized gas. These are often labeled "hospital" ventilators as opposed to "portable" ventilators because of this obligation. However, there are some older models of ventilators, appropriately named portable gas-powered ventilators, which used portable tanks of compressed gas both to drive ventilation and to provide the gas mixture that was inhaled.

The final group of ventilators in the above list relies entirely on electricity for both the controls and the development of the inspiratory flow by a turbine. The turbine takes in the ambient air and compresses it. If supplemental oxygen is needed, an external source such as an oxygen tank can be attached to a separate oxygen fitting. These portable ventilators require a lot more electricity to run the turbine and compress the air than the hospital ventilators, which use compressed gas. To make them portable, manufacturers have developed batteries which can power the ventilator for hours making them ideal for use in a transport setting. Not requiring the consistent use of compressed gas also makes it such that they are suitable for use in the home in chronically ventilated patients.

Another group of ventilators are "anesthesia ventilators," which have specific functions related to the delivery of anesthetic gases as well as maneuvers performed in the operating room in addition to more typical ventilator processes. However, a discussion of this type of ventilator is outside the scope of this chapter.

The next component of the ventilator system is the system of controls. The ventilator has to take the compressed gas and deliver it to the patient. It does this by adjusting various solenoid valves controlled by the onboard computer. These valves may help to blend gases (if 100% oxygen is being used) and deliver the flow required for the different modes of ventilation. The monitoring system consists of various sensors throughout the ventilator system designed to analyze, monitor, and adapt the pressure and flow of gas. Finally, the safety systems include filters designed to keep the patient safe as well as alarms which may alert providers to changes from the sensors but which may also identify when systems are malfunctioning or failing. More discussion on the alarms will be undertaken in the troubleshooting section.

The ventilator transfers the precisely controlled flow of gas via a system of tubing connecting the ventilator to the patient known as the ventilator circuit. The circuit can have one limb or two, will often incorporate some means of providing humidification, may have adapters for delivering inhaled medications or providing inline suction, and may have pressure and/or flow sensors. In the literature, there are numerous naming conventions for these various circuit setups adding to the complexity. For the purposes of this textbook discussion, there are two major types of ventilator circuits: dual limb and single limb. Figures 27.1 and 27.2 provide examples of portable ventilators, circuits, and active humidification.

The Circuit

A dual limb ventilator circuit consists of an inspiratory limb and an expiratory limb. At one end, the two limbs are connected to the ventilator via the inspiratory and expiratory ports. At the other end, the two limbs are connected to each other and the patient's artificial airway via a "wye" in the tubing. Gas travels from the ventilator through the inspiratory limb to the patient and then on exhalation travels back to the ventilator through the expiratory limb. The ventilator will typically measure tidal volumes by measuring the flow of gas in and out of the ventilator, but a flow sensor can also be placed at the level of the "y-piece."

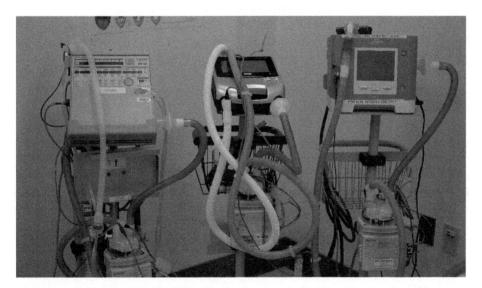

Figure 27.1 Examples of three portable ventilators, circuits, and active humidification. (*Source:* Courtesy of Michael Duff, RRT, Department of Respiratory Care, The Children's Hospital of Philadelphia, Philadelphia.)

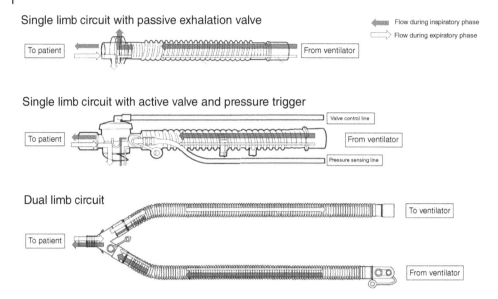

Figure 27.2 Examples of ventilator circuits showing flow during phases of respiration. (*Source:* Courtesy of Richard Lin, modified from diagrams from Philips Respironics and Hudson RCI.)

The major benefit of this circuit is the ability to more precisely measure and control flows and pressures.

A single limb ventilator circuit consists of a single stretch of tubing connecting the patient to the ventilator. There are two types of single limb circuits: passively vented circuits and actively vented circuits. A passively vented circuit is one where exhalation occurs via an intentional leak in the circuit. This leak is an exhalation port in the tubing or swivel connector. The benefit of this type of circuit is that it is simple and can be more attractive to patients since it is flexible and moves more easily. The ventilator can compensate very well for leaks in the system by increasing flows through the tubing. A limitation of this type of circuit is that the ventilator is not measuring inhaled or exhaled tidal volumes but instead is calculating them by a computer algorithm. Under some circumstances, such as the presence of high leak, ventilators, which use algorithms to calculate volumes and adjust for leak in single limb circuits, can have diminished accuracy.

The other type of single limb ventilator circuit is an actively vented circuit, also known as an active circuit. These circuits have a non-rebreathing expiratory valve in place, which opens on exhalation and closes on inspiration. The valve can produce a positive end expiratory pressure (PEEP) and can be in line with the single limb tubing or can be attached via a "T" in the tubing. The benefits of this circuit setup are that inspiratory flows can be measured and controlled more precisely and supplemental oxygen can be delivered at a more consistent level.

Humidification

In addition to delivering gas mixtures of air, oxygen, and other medical gases to the patient's airway, the ventilator circuit incorporates a source of humidification. The role of the humidifier is to replace the function of the patient's bypassed upper airway by heating and humidifying the inspired gases. It is considered absolutely necessary for invasive ventilation with an artificial airway. When there is suboptimal humidification, the airway mucosa can become irritated from being dry, lead to thickened secretions, and negatively impact mucociliary clearance. This can result in inspissated secretions, bronchospasm, atelectasis, and, in severe cases, mucus plugs obstructing the airway.

There are two general types of humidification: active humidification with a heated humidification system and passive humidification with a heat and moisture exchanger (HME). Heated humidification systems actively increase the temperature and water vapor content of the inspired gas. There are a number of different types of active humidification systems with different mechanisms. One that is frequently used has the ventilator flow pass over a container of water on top of a heater. The gas flowing over the top of the water is then heated and humidified. While many of these systems are capable of reaching higher temperatures, the suggested goal is gas with a temperature of 37°C and 100% relative humidity at the circuit wye for invasively ventilated patients.

Passive humidification is achieved through an HME. They are said to be passive because the heat and moisture is stored in a filter as the exhaled gas passes through it. When fresh inspired gas passes back through the filter, it is subsequently warmed and humidified. HMEs are generally made of paper or foam and can be hydrophobic, hygroscopic, filtered, or have some combination of these properties. Hygroscopic HMEs are impregnated with a salt like calcium chloride to enhance the water retention capabilities. Figure 27.3 depicts the different forms of humidification.

There have been a number of studies in mostly adult populations demonstrating no significant difference in terms of pneumonia, airway blockage, and overall mortality between using an inline HME and heated humidity for mechanically ventilated patients. Nonetheless, the HME is generally regarded as suboptimal for continuous use because of its reduced efficiency. While it provides some level of humidification, it may be best used intermittently or temporarily, particularly in smaller patients who are at more risk for plugging due to secretions. It can be used to supplement the heated humidification systems, for instance, when the heated humidification systems need to be changed out for regular maintenance or cleaned. In the case that the patient may be transported within the hospital or may be traveling outside of the home, the HME systems are certainly more portable. It may also be an appropriate choice in the operating room for short procedures when the reduced humidity is unlikely to negatively affect the patient.

The Patient Interface or Artificial Airway

With invasive mechanical ventilation, a catheter or tube is placed in the patient's trachea to provide a patent path for gas exchange. In most cases, an endotracheal tube is the first artificial airway to be placed. Typically, if a patient cannot be weaned off mechanical ventilation after some time, a tracheostomy is recommended to replace the endotracheal tube. Advantages of tracheostomy tube placement include reduced risk of laryngeal damage, laryngeal stenosis, and decreased instances of voice injury. They are discussed extensively in a separate chapter. For adults requiring mechanical ventilation, both endotracheal and tracheostomy tubes are often cuffed, meaning they are surrounded with a small balloon which can be inflated with air or liquid to form a seal with the tracheal wall and prevent leak of gas or help to prevent aspiration.

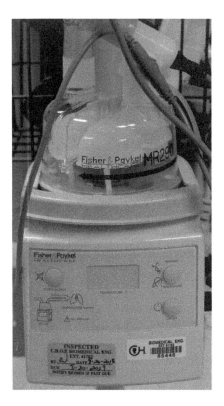

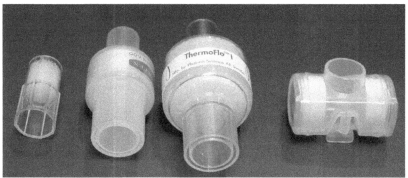

Figure 27.3 Forms of humidification: The first is an active humidifier, which requires AC power. The other set of four from left to right are a neonatal HME, two styles of general-use HME, and an HME which allows access for suctioning and has a port for oxygen administration. (*Source:* Courtesy of Michael Duff, RRT, Department of Respiratory Care, The Children's Hospital of Philadelphia, Philadelphia.)

In neonatal and pediatric patients, the endotracheal and tracheostomy tubes used are frequently uncuffed in order to prevent damage to the trachea which might result in scarring and eventually stenosis. If, however, the patient develops stiffer lungs requiring high ventilator settings, there may be significant enough leak to require the use of a cuffed tracheal tube to minimize airway leaking and ensure adequate ventilation.

Case Vignette

A five-year-old girl with a static encephalopathy secondary to a hypoxic ischemic event at birth arrives in the emergency room with the chief complaint of "ventilator alarms." She has chronic respiratory failure and a cuffed tracheostomy because of peristomal leak when she sleeps. She has generally been stable on her home vent settings without supplemental oxygen for the last few years. Her family and home nurse report that the high pressure alarm has been going off for the last couple of hours and that she has been breathing much faster than usual over the same time period. All of this seemed to start after she came home from school and was getting ready to go to bed. The family denies fevers, cough, and change in quality or quantity of secretions. They performed a tracheostomy change three days ago without difficulty.

Her vital signs in the emergency department are temperature of 37° C, heart rate of 140, respiratory rate of 55, blood pressure of 90/65, and pulse oximetry 98% on her home ventilator with 21% FiO_2. Her end-tidal carbon dioxide level is 30 mm Hg.

Her exam is notable for being in mild–moderate respiratory distress with tachypnea and subcostal retractions. Her chest has an increased diameter. There are bilateral breath sounds revealing coarse rhonchi on auscultation of her chest. Her respirations are rather erratic.

Disconnecting her from the ventilator to use a self-inflating bag for manual ventilation reveals a hiss of air, and she is easy to ventilate manually. After she is switched to a hospital ventilator on her home settings, her vital signs normalize. Further inspection of the ventilator circuit reveals significant condensation in the tubing. When asked more about the issue, the parents note that they recently installed a new air conditioning unit in the patient's room. This new draft of cool air likely caused the increased condensation or "rain out" in the ventilator circuit. This resulted in obstruction to ventilator flows, high peak pressures, and excessive triggering. The excessive triggering resulted in the hyperventilation driving the end tidal carbon dioxide down, and dynamic hyperinflation increased as a result of inadequate time to exhale. The hiss of air as the patient was disconnected from the ventilator was the release of that hyperinflation. After draining the excess water from the ventilator circuit, the patient was able to be ventilated appropriately with her home ventilator and was discharged home. The family was instructed on how to clear condensation from the tubing without accidentally spilling it down the tracheostomy tube. They were given directions intended to decrease the amount of condensation in the tubing. This included increasing the heat on the humidifier, turning down the air conditioning in the patient's bedroom, and aiming the draft away from the ventilator circuit. The medical team could have also ordered heated tubing or insulation for the circuit for the patient.

Troubleshooting

General

Managing a patient in respiratory failure often presents challenges. Many of the issues are equipment related. Successful troubleshooting mechanical ventilation requires rapid assessment of both the patient and ventilator system. Prior to making adjustments to the ventilator settings, the focus should initially be on the patient and the severity of distress and stability of their condition. If in acute distress, the patient can always be disconnected from the mechanical ventilator circuit and placed on "human" ventilation – that is, positive pressure ventilation provided by manually squeezing a flow-inflating or self-inflating resuscitation bag with ambient air or supplemental oxygen as needed until further evaluation of the patient and ventilator can be made. This maneuver can also aid the astute provider by helping to determine the patient's needs in terms of ventilator support, particularly with a flow-inflating bag. If the patient is easily manually ventilated once disconnected from the ventilator circuit, the problem may lie in the ventilator and/or circuit. If the patient continues to be in distress with manual resuscitation, it may signal that there was an acute change in the patient's condition such as bronchospasm or pneumothorax, or with the interface such as displacement or obstruction of the endotracheal tube. Once the patient is stabilized, the provider can conduct a more detailed examination of the ventilator, circuit, and patient for more clues on the origin of the malfunction. Figure 27.4 summarizes the troubleshooting steps for a ventilated patient with a tracheostomy in respiratory distress and Figure 27.5 describes different types of resuscitation bags.

Ventilator

Problems with the ventilator can result in significant morbidity including patient discomfort, hypoxemia, hypoventilation, hyperventilation, respiratory failure, and even death. Issues can range from mechanical malfunctions to a breakdown of patient-ventilator coordination and synchrony. Routine monitoring is vital to identify equipment problems, check settings, and observe the harmony (or disharmony) between patient and machine.

The mechanical ventilator is a life-sustaining system, and failure of this system could result in serious morbidity or death. Thus, many precautions are taken to ensure that mechanical ventilators are highly reliable, and they are designed with many fail-safe measures such that typically no single point of failure can endanger the patient. This includes mechanisms such as audible and visual alarms to alert providers to problems and redundancy in various systems, including the electrical power supply.

Given that most modern ventilators require electricity to at least control the valves and flows of the ventilator or, as in portable ventilators, to compress the ambient air, they typically have an internal battery to act as a back-up power source to continue to provide ventilation in the event of a power outage or electrical disconnection. The internal backup battery or external batteries should be able to supply electrical power for some time in the event of a disconnection, especially with some of the modern portable ventilators. However, battery power runs out faster when ventilators require higher settings, particularly higher PEEPs and respiratory rates. This can be a particular challenge with certain patient populations such as children with severe bronchopulmonary dysplasia and chronic respiratory failure who may require especially high levels of PEEP and higher respiratory rates for adequate gas exchange. If a ventilator alarms for electrical disconnection, low battery, low gas source pressure, or stops functioning, check the power source. The electrical cord may have become disconnected or the battery may need to charged.

Another safety feature and redundancy in mechanical ventilation systems is the asphyxia valve. This is a valve that could prevent the patient from asphyxiating due to ventilator

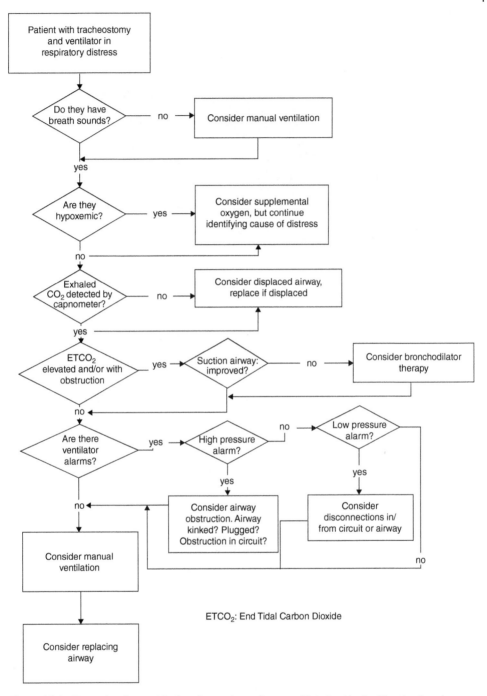

Figure 27.4 Example of a troubleshooting pathway for a ventilated patient with a tracheostomy in respiratory distress. (*Source:* Courtesy of Richard Lin.)

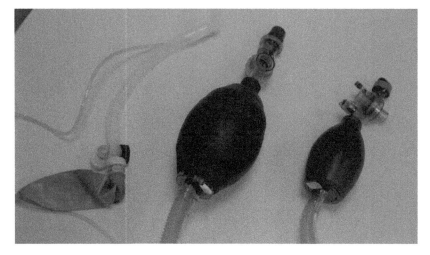

Figure 27.5 Examples of resuscitation bags – the left is a Mapleson D circuit, the other two are different sized self-inflating bags. The advantage of the Mapleson circuit is that it is easier to maintain a distending pressure (PEEP); however, it requires a source of gas flow. The advantage of the self-inflating bags is that they do not need a gas source (unless oxygen enrichment is required); however, it is harder to maintain an elevated PEEP. (*Source:* Courtesy of Michael Duff, RRT, Department of Respiratory Care, The Children's Hospital of Philadelphia, Philadelphia.)

malfunction. Should the ventilator stop functioning and air flow cease, ambient room air can be entrained through the valve. In hospital ventilators, this valve is typically controlled electronically and will remain closed so long as the electrical system is operational on the ventilator. On portable ventilators, however, this could be a source of entraining ambient air into the circuit if demand from the patient is great enough or there is a drop in the pressures within the ventilator to below that of the ambient air. If this were to happen, it could lower the fraction of inspired oxygen, if supplemental oxygen was being used.

Ventilators that require a compressed gas source require certain minimum flow rates or minimum pressures as detailed in their individual service manuals. These connections to the compressed gas source need to be maintained as does the pressure of the supplied gas. The connections to compressed gasses should be checked as they can become disconnected. And while it is extremely uncommon, if the central supply of compressed gas was not adequate or able to be maintained above a certain threshold, the ventilator might alarm indicating that the gas supply pressure was inadequate. An alternative could be to replace the connection with a high-pressure gas cylinder and regulator if there are concerns about the central supply.

Portable ventilators, in order to compress sufficient amounts of air, require consistent air flow through the intake filter to the turbine. Should this filter become excessively obstructed, it could present a problem. Aside from potentially not providing necessary flows, it could lead to the gas coming out of the ventilator being much warmer than usual. The care and instruction manuals for many ventilators recommend checking the filters on portable ventilators daily, cleaning and allowing them to dry fully before replacing if they are soiled, and exchanging them with new filters every couple of years or if damaged. Most durable equipment suppliers replace them more often. Figure 27.6 shows a soiled, partially occluded intake filter.

Figure 27.6 Example of soiled partially occluded intake filter. (*Source:* Courtesy of Michael Duff, RRT, Department of Respiratory Care, The Children's Hospital of Philadelphia, Philadelphia.)

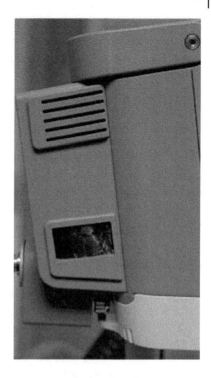

Circuit

The ventilator circuit can also be a source of problems. Circuit tubing is generally constructed of plastic and has a corrugated shape, which helps to hold its shape and prevent kinking. However, it can still be bent or compressed and could lead to obstruction of ventilator flows. This might cause high-pressure alarms or issues with triggering the ventilator. On the other hand, instead of too much resistance, there could be too much leak. This can be caused by a disconnection or a loose connection somewhere along the circuit or potentially caused by broken or cracked tubing. This could lead to low volume alarms or low pressure alarms and if not corrected quickly could lead to hypoventilation. Careful examination of the circuit will generally reveal any defects in the tubing or its connections. A common time for this problem to arise is immediately after the circuit tubing has been replaced.

Passively vented circuits are designed with intentional leaks. Ventilators will compensate for changes in leak from a passive circuit by increasing or decreasing flows. However, if low-flow supplemental oxygen is being blended into a passively vented circuit, such as with a portable or home ventilator, there is the potential to dilute the supplemental oxygen that is being added into the circuit as it mixes with a greater flow of ambient air. This potential issue with passive circuits needs to be kept in mind with patients who are dependent on supplemental oxygen.

Another issue with single limb circuits is that there is only one limb for both inspiration and exhalation; thus, there is the risk of rebreathing carbon dioxide. To clear the exhaled gas containing higher levels of carbon dioxide out of the expiratory valve, the circuit is flushed with a continuous flow of fresh gas. The amount of flow will depend on the leak characteristics of the valve and on the PEEP setting. If this flow is not sufficient, rebreathing of carbon dioxide can occur; thus, passive circuits require at least some minimal level of PEEP. More commonly, unintentional obstruction of the expiratory valve by something like a blanket or stuffed animal can result in rebreathing and impaired clearance of carbon dioxide.

Many circuit setups also have an expiratory filter to collect moisture and prevent bacterial colonization. These filters can become waterlogged if there is a lot of condensation in the tubing but can also become occluded in the setting of continuous nebulized medications. This can increase resistance in the tubing and result in high-pressure alarms.

Resistance can also be increased by adding additional lengths of tubing. This might be necessary from a logistical standpoint during transport of a patient, for example, to undergo computed tomography imaging. Resistance is proportional to the length of tubing; thus, adding additional lengths of tubing will increase the resistance in the tubing. If additional lengths of tubing are going to be added, this should be taken into account and the patient's respiratory status monitored for the duration of time that the longer length of tubing is needed.

Humidification

The most common issue with an active humidification setup is that the heated humidification system needs to be regularly monitored to see that it is constantly providing the right temperature and amount of humidity. In order to do so, it frequently needs to be maintained and refilled with fresh sterile water.

A potential problem with the active humidification system is excessive temperature. Thermal injury can result from sustained elevated temperatures above 41°C, although one study found that damage was only seen at a temperature near 80°C for 11 hours. Air that is not hot enough to cause a thermal injury could still be too warm. Inspired air with temperatures higher than 37°C and 100% relative humidity may result in significant condensation, which can affect mucociliary clearance by excessively thinning secretions particularly at the pericellular fluid layer. This occurs because warmer air is able to carry more water. This can also be problematic in the circuit, as the excess water can end up condensing and collecting in the tubing. Fluid in the tubing can result in obstruction, increased resistance to flows, which can result in auto-cycling and patient-ventilator dyssynchrony, and even accidental aspiration should the fluid drain toward the patient's artificial airway. On rare occasions, external covering on a heated circuit can result in damage to the integrity of the circuit.

If, on the other hand, the temperature is too low, the pulmonary secretions can become too thick and potentially more difficult to suction. Ciliary function in the airways is also thought to suffer in the setting of lower airway temperatures. HMEs tend to retain heat less effectively than an active humidification system, and the effect of temperature on ciliary function is a reason to limit the extent or duration of use.

The goal of humidification is to find the right temperature and the right amount of humidification for the patient at that time and in that environment. These settings may need to be adjusted throughout the year as seasons change and temperatures and relative humidities vary. Insulation around tubing or heated tubing may help prevent or reduce excessive condensation. Additionally, an investigation of the environment may be helpful to identify, for example, a cause of excessive condensation due to a draft from a fan or air conditioner directed at the ventilator circuit. Excessive condensation can be collected in a water trap or the circuit can be momentarily disconnected, and it can be drained out of the system.

An issue specific to the use of the HME is that they can become easily soiled and they may need to be changed frequently, particularly if the patient is ill and producing copious secretions. By adding the HME in the circuit (inline), it also increases resistance to the airway and increases dead space, which may worsen the work of breathing for some patients. Lastly, if there is a circuit disconnection but the HME remains on the circuit, there is the possibility that the disconnect alarm may not sound as there is increased resistance through the HME.

Artificial Airway

When initially placed, there are several methods of ensuring that the endotracheal tube is placed in the correct location within the trachea. If the endotracheal tube is placed correctly with its distal lumen in the trachea but above the level of the carina, one should hear equal breath sounds bilaterally when the patient is ventilated. If the endotracheal tube is too deep, it may enter either mainstem bronchus, but usually the right mainstem bronchus, and there may be discrepancy between breath sounds bilaterally as one lung is preferentially ventilated. If the endotracheal tube is placed in the correct location, the air that is being exhaled will contain carbon dioxide, and attaching a capnograph to the endotracheal tube system can help determine if the lungs are being ventilated. After its initial placement is established, the location of the tube should be confirmed by chest radiograph and adjusted as necessary. Endotracheal tubes can be displaced during coughing, manipulation or movement of the patient, or during other routine care. It is very important that these tubes be properly secured and routinely monitored.

Endotracheal tubes can obstruct, thus reducing or completely disrupting ventilation. This can lead to high pressure alarms, and the patient may have a reduction in oxyhemoglobin saturation such that the pulse oximeter alarms as well. Common reasons for obstruction are mucus plugging within the tube, external compression from a mass, a kink in the tubing, or biting the tube. Attempting to pass a suction catheter can act as a means of helping to diagnose the problem – if unable to pass the tubing, there may be something obstructing the tube – and to potentially treat the problem if there are obstructive secretions. A so-called bite block, a piece of plastic placed in the mouth or around the endotracheal tube designed to protect and reinforce an endotracheal tube, can be utilized to prevent external compression from biting.

Leak is another common problem at the artificial airway site. Leak is air leaving the patient-ventilator circuit. If large enough, this can activate a number of alarms including low pressure, low minute ventilation, low exhaled volumes. It can also lead to hypoventilation, resulting in oxyhemoglobin desaturation. Leak can contribute to dysynchrony and autocycling. Leak can be produced from anywhere in the circuit but most commonly is found arising from the mouth in patients who have oral endotracheal intubation or from the mouth and/or around the stoma in patients with a tracheostomy. Leak from the mouth in patients with a tracheostomy may occur more frequently when asleep or when attempting to speak or cough. It can also be exacerbated in patients who have restrictive disease and stiff chest walls as the air flow follows the path of least resistance. Treating the leak can be accomplished by inflating a cuff if the endotracheal or tracheotomy tube has one or by increasing the size of the endotracheal tube or tracheostomy tube. Repositioning the patient or adding gauze padding around the tracheostomy stoma can help reduce leak from the tracheostomy stoma itself. Settings on the ventilator can be adjusted to help with leak or to help overcome leak. Strategies for adjusting the ventilator settings will vary based on the patient's physiology and the cause of the leak. However, if they are going to be adjusted to help compensate for a leak, it should first be ascertained whether or not the leak is persistent. Increasing mechanical ventilation because of an intermittent leak could lead to unnecessary hyperventilation.

Patient and Ventilator Relationship: Synchrony

The purpose of the mechanical ventilator is to help support gas exchange in patients in respiratory failure by aiding and supporting the work of breathing. However, there are situations when the ventilator may not be as supportive as intended and may work counterproductively with the patient. This is termed *ventilator asynchrony*. Taken to its extreme, this can be witnessed as "bucking" or "fighting" the ventilator, but there are also many more subtle forms of asynchrony that demonstrate competition between the patient and the ventilator instead of cooperation. Ventilator asynchrony has been linked to several clinical issues such as dyspnea, increased work of breathing, need for more sedation, higher costs, delayed or prolonged weaning, and extended length of hospitalization. Some degree of ventilator asynchrony is certainly ubiquitous, and the exact amount of asynchrony which becomes pathologic is uncertain. Nonetheless, it is important to be aware of the potential problems and methods for correction.

Trigger Asynchrony

Problems with asynchrony are best divided up by the phase of the breath delivered by the mechanical ventilator: trigger, flow, and cycle. A breath from the ventilator is triggered by a drop in circuit pressure, known as a pressure trigger, or a change in the underlying circuit bias flow, known as a flow trigger. A problem exists when the ventilator triggers excessively or does not trigger at all. Both can be uncomfortable or distressing to the patient in addition to impacting their care and recovery.

There are two main reasons for missed or delayed triggers: Poor matching of sensitivity of the ventilator to the patient and intrinsic PEEP. Poor matching occurs when the degree of patient effort is less than the threshold for triggering a breath and effectively goes unnoticed by the ventilator. Trigger sensitivity is an adjustable setting. It is necessary to fine-tune the trigger sensitivity to the patient. And, one does not want the most sensitive setting at all times or for all patients because this may lead to inappropriate or excessive triggering. A patient with neuromuscular weakness or reduced respiratory drive may need a more sensitive setting than an otherwise healthy patient intubated for a more acute issue. Additionally, some of the smallest patients, such as the extremely premature infants in the neonatal intensive care units, may have a hard time generating sufficient flows to trigger even the most sensitive ventilators.

Intrinsic PEEP is the result of dynamic hyperinflation. Factors such as an increased resistance to expiratory flow, short expiratory time, reduced elastic recoil, or other states of increased ventilatory demand can lead to dynamic hyperinflation. When dynamic hyperinflation is present, the end expiratory lung volume is greater than the passive functional residual capacity or the end expiratory lung volume decided by the ventilator determined "external" PEEP. Elastic recoil pressure at end expiration is thus higher than the ventilator determined PEEP, and the difference between these two pressures is the intrinsic PEEP. Clinically, the respiratory muscles have to first generate enough force to overcome the intrinsic PEEP before they can alter circuit pressure or flow in order to trigger the ventilator. The increased force necessary can lead to missed triggers or delayed triggers. Leung et al. used esophageal pressure measurements to demonstrate that ventilatory muscle loaded is increased for missed triggers compared to properly triggered breaths.

Lastly, there are "auto-triggered" breaths that are neither initiated by the patient nor a mandatory scheduled breath determined by the set respiratory frequency. A number of factors can contribute to the ventilator triggering, including leaks in the ventilator system, condensation in the tubing, or improper sensitivity settings. Additionally, changes in intrathoracic pressure caused by cardiac oscillation in patients with large stroke volumes can be enough to trigger the ventilator if the settings are sensitive enough. These additional breaths can result in a respiratory alkalosis or can worsen dynamic hyperinflation and intrinsic PEEP by breath stacking potentially worsening optimal triggering. Another phenomenon closely related to auto-triggering is called entrainment. Entrainment is what appears to be a "spontaneous" effort triggering a ventilator-delivered breath that is elicited shortly following a machine-triggered breath. It is thought to be mediated through vagal pathways and mechanical stretch receptors. This will often occur in heavily sedated patients with high ventilator settings. Notably, this phenomenon can be seen in patients who have cessation of neurological function, leading to lack of apnea on the "brain death" exam with the appearance of apparent spontaneous breaths on the ventilator.

Identifying triggering issues can be performed with esophageal pressure monitoring, which is used as a surrogate for pleural pressure. Changes in esophageal pressure parallel changes in pleural pressure. When coupled with flow curves, one can clearly identify missed triggers, delayed triggers, and triggered breaths occurring without patient effort. However, esophageal pressure monitoring is not a standard clinical practice. Triggering asynchrony may be able to be inferred by inspecting the flow waveform and observing the patient's diaphragm motion. Momentary reductions or reversals in expiratory flow followed by resumption of expiratory flow that does not trigger a ventilator breath can signal a patient effort that failed to trigger the ventilator.

To improve trigger synchrony, the triggering mode can be changed from a flow trigger to pressure trigger or vice versa. If there are frequent missed efforts, the trigger can be made more sensitive, or if there is excessive triggering, the sensitivity can be reduced. If the problem is missed efforts because of intrinsic PEEP, attempts can be made to reduce the amount of dynamic hyperinflation by adjusting the external PEEP applied by the ventilator to better match the intrinsic PEEP and reduce the amount of elastic recoil pressure that needs to be overcome to trigger a breath.

Flow Asynchrony

The second phase of the ventilator breath cycle is the flow. A patient effort is started by diaphragmatic contraction. Once the ventilator is triggered, the contraction of the diaphragm continues through the breath. If ventilator flow is synchronous, the ventilator will help to support and assist this effort. If asynchronous, excessive load can be applied to the respiratory muscles and this is the basis for dyssynchrony during this phase.

Flow asynchrony can arise from inadequate flow delivery or excessive flow delivery. Inadequate flow delivery occurs when inspiratory flow demands are high or flow delivery is set too low. In normal subjects exposed to increasing inspired carbon dioxide, the primary determinant of their work of breathing was the set flow on the ventilator, and when that flow was reduced, work of breathing increased. Excessive flow can also be a problem. If flows are too fast or rise time too rapid on pressure control settings, lung expansion can occur more quickly than what is desired by the patient and may even result in the ventilatory control center abruptly aborting or fighting the inspiratory flow via the Hering–Breuer Reflex.

Flow asynchrony tends to occur more frequently in volume-targeted modes that are less flexible and deliver a fixed flow rather than pressure-targeted breaths when flow can vary with effort. Troubleshooting could involve changing from a volume-targeted mode to a pressure-targeted mode or adjusting the flow rates accordingly.

Cycle Asynchrony

The end of the ventilator breath is the cycle phase. The ventilator will cycle from inspiration to expiration with termination of flow at the end of the inspiratory phase. Cycle asynchrony occurs when the ventilator terminates the inspiratory portion of the breath discordantly with the patient. It is consists of two issues: delayed termination and premature termination.

Delayed termination occurs when the ventilator continues the inspiratory portion of the breath longer than the patient desires. This can result in increased work of breathing through the use of accessory muscles of exhalation, an increase in elastic recoil, and subsequently dynamic hyperinflation and the need for a greater inspiratory effort to trigger the ventilator or even missed or delayed inspiratory triggers. This can be seen as a "pressure spike" at the end of the breath coinciding with the zero flow point. The astute clinician might also notice accessory muscles being used at the end of inhalation.

Premature termination can also be a problem. Premature termination is when the inspiratory phase of the ventilator breath terminates earlier than the patient desires. In one study of pressure-supported ventilation, adjusting the termination criteria such that the flows terminated earlier resulted in reduced tidal volumes, increased respiratory rates, increased work of breathing, and double triggering. To identify premature termination, one can look for an abrupt (as opposed to gradual) reversal of flow in the flow and airway pressure tracings, as these findings would indicate continued inspiratory effort from the patient. Double triggers may also be seen if the maintained inspiratory effort is sufficient enough.

Troubleshooting cycle asynchrony involves adjusting the length of time for inspiration. On mandatory breaths from the ventilator, this might require adjusting the inspiratory times either shorter or longer. For pressure-supported breaths, this might mean adjusting the settings such that the breath flow cycles at a higher percentage of peak flow to terminate inspiration earlier or at a lower percentage of peak flow to terminate inspiration later. The goal though is to match the patient's current respiratory mechanics, and in periods of illness and recovery, this may be a moving target.

Ventilator Alarms

All mechanical ventilators will have elaborate systems of safety alarms to alert the patient and/or medical practitioner to a variety of issues. The specific alarm options and terminology will vary depending on the brand and/or model of mechanical ventilator, but the larger concepts are generally the same from ventilator to ventilator. One should know though that there is not yet a standard nomenclature for ventilator alarms. In this chapter, we may refer to a "high pressure alarm," which on a specific brand of ventilator may be labeled "high peak pressure" or some other terminology. If there is confusion, it is recommended to cross-reference this chapter with the instruction manual of the mechanical ventilator.

When an alarm sounds, it is absolutely necessary to evaluate the patient first to ensure safety. It may even be necessary to provide an alternate means of ventilation while investigating the alarm. However, some of these alarms will not be for true emergencies. In hospitals and intensive care units, nuisance alarms are a large problem and a safety risk. And vigilance to these frequent alarms is one of the factors thought to lead to exhaustion and burnout, especially among intensive care unit nurses and caregivers for technology-dependent patients. There is the thought that a way to combat nuisance alarms is to reduce the number of false alarms by setting alarm parameters that make the most sense for the patient. Additionally, this author feels that caregivers who are comfortable with the equipment and the alarms we are discussing today may have less burnout if they are rapidly able to assess patients and quickly identify problems. The rest of this section details many of the common causes of alarms.

High Pressure Alarms

This alarm might be called a high peak pressure alarm or a high inspiratory pressure alarm. This alarm sounds when the ventilator pressure reaches or exceeds a previously adjusted upper pressure limit. Generally speaking, this alarm results in a bleeding of flow out of the ventilator away from the patient so that the patient doesn't see pressures higher than this limit. On many ventilators, the bleeding or leak begins at a level about 5 cm H_2O below the preset limit.

This alarm may sound if pressures go up because the patient is in a volume-targeted mode and their pulmonary compliance changed (e.g. due to bronchospasm and pneumothorax) and now higher pressures are required to achieve the same volumes. It may also go off if there is some sort of obstruction or increased resistance in the ventilator circuit or in the patient. Some examples include a mucus plug in the airways, a kink in the endotracheal tube or circuit, or excessive condensation in the ventilator circuit. The patient can also cause the high pressure alarm to go off with excessive movement, cough, Valsalva maneuver, or dyssynchrony.

When troubleshooting this alarm, it is important to examine the patient to see what secretions are like and if there are sounds of obstruction such as wheeze on auscultation. Other actions that the patient is taking might help provide clues such as if they are coughing or bearing down. Chest physiotherapy and suctioning the artificial airway can help with identifying and possibly correcting obstruction to the tracheal tube. Lastly, observing that the ventilator settings make sense and fit the patient's respiratory pattern can help correct the issue.

Some ventilators will also have high PEEP alarms, indicating that the pressure at the end of exhalation is too high. This could be due to incomplete emptying, which often occurs in patients with status asthmaticus and respiratory failure who need long exhale times because of the expiratory resistance to flow. They often need a lower respiratory rate to allow for longer time spent in exhalation.

Low Pressure Alarms

This alarm might be called a low peak pressure alarm or low inspiratory pressure alarm on different ventilators. There may also be a separate alarm for low PEEP. This alarm will sound when the pressures during inspiration or at the end of exhalation are below the predetermined alarm setting.

Low pressure alarms often will sound when there is a leak in the ventilator circuit or if there is a disconnection. Leaks in the ventilator circuit can be due to loose connections, faulty exhalation or PEEP valves, leak from the patient's mouth or around the tracheostomy stoma, faulty filters, or even from cracked tubing. The most urgent source of leak is a dislodged endotracheal or tracheostomy tube, as this can lead to hypoventilation and hypoxemia acutely. After confirming that the artificial airway is not dislodged, one of the best ways to investigate this alarm is to examine for leaks or disconnections, starting at the patient and following the circuit back to the ventilator. If a disconnection or crack in the tubing is not found, the leak may be positional and may stop with adjustment in the patient's position. Other times, inflation of the cuff on the endotracheal or tracheostomy tube may be needed.

It is important to note that this alarm will not always sound when there is a disconnection. It is possible to have a circuit disconnected but to have either enough obstruction or occlusion of the circuit that the ventilator perceives some threshold of pressure. Patients with smaller endotracheal tubes or tracheostomy tubes may be at higher risk of this, given the resistance of the smaller diameter of the tubes. Many ventilators have other alarms that help with identifying disconnection knowing that this one is not perfectly sensitive, yet another example of how ventilators are built with redundancy and safety in mind.

High Exhaled Minute Volume Alarm

This alarm is triggered when the patient's minute ventilation (typically measured by exhaled tidal volume) exceeds the preset threshold. This might occur when the patient is tachypneic. Potential etiologies include anxiety, poor pain control, hypoxemia, metabolic acidosis, or a response to exertion. Like with all alarms, it is important to assess your patient and look for potential causes.

Low Exhaled Minute Volume Alarm

This alarm sounds when the minute ventilation is below the threshold set. The causes are the same that cause low pressure alarms such as leaks and disconnection. This alarm functions as a redundant safety alarm for leaks and disconnections.

Apnea Alarm

Apnea alarms will trigger when the length of time between breaths exceeds a preset interval. Some ventilators such as the LTV will start backup ventilation with a preset apnea ventilation mode and prescribed respiratory rate until the alarm is canceled or the patient triggers two consecutive breaths. This alarm typically sounds when the patient has an episode of apnea, the respiratory rate has decreased, or when they become disconnected from the ventilator. If this alarm is being triggered, it is important to fully assess the patient and see if the episodes of apnea are truly apnea by looking for respiratory effort from the patient that the ventilator might not be registering. It is possible for this alarm to trigger because there is enough leak that the ventilator is not sensing the patient's efforts. If this is the case, fixing any potential leak in the circuit or around the artificial airway can help. Additionally, adjusting the trigger to make it more sensitive might help reduce alarms.

Disconnect Alarm

Some ventilators will have a disconnect alarm that can alert caregivers to disconnections in the circuit. On the LTV, there is a sensing line that if occluded, kinked, or disconnected will alarm because it does not appreciate an appropriate pressure change at the beginning of inspiration. Troubleshooting this alarm requires an immediate response to determine if the patient has become disconnected from the ventilator circuit. We recommend quickly assessing the patient and determining if an alternative mode of ventilation is needed prior to examining the circuit looking for disconnections or problems with the sensing line.

Low Power/Low Battery Alarm

If there is an inadequate source of electrical power, this alarm will trigger. Many times, this is simply alerting the caregiver that the electrical cord is not firmly or completely connected either at the ventilator or at the connection with the electrical outlet. It is important to check the electrical connections. If one cannot find the source of the problem, there may be an internal problem with the ventilator, and switching to a new ventilator may be necessary until the alarming ventilator can be serviced.

If the amount of charge left in the battery is low, similar alarms may sound. Typically, the battery will start alarming when the charge reaches a level at which the ventilator battery will continue to operate but is close to empty, thus allowing caregivers a few minutes to plug the ventilator into an electrical outlet. Again, based on ventilator settings and patient demand, this amount of time may vary, so it is important to quickly identify where the portable ventilator can be plugged in and charged when this alarm sounds.

Conclusion

Patients with respiratory failure requiring invasive ventilation, whether acutely or chronically, can have a multitude of medical problems which bring them to seek care. In this chapter, many of the obstacles that can arise from this sophisticated and varied life-supporting equipment were identified. Technology though will continue to advance and new equipment will enter the sphere. While many of the principles and ideas discussed in this chapter will likely remain relevant, it will be vitally important to prepare for and review new equipment in order to continue to provide the best care.

Further Reading

1 Baker, D.J. (2016). *Basic Principles of Mechanical Ventilation. Artificial Ventilation: A Basic Clinical Guide*, 107–131. Cham: Springer International Publishing.

2 Branson, R.D. and Chatburn, R.L. (1992). Technical description and classification of modes of ventilator operation. *Respir. Care* 37 (9): 1026–1044. Epub 1992/09/01. PubMed PMID: 10183731.

3 Baker, D.J. (2016). *Artificial Ventilation A Basic Clinical Guide*. Switzerland: Springer International Publishing AG.

4 Lujan, M., Sogo, A., Pomares, X. et al. (2013). Effect of leak and breathing pattern on the accuracy of tidal volume estimation by commercial home ventilators: a bench study. *Respir. Care* 58 (5): 770–777. https://doi.org/10.4187/respcare.02010. Epub 2012/10/12. PubMed PMID: 23051878.

5 Williams, R., Rankin, N., Smith, T. et al. (1996). Relationship between the humidity and temperature of inspired gas and the function of the airway mucosa. *Crit. Care Med.* 24 (11): 1920–1929. https://doi.org/10.1097/00003246-199611000-00025. Epub 1996/11/01. PMID: 8917046.

6 Gillies, D., Todd, D.A., Foster, J.P., and Batuwitage, B.T. (2017). Heat and moisture exchangers versus heated humidifiers for mechanically ventilated adults and children. *Cochrane Database Syst. Rev.* (9): CD004711. https://doi.org/10.1002/14651858.CD004711. pub3. Epub 2017/09/15. PMID: 28905374; PubMed Central PMCID: PMCPMC6483749.

7 Durbin, C.G. Jr. (2005). Indications for and timing of tracheostomy. *Respir. Care* 50 (4): 483–487. Epub 2005/04/06. PMID: 15807910.

8 Haas, C.F., Eakin, R.M., Konkle, M.A., and Blank, R. (2014). Endotracheal tubes: old and new. *Respir. Care* 59 (6): 933–952; discussion 52-5. doi: https://doi.org/10.4187/respcare.02868. Epub 2014/06/04. PMID: 24891200.

9 Campbell, R.S., Johannigman, J.A., Branson, R.D. et al. (2002). Battery duration of portable ventilators: effects of control variable, positive end-expiratory pressure, and inspired oxygen concentration. *Respir. Care* 47 (10): 1173–1183. Epub 2002/10/02. PMID: 12354337.

10 Blakeman, T.C., Toth, P., Rodriquez, D., and Branson, R.D. (2010). Mechanical ventilators in the hot zone: effects of a CBRN filter on patient protection and battery life. *Resuscitation* 81 (9): 1148–1151. https://doi.org/10.1016/j.resuscitation.2010.05.006. Epub 2010/08/25. PMID: 20732606.

11 Lloyd, E. (1990). Airway warming in the treatment of accidental hypothermia: a review. *J. Wilderness Med.* 1 (2): 65–78.

12 American Association for Respiratory Care, Restrepo, R.D., and Walsh, B.K. (2012). Humidification during invasive and noninvasive mechanical ventilation: 2012. *Respir. Care* 57 (5): 782–788. https://doi.org/10.4187/respcare.01766. Epub 2012/05/02. PMID: 22546299.

13 Nilsestuen, J.O. and Hargett, K.D. (2005). Using ventilator graphics to identify patient-ventilator asynchrony. *Respir. Care* 50 (2): 202–234; discussion 32-4. Epub 2005/02/05. PMID: 15691392.

14 Leung, P., Jubran, A., and Tobin, M.J. (1997). Comparison of assisted ventilator modes on triggering, patient effort, and dyspnea. *Am. J. Respir. Crit. Care Med.* 155 (6): 1940–1948. https://doi.org/10.1164/ajrccm.155.6.9196100. Epub 1997/06/01. PMID: 9196100.

15 Marini, J.J., Capps, J.S., and Culver, B.H. (1985). The inspiratory work of breathing during assisted mechanical ventilation. *Chest* 87 (5): 612–618. https://doi.org/10.1378/chest.87.5.612. Epub 1985/05/01. PMID: 3987373.

16 Tokioka, H., Tanaka, T., Ishizu, T. et al. (2001). The effect of breath termination criterion on breathing patterns and the work of breathing during pressure support ventilation. *Anesth. Analg.* 92 (1): 161–165. https://doi.org/10.1097/00000539-200101000-00031. Epub 2001/01/03. PMID: 11133620.

17 Ruskin, K.J. and Hueske-Kraus, D. (2015). Alarm fatigue: impacts on patient safety. *Curr. Opin. Anaesthesiol.* 28 (6): 685–690. https://doi.org/10.1097/ACO.0000000000000260. Epub 2015/11/06. PMID: 26539788.

28

Respiratory Medication Devices

Natalie Napolitano[1] and James B. Fink[2,3,4]

[1] *Department of Respiratory Care Services, Children's Hospital of Philadelphia, Philadelphia, PA, USA*
[2] *Aerogen Pharma Corporation, San Mateo, CA, USA*
[3] *Rush Medical School, Chicago, IL, USA*
[4] *Texas State University, Round Rock, TX, USA*

Introduction

Inhaled respiratory medications are a frontline therapy for patients presenting to the acute care setting with complaints of respiratory distress. Medical aerosols have the advantage of providing local topical administration to the airways, with reduced systemic effects and faster response time than other routes of administration with the exception of the intravenous route. In addition, aerosol therapy has been used for administration of drugs for systemic effect due to their absorption through the lung air-blood barrier.

Of the many drugs administered as aerosols to acutely ill patients (Table 28.1), the most common during the first few hours of care in the Emergency Department (ED) or intensive care unit (ICU) are short-acting bronchodilators, vasoconstrictors, and mucokinetics, to relieve airway obstruction and decrease work of breathing. Inhaled steroids and other anti-inflammatory agents by aerosol require hours to have an effect on reversible obstructive airways disease and thus are secondary to parenteral administration in the ED and ICU. Similarly, inhaled antibiotics and antivirals are seldom first-line treatment in the ED and are often reserved until cultures have been obtained. Pulmonary vasodilators such as inhaled prostacyclins and nitric oxide are not a first-line treatment upon presentation.

Equipment/Device and Interface Options

Patients with previously diagnosed respiratory problems are often prescribed inhaled medications for use at home with a combination of dry powder inhalers (DPIs), pressurized metered dose inhaler (pMDI), soft mist inhaler (SMI) (Figure 28.1), or a small volume jet nebulizer (SVN) (Figure 28.2). It is uncommon to integrate devices from home for initial

Emergency Management of the Hi-Tech Patient in Acute and Critical Care, First Edition. Edited by
Ioannis Koutroulis, Nicholas Tsarouhas, Richard J. Lin, Jill C. Posner, Michael Seneff, and Robert Shesser.
© 2021 John Wiley & Sons Ltd. Published 2021 by John Wiley & Sons Ltd.

Table 28.1 Medications via aerosol for acutely Ill patients.

Medication class	Examples	Disease management for	Examples of available delivery routes
Bronchodilators (beta agonists, cholinergics)	Albuterol, ipratropium	Lower airway obstruction (asthma, bronchiolitis)	JN, VMN, USN, pMDI, SMI, DPI
Vasoconstrictors	Racemic epinephrine	Extrathoracic airway obstruction (laryngotracheobronchitis, angioedema)	JN, USN, VMN
Expectorant Mucolytics	Hypertonic saline, Dornase alfa	Cystic fibrosis, asthma, chronic obstructive pulmonary disease	JN, USN, VMN
Anticoagulants, thrombolytics	Heparin, alteplase	Airway burns, plastic bronchitis	JN, USN, VMN
Anti-inflammatory (steroids, mast cell stabilizers)	Fluticasone, budesonide, cromylyn	Asthma, cystic fibrosis, chronic obstructive pulmonary disease	JN, USN, VMN, pMDI, DPI, SMI
Anti-infectives (antibiotics, antivirals)	Tobramycin, ribavirin	Bronchiectasis, viral pneumonitis	JN, USN, VMN, SMI
Prostanoids	Epoprostenol	Pulmonary hypertension	JN, USN, VMN, SMI

Notes:
DPI – Dry Powder Inhaler.
pMDI – pressurized Meter Dose Inhaler.
SMI – Soft Mist Inhaler.
JN – Jet Nebulizer (includes Small Volume Jet Nebulizer (SVN) and Large Volume Nebulizer (LVN))
USN – Ultrasonic Nebulizer.
VMN – Vibrating Mesh Nebulizer.

treatment in the ED/ICU. Patients presenting to the ED with acute respiratory distress are commonly triaged with a standard initial treatment, which may include oxygen therapy and inhaled short-acting bronchodilators.

Jet Nebulizers

Small volume jet nebulizers (SVN) (Figure 28.2) have been in use since the 1930s and are an example of single dose jet nebulizers (JN). They tend to be inexpensive and are often purchased by institutions as a commodity, in range of US$1.00.

A JN consists of a medication cup with an inlet for gas (jet), which directs gas over a capillary tube or conduit, generating a negative pressure that draws medication from the reservoir to be sheared into particles, which can range from 0.1 to 100 μm in diameter. The gas stream directs the aerosol to one or more surfaces or baffles where larger particles impact and drip back into the reservoir, while smaller particles are emitted as an aerosol from the nebulizer. JN are designed to operate at specific gas flow rates, typically in a range of 6–10 l/min, determined by the manufacturer to produce the desired particle size.

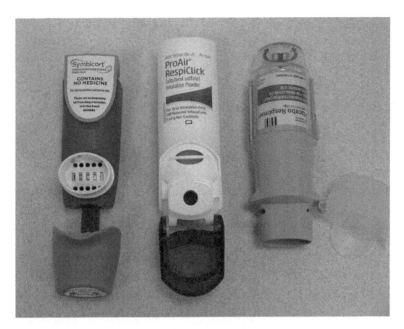

Figure 28.1 Three examples of self-contained aerosolized medication devices: metered dose inhaler (MDI), dry powder inhaler (DPI), and soft mist inhaler (SMI). (*Source:* Michael Duff, RRT, Department of Respiratory Care, The Children's Hospital of Philadelphia, Philadelphia, PA 19104)

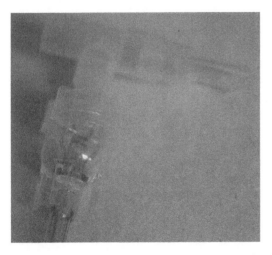

Figure 28.2 Jet nebulizer (JN). (*Source:* Michael Duff, RRT, Department of Respiratory Care, The Children's Hospital of Philadelphia, Philadelphia, PA 19104)

Residual drug of 0.8–1.2 ml never leaves the nebulizer, so the therapy is considered complete when the nebulizer begins to sputter. The duration of a typical treatment from a 3.0 ml unit dose of albuterol is 10–20 minutes. Continuous aerosol emitted from the device is inhaled during inspiration or passes by the patient to the atmosphere during the rest of the breathing cycle. Aerosol delivery efficiency varies with JN between a 4 and 12% lung dose.

The common SVN can be used with a mouthpiece, mask, and other interfaces. No SVNs were designed for infants or small children, with masks providing an interface in a range of sizes and shapes to fit. A tight fit of mask to face is essential for efficient drug delivery. Children that are fussing or crying receive virtually no aerosol to the lung, and up to 47% of children will not tolerate a mask without fussing, especially in the ED. Alternate options include "blow by" in which the stream of aerosol is pointed at the child's face, which may cause less agitation but also delivers much less aerosol and is not recommended. Aerosol hoods and tents work as well as masks but are not commonly used. The delivery of aerosol via nasal cannula (NC) with low and high flow oxygen has shown promise to be effective in all size patients (discussed later in the chapter).

As an alternative to multiple, end-to-end, serial doses of bronchodilator via SVN, it may be preferable to administer a large dose of a bronchodilator over several hours by generating a continuous aerosol, which runs for an extended period of time. Large volume nebulizers (LVNs) can be used to deliver medications over a period of hours for therapies such as continuous albuterol for status asthmaticus. LVNs can hold from 20 to 120 ml, enabling them to provide therapy for four hours or longer. Some LVNs have a port to allow continuous feed via bag or syringe pump.

Breath-Actuated/Enhanced Nebulizers

Breath-actuated (or enhanced) nebulizers are vented with a one-way valve in the mouthpiece or mask, reducing the loss of continuous aerosol to atmosphere, increasing inhaled dose marginally over simple SVNs. Breath-actuated nebulizers (BANs) are triggered by the patient's inspiratory flow and the aerosol is only emitted during inspiration. These nebulizers must be used with a valved mouthpiece or valved mask and thus cannot be used in conjunction with invasive and noninvasive ventilators. In small children, BANs might not actuate until late in the inspiratory cycle, delivering less drug than simple continuous JNs. Since BANs only produce aerosol during the patient's inspiration, they can increase inhaled dose by up to three fold over JNs, but require three times longer to administer the same dose volume. One company promotes using BANs with undiluted albuterol to provide effective dosing in fewer total breaths; BANs and breath-enhanced nebulizers are more expensive than simple SVNs and have limited clinical data showing improved response. Manual breath synchronized JNs require a patient to depress a lever during inspiration, with similar benefits and problems as BAN, with the added risk of poor hand–breath coordination in a patient who is in respiratory distress.

Ultrasonic and Vibrating Mesh Nebulizers

Ultrasonic nebulizers (USNs) were introduced in the 1960s. They use electrical stimulation of a piezo ceramic element to vibrate at 1.5–3 MHz and are focused to produce a standing wave at the surface of the medication, which generates an aerosol. These devices tend to generate considerable heat and, therefore, are not suitable for enzymatic medications such as dornase alfa. They also tend to generate small particle sizes and thus are not suitable for suspensions. These nebulizers are no longer commonly used in the ED.

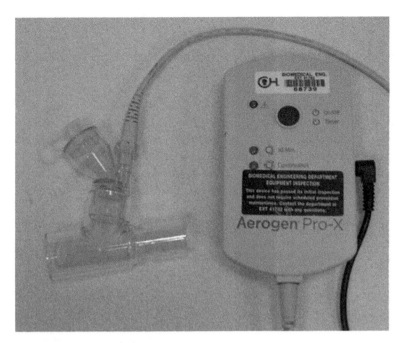

Figure 28.3 Vibrating mesh nebulizer: On the left is an 'in-line' type mesh nebulizer which would be used to deliver aerosol via a ventilator circuit. On the right is an electronic controller which causes the mesh to vibrate. (*Source*: Michael Duff, RRT, Department of Respiratory Care, The Children's Hospital of Philadelphia, Philadelphia, PA 19104)

Vibrating mesh nebulizers (VMNs) generate aerosols by forcing the liquid through multiple mesh plates (Figure 28.3). They are powered by electricity (battery or an AC power supply). VMNs generate small and consistent particle sizes (4–6 μm), do not add any extra flow to ventilator circuitry, are silent, and tend to have shorter treatment times with minimal residual volume, thus providing greater amounts of medication to the patient. Mesh and ultrasonic nebulizers provide similar aerosol delivery to ventilator dependent patients. Recently, the use of VMNs with a valved chamber has shown to increase inhaled dose and reduce time in the ED with COPD patients.

Inhalers

Pressurized metered dose inhalers, or pMDIs, are the most common medical aerosol device in the world. They are propellant powered, compact, and disposable, making them a popular way for patients to receive inhaled medications.

Although simple to use, pMDIs require "hand–breath" coordination to make sure that the time of actuation of the pMDI is at the beginning of inspiration. The patient is encouraged to hold their breath for 5–10 seconds after inhalation to ensure maximal deposition. This can be difficult for patients in respiratory distress. As simple as the pMDI is, up to 69% of patients and clinicians do not operate them properly. Even with proper use, up to 80–90% of the aerosol deposits in the mouth and upper airway, with only 10% reaching the lungs.

SMIs are designed for ambulatory patients with spontaneous breathing incorporating manual actuation and relatively long aerosol release/generation times. As with other inhalers, they may not be the more reliable option during exacerbation. The range of drugs available in SMI format has increased, and some may be of benefit for acutely ill patients.

DPIs are commonly prescribed for patients with chronic respiratory disease. Combination long-acting bronchodilator-anti-inflammatory medications are more readily available via DPIs than as nebulizer solutions or non-dry powder inhalers. DPIs are passive, requiring the patient's inspiratory force to dispense medication. Inability to generate the minimum necessary inspiratory pressures for the required time results in reduced delivered dose. DPIs are not an option for children under the age of five years even under the best of conditions. For patients presenting with respiratory distress, there is reasonable concern of whether they can adequately operate the device. Consequently, the use of DPI is rare in the ED or ICU, until the patient stabilizes and is capable of returning to his/her prescribed medications for home. There is currently no reliable way of administering DPIs during ventilatory support.

Accessory Devices

For younger (and older) patients, the use of spacers or valved holding chambers (VHCs) may maximize benefit of the pMDI. A spacer provides distance between the pMDI and the patient so that the aerosol speed slows and evaporation occurs, reducing particle size and velocity before it reaches the mouth so that the patient can inhale more medication with less oral deposition (approximately 10%). A VHC holds the medication suspended in the chamber even when the patient exhales, requiring no coordination of breath and actuation to achieve a high level of deposition of medication, while valves act as a baffle reducing oropharyngeal deposition to 1% (Figure 28.4). When a slow, deep breath is not possible to clear the chamber with one breath, taking three to six breaths to clear aerosol from a single actuation in the chamber is an effective alternative. In acute care, pMDI with VHC is highly recommended for all patients.

Breath-Actuated pMDIs

Some metered dose inhalers (MDIs) are triggered with the negative pressure of inhalation. This requires an inspiratory flow of 20 l/min or higher to trigger, which may not be achievable by small children or patients in respiratory distress.

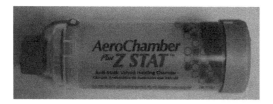

Figure 28.4 Valved holding chamber. (*Source:* Michael Duff, RRT, Department of Respiratory Care, The Children's Hospital of Philadelphia, Philadelphia, PA 19104)

Dose Counters

pMDIs contain 60–200 doses, and administration beyond that number has little to no effect. It is difficult to identify by sight and sound when all label doses have been administered. The most reliable method is to track actuations, which could be a simple as piece of tape placed on the box or canister with a slash mark added with each puff used. Manufacturers in the US are now required to provide counters on new MDIs introduced in the market to aid in the reliability of knowing how many medicated actuations are left in a canister. There are some accessory devices which make pMDIs "smart" by allowing the user to send actuation events via Bluetooth to a device such as a tablet or smartphone for tracking pMDI use.

Interface

Mouthpiece and Mask

Most nebulizers and inhalers use a mouthpiece to interface with the patient. For longer treatments, smaller patients (less than 12 month of age) who are obligate nose breathers, and older patients who have trouble using a mouthpiece, the mask is the obvious option. A poorly fitting mask does not deliver much aerosol, and the use of mask with an agitated child (which occurs up to 49% of the time) delivers even less.

Nasal Cannula

NCs are commonly used to deliver both low flow and high flow oxygen and are more comfortable and easily tolerated than masks. Trans-nasal pulmonary delivery of aerosol is currently used in 23% of ICUs worldwide. For patients receiving high flow nasal oxygen, aerosol administration through the cannula is more efficient than administering aerosol devices over the cannula and less disruptive than interrupting oxygen therapy during aerosol administration.

Aerosol delivery via NC is greatest at low and medium gas flows, being comparable to standard nebulizer therapy. At higher gas flows, inhaled dose decreases but may still provide sufficient efficiency to have clinical effect. Lie et al. demonstrated that asthma and COPD patients who responded to albuterol in the pulmonary function test lab also showed optimal bronchodilator response with aerosol via high-flow nasal cannula at 30 and 50 l/min using the standard unit doses of albuterol. Greater doses may be required with more severe exacerbation.

Mechanical Ventilation

JNs, pMDI, Ultrasonic Nebulizer (USN), and VMN are used with conventional mechanical ventilation. In general, when placed in the inspiratory limb of a circuit close to a patient, JN is less efficient (3%) than pMDI with spacer adapter (Figure 28.5), USN, and VMN (all between 12 and 17%). In addition, JNs add 6–10 l/min of gas flow to the circuit, which can change ventilator parameters, especially with children. For ventilators with bias flow up to 6 l/min, a JN or VMN placed at the inlet of humidifier is more efficient with adult and

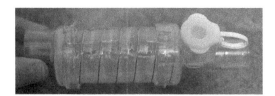

Figure 28.5 Spacer used for delivery with mechanical ventilation. (*Source:* Michael Duff, RRT, Department of Respiratory Care, The Children's Hospital of Philadelphia, Philadelphia, PA 19104)

pediatric patients. However, for infant ventilation, device placement in the inspiratory limb, proximal to the patient, is best.

Similar to the pMDI, an adapter to prevent leaks is required to attach an SMI to a ventilator circuit. However, unlike the pMDI, there are few commercial adapters available for SMI and information on their delivered dose efficiency is limited. Dose efficiency is typically greater than 50% in spontaneously breathing patients. This is reduced to a range of 2–30% in mechanically ventilated patients, depending on adapter design.

Noninvasive Ventilation

A variety of aerosol devices has been characterized during the administration of noninvasive ventilation (NIV). For NIV using turbines and vented masks with single limb circuits, aerosol generators should be placed between the fixed leak and the patient. This delivers >twofold more aerosol independent of the device. Both VMN and pMDI are over two fold more efficient than JN.

For NIV administered with closed (nonvented) masks and a standard two limb ventilator circuit, the aerosol device should be placed in the inspiratory limb of the circuit, either proximal to the patient or before or after the humidifier.

High-frequency Oscillation

There are two devices that deliver aerosolized medication in conjunction with high-frequency oscillations with the purpose of delivering medication and airway clearance therapies simultaneously. Both intrapulmonary percussive ventilation (Percussionaire Corporation) and Metaneb (Hillrom, US) provide aerosol with continuous high-frequency oscillations at the airway, whether with mouthpiece or mask or integrated with a mechanical ventilator. Independent of benefits of the airway oscillation, the design and position of the JN is not efficient (<2% inhaled dose) so should not be considered as a first-line device for aerosol administration in the ED or ICU. As with high-frequency oscillatory ventilation, the VMN is more efficient than JN, and placement of the aerosol device between the circuit and patient airway is the most efficient, with a delivered dose ranging from 18 to 30%.

Management

Dosing Strategies for Aerosols

Most drugs for inhalation are approved based on clinical trials of not-very-sick patients at home. When these patients present during exacerbation, many have been using their inhalers and nebulizers at home before coming to the hospital with little to no effect. It has become clear that during exacerbation, the same drugs can work, but may require different doses, frequency, and even delivery devices to achieve therapeutic goals.

A standard albuterol dose of pMDI of one to two puffs may be sufficient at home, but for ill patients, dosing strategies of administering up to 12 puffs per hour have been recommended for pediatric patients before coming to the ED. Similarly, nebulizer treatments of 2.5 mg q 20 minutes three times or weight-based continuous administration are now part of the standards for treatment of pediatric asthma. During mechanical ventilation, in stable COPD patients, four puffs from the pMDI with spacer showed 10–20% reduction in passive airway resistance. There was no improvement with up to 18 additional actuations. However, during severe airway obstruction, higher doses might be warranted.

No medical aerosols have been approved for use in mechanically ventilated patients, whether adult or infant. This provides a dilemma for the clinician to provide an otherwise effective drug in an off-label manner. Bench testing, pharmacokinetics, pharmacodynamics, and radiolabeled imaging of aerosols have helped to understand aerosol drug delivery with a variety of devices in the acute care environment. Quantifying the efficiency of the aerosol systems used in the ED or ICU provides insights as to the dose required to achieve the desired "targeted" lung dose. For a medication such as inhaled tobramycin, which is approved for administration using a nebulizer with 12% lung dose efficiency at home, the clinician can either choose an aerosol delivery system that meets or exceeds that delivery efficiency such VMN, USN, or pMDI (each around 17% *in vitro*) or increase the dosage up to threefold for use with JN delivering only 4%.

Bronchodilators

For short-acting bronchodilators which can show benefits in as little as five minutes, it is common to initially triage with a JN with standard dose of 2.5–5 mg. For treatment of acute asthma, the combination of albuterol with ipratropium bromide has shown benefit with both adults and children.

If symptoms persist despite initial treatment, and FEV1 or PEFR of less than 50% is predicted, several strategies have been described:

1) Repeat nebulizer treatment at 15- to 20-minute intervals until symptoms resolve.
2) Continuous nebulization delivering the equivalent cumulative dose per hour of the SVN treatments – doses of 10, 20, and 30 mg/h – have been described.
3) Using pMDI with VHC, provide up to 5 puffs at one-minute intervals, wait five minutes, then proceed to give one puff each minute up to a total of 12 puffs.

When intermittent high-dose bronchodilators fail to reduce symptoms, continuous nebulization has the advantage of providing therapy over an extended period of time while reducing the staff time required for back-to-back SVN treatments.

For other medical aerosols, where response times are longer, the best strategy is to select devices capable of delivering similar or greater lung doses than what can be achieved with the approved label for the drug. It is reasonable to assume that most pMDIs and nebulizers were approved with systems delivering around 10–12% of dose. If you are using a system that only delivers 4% (JN on ventilator), you might want to use a larger nominal dose in the nebulizer to achieve the "target" lung dose used in the ambulatory setting.

Device Selection

A range of aerosol devices work as long as they are used properly by the patient and are tolerated. Less efficient systems, like JN, may require higher doses and more frequent administration. Interfaces and adapters are critical for effective performance.

Complications/Emergencies

Complications of aerosol medication delivery can be categorized as side effects of the medication, failure to consistently and effectively administer, and problems associated with fugitive aerosol emission.

Failure to administer is of primal concern. If an aerosol device is not used properly, it may fail to administer the prescribed medication. This could be as simple as actuating a pMDI or SMI when the patient is exhaling or having a nebulizer that stops nebulizing before the full dose is administered. More commonly, we find patients receiving aerosol by mouthpiece with the nebulizer not in the patient's mouth, or a mask that is not properly positioned on his/her face. No aerosol device has alarms monitoring output or patient interface, so the clinical team must directly and frequently observe the device and patient to make sure that the device is making aerosol and that the patient is inhaling it throughout the course of administration.

Fugitive aerosols can pose a direct and indirect risk to patients, health care workers, and the environment. With only a small percent of aerosol inhaled, it is important to reduce the amount of aerosol that enters the surrounding environment. Simple filters can contain fugitive aerosol produced by continuous nebulizers, and the use of filters in the expiratory limb of ventilator circuits can protect sensitive sensors from aerosol accumulation and reduce fugitive emissions by more than 50%.

Infection Risks and Maintenance

JN and USN have open medication reservoirs, which can collect contaminated condensate or secretions, contaminating medications being nebulized. These devices should be replaced, rinsed, washed, air dried, disinfected, and/or sterilized after each dose. In contrast, pMDI and VMNs are not prone to such contamination, with CDC recommendations that they do not require cleaning after each dose.

Further Reading

1 Ari, A. (2015 Jun). Aerosol therapy in pulmonary critical care. *Respiratory Care* 60 (6): 858–874.

2 Ari, A. and Fink, J.B. (2016). Aerosol delivery devices for the treatment of adult patients in acute and critical care. *Current Pharmaceutical Biotechnology* 17 (14): 1268–1277.

3 Ari, A. and Fink, J. (2017). Humidity and aerosol devices. In: *Mosby's Respiratory Care Equipment*, 10e (ed. J.M. Cairo), 156–200. St. Lois: Elsevier Mosby.

4 Fink, J. and Ari, A. (2013). Aerosols and administration of medication. In: *Neonatal and Pediatric Respiratory Care*, 4e (ed. B.K. Walsh), 163–195. St. Louis, MO: Elsevier Saunders.

5 Ari, A. (2016 Aug). Drug delivery interfaces: a way to optimize inhalation therapy in spontaneously breathing children. *World Journal of Clinical Pediatrics* 5 (3): 281–287.

6 Lin, H.L., Wan, G.H., Chen, Y.H. et al. (2012 Nov). Influence of nebulizer type with different pediatric aerosol masks on drug deposition in a model of spontaneously breathing small child. *Respiratory Care* 57 (11): 1894–1900.

7 Ari, A., Atalay, O.T., Harwood, R. et al. (2010 Jul). Influence of nebulizer type position and bias flow on aerosol drug delivery in simulated pediatric and adult lung models during mechanical ventilation. *Respiratory Care* 55 (7): 845–851.

8 Dunne, R.B. and Shortt, S. (2018 Apr). Comparison of bronchodilator administration with vibrating mesh nebulizer and standard jet nebulizer in the emergency department. *The American Journal of Emergency Medicine* 36 (4): 641–646.

9 Ari, A. and Fink, J.B. (2016 Apr). Differential medical aerosol device and interface selection in patients during spontaneous, conventional mechanical and noninvasive ventilation. *Journal of Aerosol Medicine and Pulmonary Drug Delivery* 29 (2): 95–106.

10 Zhang, Z., Xu, P., Fang, Q. et al. (2019 Aug). On behalf of China Union of Respiratory Care (CURC). Practice pattern of aerosol therapy among patients undergoing mechanical ventilation in mainland China: a web-based survey involving 447 hospitals. *PLoS One* 14 (8): e0221577. eCollection 2019.

11 Alcoforado, L., Ari, A., Barcelar, J.M. et al. (2019 Jul). Impact of gas flow and humidity on trans-nasal aerosol deposition via nasal cannula in adults: a randomized cross-over study. *Pharmaceutics* 11: 320.

12 Li, J., Zhao, M., Hadeer, M. et al. (2019). Dose response to transnasal pulmonary administration of bronchodilator aerosols via nasal high-flow therapy in adults with stable chronic obstructive pulmonary disease and asthma. *Respiration* 98 (5): 401–409. Epub ahead of print 2019 Aug 30.

13 DiBlasi, R.M., Crotwell, D.N., Shen, S. et al. (2016 Mar). Iloprost drug delivery during infant conventional and high frequency oscillatory ventilation. *Pulmonary Circulation* 6 (1): 63–69.

14 Dellweg, D., Wachtel, H., Höhn, E. et al. (2011 Dec). *In vitro* validation of a Respimat® adapter for delivery of inhaled bronchodilators during mechanical ventilation. *Journal of Aerosol Medicine and Pulmonary Drug Delivery* 24 (6): 285–292.

15 Michotte, J.B., Jossen, E., Roeseler, J. et al. (2014 Dec). *In vitro* comparison of five nebulizers during noninvasive ventilation: analysis of inhaled and lost doses. *Journal of Aerosol Medicine and Pulmonary Drug Delivery* 27 (6): 430–440.

16 Galindo-Filho, V.C., Alcoforado, L., Rattes, C. et al. (2019 Jul). A mesh nebulizer is more effective than jet nebulizer to nebulize bronchodilators during non-invasive ventilation of subjects with COPD: a randomized controlled trial with radiolabeled aerosols. *Respiratory Medicine* 153: 60–67.

17 Velasco, J. and Berlinski, A. (2018 Feb). Albuterol delivery efficiency in a pediatric model of noninvasive ventilation with double-limb circuit. *Respiratory Care* 63 (2): 141–146.

18 Li, J., Elshafei, A.A., Gong, L., and Fink, J.B. (2019). Aerosol delivery during continuous high frequency oscillation for simulated adults during quiet and distressed spontaneous breathing. *Respiratory Care 64* (Suppl 10): 3229835.

19 Fang, T.P., Ling, H.L., Chiu, S.H. et al. (2016 Oct). Aerosol delivery using jet nebulizer and vibrating mesh nebulizer during high frequency oscillatory ventilation: an *in vitro* comparison. *Journal of Aerosol Medicine Pulmonary Drug Delivery* 29 (5): 447–453.

20 Ari, A. and Fink, J.B. (2012 June). Off-label use of nebulized medications in respiratory care. *Treatment Strategies – Respiratory* 3 (1): 41–44.

21 Reddel, H.K., Bateman, E.D., Becker, A. et al. (2015 Sep). A summary of the new GINA strategy: a roadmap to asthma control. *The European Respiratory Journal* 46 (3): 622–639.

22 Kirkland, S.W., Vandenberghe, C., Voaklander, B. et al. (2017 Jan). Combined inhaled beta-agonist and anticholinergic agents for emergency management in adults with asthma. *Cochrane Database Systematic Review* (1): CD001284. https://doi.org/10.1002/14651858. CD001284.pub2.

23 Ari, A., Fink, J., Harwood, R., and Pilbeam, S. (2016). Secondhand aerosol exposure during mechanical ventilation with and without expiratory filters: an in-vitro study. *Indian Journal of Respiratory Care* 5 (1): 677–682.

24 Saeed, H., Mohsen, M., Fink, J.B. et al. (2017). Fill volume, humidification and heat effects on aerosol delivery and fugitive emission during noninvasive ventilation. *Journal of Drug Delivery Science Technology* 39: 372–378.

25 Seto, W.H. (2015 Apr). Airborne transmission and precautions: facts and myths. *The Journal of Hospital Infection* 89 (4): 225–228.

29

Secretion Clearance Devices

Amanda J. Nickel[1], Daniel Dawson[1], and Oscar H. Mayer[2,3]

[1] Department of Respiratory Care Services, Children's Hospital of Philadelphia, Philadelphia, PA, USA
[2] Division of Pulmonary and Sleep Medicine, Children's Hospital of Philadelphia, Philadelphia, PA, USA
[3] Department of Pediatrics, Perelman School of Medicine at the University of Pennsylvania, Philadelphia, PA, USA

Before discussing how to support ineffective airway clearance, it is important to first describe normal airway clearance, which is facilitated by two physiologic mechanisms. The mucociliary escalator is composed of cilia that line the airways and beat at a frequency of 8–20 hertz to propel secretions from distal to proximal airways. Cilia along the airway epithelium are designed to trap foreign matter and mobilize fluid and mucus cephalad to maintain a healthy respiratory tract. Average production is 10–100 ml of secretions per day, which are expelled from the airways by coughing. A cough is a four-phase maneuver that requires both inspiratory and expiratory muscle strength, but also coordination of each maneuver.

1) Full inspiration
2) Forceful exhalation
3) Transient glottic closing that causes increased intrathoracic pressure
4) Explosive high flow exhalation after glottic opening

Management of both acute and chronic pulmonary illnesses often requires assisted airway intervention to promote effective cough, aid in the mobilization of secretions, improve atelectasis and airway collapse, which in turn can improve lung mechanics and reduce respiratory load, and facilitate adequate gas exchange. It is important to use a strategy for airway clearance appropriate to the patient's capability and condition. There are clinical scenarios where the cough is ineffective and needs to be augmented as with mechanical insufflation–exsufflation (the so-called cough assist), while, in other situations, the cough is effective, but the secretions are thick or adherent and mucus mobilization therapies may be needed.

The strategies used to facilitate secretion clearance depend on the nature of the patient's disease state. Table 29.1 summarizes some of the pathophysiologic issues, therapeutic approaches, devices, and medications used to assist patients. Many of these devices are discussed below. Inhaled medications are also discussed in a separate chapter on respiratory medications.

Emergency Management of the Hi-Tech Patient in Acute and Critical Care, First Edition. Edited by Ioannis Koutroulis, Nicholas Tsarouhas, Richard J. Lin, Jill C. Posner, Michael Seneff, and Robert Shesser.
© 2021 John Wiley & Sons Ltd. Published 2021 by John Wiley & Sons Ltd.

Table 29.1 Pathophysiologies in secretion clearance and methods, devices, and medications for assisting.

Pathophysiologic issue	Intervention	Device/medication
Inadequate cough	Cough replacement therapies	Cough assist devices
Failure of transport mechanics	Postural drainage and percussion	Percussors, pneumatic percussors
	Mechanized external therapies	HFCWO
	Mechanized internal therapies	IPV, Metaneb, Flutter, Acapella
Altered respiratory mechanics	Active cycle breathing, autogenic drainage, forced expiratory techniques	
	Lung expansion and recruitment	Incentive spirometry, IPPB, CPAP, EPAP, PEP
Abnormal secretion characteristics	mucolytics	Dornase alfa, N-acetylcysteine
	Expectorants	Hypertonic saline
	mucokinetics, mucoregulators	

Cough Augmentation

Mechanical insufflation/exsufflation

It is frequently also known as a CoughAssist® (Emerson, Philips Respironics). The CoughAssist supports coughing for patients unable to adequately generate enough force to cough effectively. This may be due to respiratory muscle weakness or the presence of an artificial airway and pharmacologic sedation. The device is connected to the patient's airway via a face mask, endotracheal tube, or tracheostomy tube. With the insufflation phase, the device applies a set positive pressure to help the patient inhale fully. After inhalation (insufflation), the cough assist is shifted to exhalation (exsufflation) using negative pressure to help expel secretions, simulating a cough. Figure 29.1 shows examples of cough assist devices.

In pediatrics, the pressures used are typically in the 30–40 cm H_2O range for both insufflation and exsufflation, though, in younger children or children naïve to the cough assist, pressures below 30 cm H_2O may be used. The choice of pressure is based both on visual assessment of chest wall motion and patient comfort/tolerance. For example, patients may have an uncomfortable sense of pharyngeal collapse when the exsufflation pressure is applied (via mask). When that occurs, the magnitude of exsufflation pressure is decreased to a more comfortable pressure.

Above all, the settings and technique used with the cough assist should result in the patient having improved airway clearance and decreased severity of respiratory illness. When prescribing a routine for airway clearance to replace an ineffective cough, it is crucial to keep in mind that the need for airway clearance during an acute illness will increase. Any airway clearance routine needs to have the flexibility to accommodate increase in

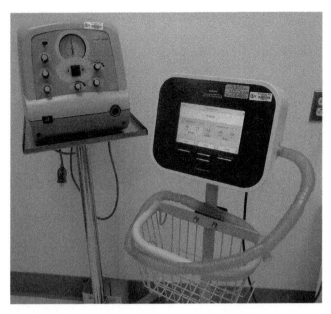

Figure 29.1 Examples of cough assist devices. (*Source:* Michael Duff, RRT, Department of Respiratory Care, The Children's Hospital of Philadelphia.)

frequency of cough assist treatments as needed and to do so at the earliest stages of an acute illness.

A typical cough assist treatment consists of five sets of five insufflation/exsufflation cycles in a row. The inhalation and exhalation phases are each two to three seconds giving time for the target pressure to be reached and held for at least one second. There is then a pause in between breaths that lasts for one to two seconds. After each set of five breaths, the airway is suctioned to remove mobilized mucus. The cough assist can be used both in patients with an artificial airway and with a natural airway. On newer cough assist devices (such as the T70), oscillations of pressure may be imposed on the inhalation phase, exhalation phase, or both. In theory, these oscillations are intended to vibrate the peripheral airways which can help to loosen secretions from the airway mucosa and make them easier to expectorate.

Patients with severe airway obstruction are at increased risk of regional pulmonary overdistention in using the cough assist, and so it is important to use the cough assist cautiously in this population.

Intermittent Positive Pressure Breathing

Intermittent positive pressure breathing (IPPB) is a method of recruiting atelectatic lung units similar to mechanical insufflation–exsufflation in that a positive pressure is applied that helps a patient inhale deeply to get air behind secretions. Exhalation, however, is driven by whatever expiratory force a patient can generate with his/her expiratory muscles on top of the elastic recoil of the lungs and chest wall. IPPB can be delivered via mouthpiece, mask, or artificial airway.

The IPPB delivery system consists of a pressure source that can be triggered by the patient (typically a ventilator or a specific IPPB machine). The pressure is gradually increased as tolerated by the patient until they reach a target exhalation volume.

IPPB facilitates deep breathing and lung recruitment, thus helping patients to mobilize and clear secretions. To further augment airway clearance, a nebulized medication can be administered during the IPPB treatment.

Peripheral Mucus Mobilization

It should be remembered that none of these modalities replace a cough and are only effective in patients with an intact cough, in conjunction with one of the above cough replacement therapies.

Manual Chest Physiotherapy – Chest Physiotherapy (CPT or Chest PT)

Chest physiotherapy (CPT) is an airway secretion clearance technique that applies external percussive forces on the chest using a cupped hand or a padded percussion cup. During the course of therapy, the patient is asked to take intermittent deep breaths and cough. In addition to percussion, postural drainage and vibration are used in conjunction with gravity to assist in clearing secretions. With postural drainage, the patient is placed in a variety of different positions so that the segmental or lobar bronchus that is being percussed is pointing downward to allow the lobe to be drained by gravity. Figure 29.2 describes different chest physiotherapy positions.

CPT is typically performed for at least 30 minutes usually two to four times daily with increased frequency when need for secretion clearance is greater during respiratory illness. Timing of therapy should be before meals or 1½ hours after eating to avoid the risk of vomiting. CPT is usually performed with cupped hands to avoid slapping the skin. Sometimes, a barrier such as a blanket is used to diffuse the force of contact. Some manufacturers, such as Portex® (Palm Cups® Percussors), make plastic percussion cups to assist with and allow for consistent delivery of manual CPT. Figure 29.3 shows examples of percussion devices. These are made of soft plastic and are designed to be held either in the caregiver's hand or via a handle. They are intended to provide percussive force in place of the caregiver's hand. Available sizes range from neonatal to adult. These percussion cups absorb the force of physiotherapy. Some manufacturers claim the device helps to provide uniform and consistent CPT from one user to the next. Sometimes, caregivers will use a small anesthesia mask as an alternative percussion device.

The pneumatic percussor is an alternative to manual CPT. Instead of using the force from a caregiver's hands, the percussion device uses a high-pressure (50 PSI) air or oxygen source to provide rapid pneumatic chest percussions. The device percusses over the chest and can deliver a variety of speeds and intensities. An example is the Fluid Flo handheld pneumatic percussor (Med Systems 2631 Ariane Drive San Diego CA.92117, www.medsystems.com). Such a percussor is not practical in the home setting since these types of

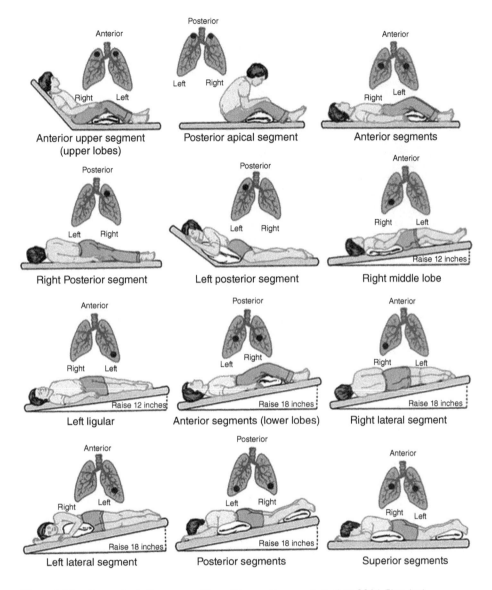

Figure 29.2 Chest physiotherapy positions. (*Source:* Kacmarek et al. © 2014, Elsevier.)

percussors require a source of compressed gas. However, there are electrically powered percussors that can be used for the same purpose.

Intrapulmonary percussive ventilation (IPV) and high-frequency chest wall oscillation (HFCWO) are two therapies that aid the mucociliary escalator by moving secretions from distal to proximal airways where they can be expelled by cough or suctioning. Oscillatory frequencies greater than 3 Hz cause shear forces on mucus in the airways and promote greater expiratory flows than inspiratory flows to favor the movement of secretions cephalad. When frequencies exceed 10 Hz, viscosity of the mucus can actually be reduced.

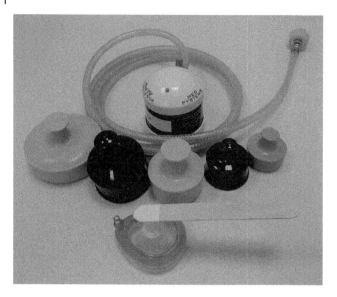

Figure 29.3 Examples of percussion devices. Top row: Pneumatic percussor. Middle row: Manual percussors of different sizes. Bottom row: Example of an anesthesia mask modified with tongue depressor to be used as a percussor. (*Source:* Michael Duff, RRT, Department of Respiratory Care, The Children's Hospital of Philadelphia.)

Evidence suggests that using frequencies between 12 and 22 Hz for a 15- to 30-minute treatment can mimic physiologic mechanisms to propel secretions toward the mouth. While much of the work validating HFCWO is in cystic fibrosis (CF), there has been some work evaluating its utility in patients with neuromuscular disease. A few case studies has reported its usefulness in other diseases; however, no recommendations exist for its regular implementation in other populations.

IPV (Percussionaire Corporation) is a form of high-frequency percussive ventilation. The IPV machine has a pneumatic circuit that functions as a cyclic pressure generator that delivers small volume percussive or high-frequency breaths ranging in frequency from 150 to 500 per minute to the airway while the patient breathes on his or her own. The treatment integrates a jet nebulizer to deliver aerosol therapy to humidify and thin respiratory secretions. Typically, the treatment involves alternating between periods of high-frequency, low-volume breaths and low-frequency, high-volume breaths. The high-frequency period helps with the mobilization of peripheral secretions, while the low-frequency period helps with the movement of secretions to the larger, more central airways. IPV therapy can be given via mouthpiece, mask, or artificial airway.

The hospital version requires a source of compressed gas (usually oxygen) to run the IPV machine. There are two home versions which have a built-in compressor to run the pneumatic circuit which generates the high-frequency percussive ventilation. The more portable version has a weaker compressor and requires a longer period of time to complete a session of treatment.

A similar device which incorporates a nebulizer and rapid positive pressure breaths is the MetaNeb manufactured by Hill ROM (Figure 29.4). The MetaNeb can treat a patient in three different ways: (i) nebulizer only, (ii) CPEP (continuous positive expiratory pressure), and (iii) CHFO (continuous high-frequency oscillation). The CPEP mode helps recruit

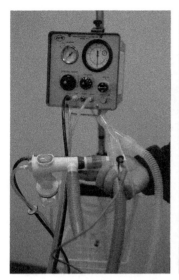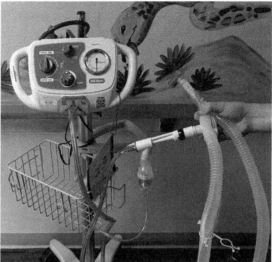

Figure 29.4   IPV (left) and Metaneb (right) machines configured to work with ventilator circuit. (*Source:* Michael Duff, RRT, Department of Respiratory Care, Children's Hospital of Philadelphia and Tricia Cunningham, RRT, Clinical Director of Respiratory Care, Voorhees Pediatric Facility.)

lung units and open airways, which helps combat atelectasis. The CHFO mode uses oscillatory pressures to facilitate the movement of secretions in a fashion similar to that of IPV. Like IPV, MetaNeb treatments can be given via mouthpiece, mask, or artificial airway, and nebulization continues during all phases of treatment. A MetaNeb treatment consists of alternating periods of CPEP and CHFO therapies until the nebulization is complete. The system is driven by gas pressure, so it is only practical for hospital use at this time. As of this writing, Hillrom has released a system called the Volara which has a self-contained compressor, which allows it to be used in the non-hospital setting. This system can do CPEP, CHFO, and nebulization therapies in a fashion similar to the MetaNeb.

HFCWO uses an inflatable vest or wrap which is secured around the upper chest. Some commercial machines available include The Vest® System, inCourage®, Smart Vest, and AffloVest®. HFCWO is connected with tubing to a generator device that creates high-frequency pneumatic pulses (Figure 29.5). The pulses from the generator rapidly inflate and partially deflate the vest, creating a vibration on the chest wall that is transmitted on to the airways. This vibration has been shown to decrease the viscosity of respiratory secretions and, in a fashion similar to IPV, create coaxial ventilation to help move secretions proximally. The settings (vibration frequency, pressure, and length of time) are determined by the personal assessment of the patient by an experienced respiratory therapist. The settings need to be customized to each patient individually with the device in place.

Handheld Devices

Not all devices used to assist with airway clearance are complex and require the assistance of a respiratory therapist or caregiver. There are several simple devices that can be self-administered by patients who have normal respiratory muscle strength.

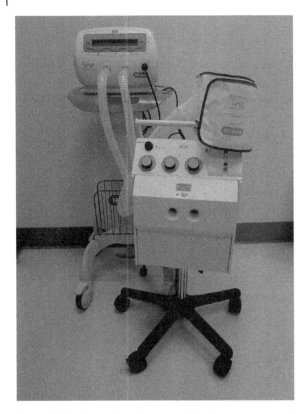

Figure 29.5 Examples of therapeutic high-frequency chest wall oscillatory machines. (*Source:* Michael Duff, RRT, Department of Respiratory Care, The Children's Hospital of Philadelphia.)

Positive expiratory pressure (PEP) therapy is helpful because it can combat atelectasis by opening distal airways which, in turn, can help with the mobilization of secretions. Devices like the TheraPEP (Smiths Medical) and Threshold PEP (Respironics) have a resistance that the patient exhales against to create the PEP. The TheraPEP can also be combined with a nebulization or MDI spacer so that aerosol therapy can be delivered with the pressure therapy.

Other devices, such as the Flutter (Aptalis), Acapella (Smiths Medical), and Aerobika (Monaghan Medical), combine PEP therapy with oscillations in pressure during exhalation to augment clearance of secretions. These are compact devices that are portable and easy for patients to use. Some examples of handheld devices used as adjuncts for clearance can be found in Figure 29.6.

Pharmacotherapy

Mucus is a combination of proteins, carbohydrates, water, and cellular debris, including white blood cells and infectious material. There are a variety of pharmacotherapies available to address different components of airway mucus and most of them can be nebulized in the devices discussed above.

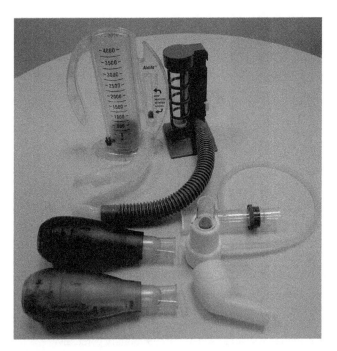

Figure 29.6 Handheld devices used as adjuncts for clearance. Top row: Two sizes of incentive spirometers. Bottom left: Two versions of Acapella devices (darker device for flows <15 lpm, lighter device for flows >15 lpm). Bottom right: Example of TheraPEP and Flutter valve. (*Source:* Michael Duff, RRT, Department of Respiratory Care, The Children's Hospital of Philadelphia.)

The medications used for secretion clearance come from extensive clinical research and experience in the treatment of CF, a disease in which the mucus becomes thick and viscous due to the absence or dysfunction of an epithelial chloride channel. N-acetylcysteine (Mucomyst®) is believed to work by destroying disulfide bonds between mucin molecules, but has largely been superseded by dornase alfa (Pulmozyme®), which cleaves DNA. This is effective in CF because the mucus is purulent and replete with neutrophilic DNA, which makes the mucus very thick. Although Pulmozyme has been shown to be efficacious in CF, it has not been shown to be effective in other conditions. It is reasonable to consider prescribing it in conditions with purulent mucus during the acute phase of therapy; however, there is no evidence to support chronic use outside of the CF population.

Hypertonic saline is an expectorant agent used to treat thick, retained secretions and is administered in 3, 7, 9, and 12% concentrations. Seven percent hypertonic saline is standard therapy in CF and functions by drawing water from the airway epithelium to hydrate secretions when delivered by nebulization. Research in CF demonstrated that the balance between effect (mucus expectoration) versus side-effect (bronchoconstriction) was optimal with the administration of 7%, though, in select situations, 9 and 12% can be used with caution. Frequently, albuterol or another bronchodilator is administered prior to hypertonic saline to minimize bronchoconstriction. While there is no evidence to support the use of nebulized hypertonic saline in patients without CF, it may be reasonable to consider it (as well as systemic hydration) when respiratory secretions are thick due to dehydration. However, it is important to keep in mind that hypertonic saline will hydrate mucus whether it is thick or has normal viscosity. In the latter situation, overuse of hypertonic saline can have the unwanted effect of producing copious thin secretions. For that reason, it needs to be used selectively and with a limited duration. Constant assessment and reevaluation of secretion characteristics is important in order to modify all airway clearance therapies accordingly.

Further Reading

1 Panitch, H.B. (2017). Respiratory implications of pediatric neuromuscular disease. *Respiratory Care* 62 (6): 826–848.

2 Mirra, V., Werner, C., and Santamaria, F. (2017). Primary ciliary dyskinesia: an update on clinical aspects, genetics, diagnosis, and future treatment strategies. *Frontiers in Pediatrics* 5 (135): 1–13.

3 McIlwaine, M., Bradley, J., Elborn, J.S., and Moran, F. (2017). Personalising airway clearance in chronic lung disease. *European Respiratory Review* 26: 1–12.

4 Ginderdeuren, F.V., Vandenplas, Y., Deneyer, M. et al. (2017). Effectiveness of airway clearance techniques in children hospitalized with acute bronchiolitis. *Pediatric Pulmonology* 52: 225–231.

5 Deakins, K. and Chatburn, R.L. (2002). A comparison of intrapulmonary percussive ventilation and conventional chest physiotherapy for the treatment of atelectasis in the pediatric patient. *Respiratory Care* 47 (10): 1162–1167.

6 Strickland, S.L., Rubin, B.K., Drescher, G.S. et al. (2013). AARC clinical practice guideline: effectiveness of nonpharmacologic airway clearance therapies in hospitalized patients. *Respiratory Care* 58 (12): 2187–2193.

7 Lee, A.L., Button, B.M., and Esta-Lee, T. (2017). Airway-clearance techniques in children and adolescents with chronic suppurative lung disease and bronchiectasis. *Frontiers in Pediatrics* 5 (2): 1–8.

8 Flume, P.A., Robinson, K.A., O'Sullivan, B.P. et al. (2009). Cystic fibrosis pulmonary guidelines: airway clearance therapies. *Respiratory Care* 54 (4): 522–537.

9 Lee, A.L., Burge, A.T., and Holland, A.E. (2015 Nov 23). Airway clearance techniques for bronchiectasis. *Cochrane Database Syst Rev.* 2015 (11): CD008351. https://doi.org/10.1002/14651858.CD008351.pub3.

10 Strickland, S.L., Rubin, B.K., Haas, C.F. et al. (2015). AARC clinical practice guideline: effectiveness of pharmacologic airway clearance therapies in hospitalized patients. *Respiratory Care* 60 (7): 1071–1077.

11 Bach, J.R. (1993 Nov). Mechanical insufflation-exsufflation. Comparison of peak expiratory flows with manually assisted and unassisted coughing techniques. *Chest* 104 (5): 1553–1562.

12 Koenig, E., Singh, B., and Wood, J. (2016). Mechanical insufflation-exsufflation for an individual with duchenne muscular dystrophy and a lower respiratory infection. *Respirology Case Reports* 5 (2): 1–3.

13 Kallet, R.H. (2013). Adjunct therapies during mechanical ventilation: airway clearance techniques, therapeutic aerosols, and gases. *Respiratory Care* 58 (6): 1053–1071.

14 Hirsch, C.A. (2017)). *CPT positions - Egan's Fundamentals of Respiratory Care, Chapter 43, Airway Clearance Therapy*. St. Louis, MO: Elsevier.

15 Lechtzin, N., Wolfe, L.F., and Frick, K.D. (2016 Jun). The impact of high-frequency chest wall oscillation on healthcare use in patients with neuromuscular diseases. *Annals of the American Thoracic Society* 13 (6): 904–909. https://doi.org/10.1513/AnnalsATS.201509-597OC.

16 Donaldson, S.H., Bennett, W.D., Zeman, K.L. et al. (2006 Jan 19). Mucus clearance and lung function in cystic fibrosis with hypertonic saline. *The New England Journal of Medicine* 354 (3): 241–250.

17 Elkins, M.R., Robinson, M., Rose, B.R. et al. (2006 Jan 19). A controlled trial of long-term inhaled hypertonic saline in patients with cystic fibrosis. *The New England Journal of Medicine* 354 (3): 229–240.

18 Gauld, L.M. (2009). Airway clearance in neuromuscular weakness. *Developmental Medicine & Child Neurology* 51: 350–355.

19 Chatburn, R.L. (2007). High-frequency assisted airway clearance. *Respiratory Care* 52 (9): 1224–1235.

20 Kacmarek, R.M., Stoller, J.K., Heuer, A.J., and Egan, D.F. (2014). *Egan's Fundamentals of Respiratory Care*, 10e, 954–957. St. Louis, Mo: Elsevier/Mosby.

30

Non-invasive Ventilation

Oscar H. Mayer[1,2] and Anthony Mozzone[3]

[1] *Division of Pulmonary and Sleep Medicine, Children's Hospital of Philadelphia, Philadelphia, PA, USA*
[2] *Department of Pediatrics, Perelman School of Medicine at the University of Pennsylvania, Philadelphia, PA, USA*
[3] *Promptcare Respiratory, King of Prussia, PA, USA*

Successful ventilation requires two components: a ventilator to produce the pressure or volume that becomes the breath and an interface through which the breath is given to the patient. Although in acute illness ventilation is achieved with the use of an endotracheal tube, in more chronic conditions, the interface can be a tracheostomy tube for invasive ventilation or a nasal, oronasal, full-face, or oral interface for non-invasive ventilation (NIV). While the physiologic titration to optimize patient ventilation and gas exchange is the central purpose of initiating ventilatory support, identifying and accommodating to a comfortable interface is absolutely critical for NIV. We will discuss both components of this process below.

Components of Non-Invasive Ventilation

Interfaces

The hardest part of NIV is finding and fitting the right mask. The team in the hospital starts this process, but the home care company is often brought in with more mask choices than the hospital may have. The choices are nasal masks, nasal pillows, or full-face masks. The choice will depend on the size, age, dexterity, and patient preference. The goal of the interface is to be comfortable for the patient and to have a good fit to the contour of their nose or face (depending on the type of mask). The fit should minimize uncontrolled leak around the mask so that a patient can get the full benefit of support from the ventilator. Uncontrolled leak will also be influenced by the tightness of the headgear which secures the mask and the pressures used to ventilate the patient.

There is a limitation on choices with smaller patients due to the lack of good, pediatric masks. There are multiple mask options for adults. Masks were limited for pediatrics because of the weight limitation on continuous positive airway pressure (CPAP) and bi-level positive airway pressure (BlPAP) machines, but manufacturers are now developing

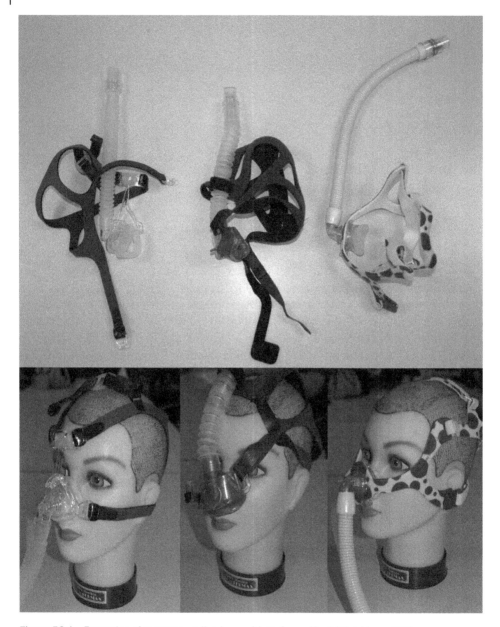

Figure 30.1 Examples of common pediatric nasal interfaces: Noni, Mini-Me, and Wisp. (*Source:* Michael Duff, RRT, Department of Respiratory Care, Children's Hospital of Philadelphia, Philadelphia, PA 19104)

more choices. Facial breakdown and anomalies also impact the decision. Mask interfaces can be secured with straps or headgear, and, sometimes, some creativity is required to adjust or select headgear components to get the best fit. Children are often provided two different styles of interface, such as pillows and nasal mask. The goal is to choose interfaces

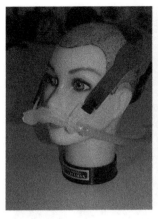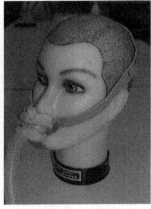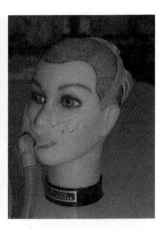

Figure 30.2 Examples of nasal pillow interfaces: SNAPP, Airfit P10, and Swift FX Bella. (*Source:* Michael Duff, RRT, Department of Respiratory Care, Children's Hospital of Philadelphia, Philadelphia, PA 19104)

that have different pressure points and alternate them to reduce the risk of irritation and breakdown. Barriers, such as Mepilex® Lite (Mölnlycke Healthcare), can be used as additional protection from pressure points of the interface on the skin.

AG Noni (AG industries), Mini-me (Sleepnet), and The Wisp Giraffe (Philips Respironics) are three of the most common and successful pediatric masks (Figure 30.1). The SNAPP (Carefusion), Nasal Aire (Innomed), AirFit P10 (ResMed), and Swift FX Bella (ResMed) are good nasal pillow options (Figure 30.2). There are some off-label choices for extremely small patients, but this is not supported by all home respiratory companies. Finding the right mask is trial and error, and this often takes a number of attempts before finding an interface that will work. A full-face mask is not recommended for children who are unable to get out of the mask on their own, and there are not many small choices for that reason. Such an interface may not be appropriate if the patient has issues with copious oral secretions or a history of gastroesophageal reflux disease.

Another nuance about interfaces is that some come in "vented" or "non-vented" versions. The distinction is important because that has implications for what kind of ventilator circuit the mask can be used with. As we will discuss below, most NIV ventilators are single limb and require the presence of a controlled leak to allow the exhaled gas to leave the circuit and not be re-breathed. Most interfaces are "vented" and have the leak built into the mask, which means that they are ready to be used with a single limb circuit. Interfaces that are "non-vented" need to have a leak valve added into the circuit if it is single limb. On the other hand, only non-vented interfaces can be used with a dual limb circuit, which is sometimes done when a patient who uses NIV becomes ill and is put on a hospital ventilator. A vented interface has too much leak to be used with a dual limb circuit, leading to patient–ventilator desynchrony due to an inability to trigger the initiation and then termination of a breath (Figure 30.3).

Having an experienced clinician with a broad understanding of the available interfaces come to work with the patient and parents to identify and fit an appropriate mask and backup mask can play a large role in identifying a good interface for the patient.

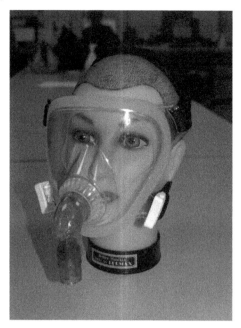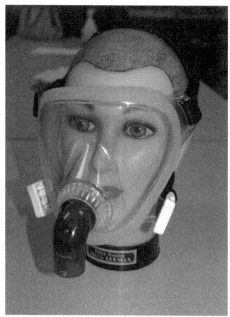

Figure 30.3 Vented and non-vented versions of the FitLife mask (Philips), an example of a full-face mask. The vent can be seen in the angled connector which is attached to the mask. (*Source:* Michael Duff, RRT, Department of Respiratory Care, Children's Hospital of Philadelphia, Philadelphia, PA 19104)

Ventilator and Circuit

Mechanical ventilation is usually described by (i) what defines the breath (pressure or volume) and (ii) the mode of ventilation, which describes how the ventilator responds to the patient's breathing effort. The breath in NIV is always defined as a pressure because of the necessary leak in NIV circuits and masks. The most common modes of non-invasive support are CPAP and BIPAP (Figure 30.4).

With CPAP, there is just one level of constant pressure that keeps the airway open, as is done in patients with obstructive sleep apnea. A common range is 4–10 cm H_2O. The ventilator adjusts flow to maintain the pressure at the prescribed setting. CPAP is not ventilatory support and, therefore, cannot be used to treat respiratory failure from hypoventilation and correct the resultant hypercarbia.

With the BIPAP mode, there are two levels of pressure: a higher one called inspiratory positive airway pressure (IPAP) and a lower one called expiratory positive airway pressure (EPAP). The ventilator stays at the EPAP until the ventilator detects a patient's respiratory effort. With the effort, the ventilator cycles to IPAP and then returns to EPAP after the patient's flow drops below a certain threshold or after a certain time period. BIPAP can be further distinguished by whether there is a backup rate (a rate below which the ventilator begins cycling breaths regardless of patient effort). If there is no backup rate and the patient only gets breaths on demand, this is often referred to as a spontaneous (S) mode. If there is a backup rate in case a patient cannot or does not trigger a breath, this is referred to as a spontaneous-timed (S-T) mode.

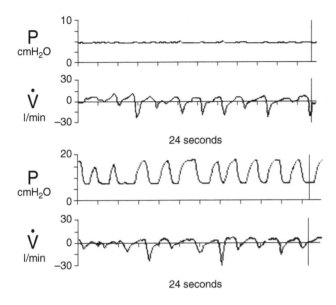

Figure 30.4 CPAP and BIPAP waveforms: tracings are pairs of pressure and flow over time. The top pair shows a patient on CPAP. The bottom pair shows the same patient on BIPAP. (*Source:* Courtesy of Richard Lin)

Beyond this, some of the newer ventilators have settings that allow automatic adjustment of the pressure used for a breath based on the way a patient is breathing. These include a volume-targeted mode like average Volume Assured Pressure Support (AVAPS) in the Trilogy® (Philips) and Intelligent Volume Assured Pressure Support in the Astral® (ResMed). These are not identical modes and are specific to their manufactured machine. They both adjust pressure settings to maintain a consistent tidal volume. This is a useful mode to use in patients with variable respiratory compliance and will adjust to the patient's needs according to the prescribed settings for tidal volume. The Trilogy also has an AVAPS A/E version which adds an auto-titrating EPAP.

MPV is the mouthpiece ventilation and this is typically used in volume or pressure without an EPAP or breath rate. This is used while awake and often when the patient is portable in a wheelchair. This gives the patient a break from the mask and can help decrease the likelihood of skin breakdown. This is often used in patients with neuromuscular disorders who have a need for diurnal ventilation (Figure 30.5).

NIV is most commonly done by dedicated portable machines that are designed for that purpose. These machines consist of a turbine to generate flow, the flow needed to achieve the prescribed pressures. There is one tube or circuit coming from the ventilator and delivering flow to the interface. For the patient to be able to exhale, there is a leak either at the mask or a leak valve in the circuit through which the patient exhales when the ventilator cycles from IPAP to EPAP (Figures 30.6 and 30.7). Traditional invasive ventilators can also be used for non-invasive support; however, one adjustment has to be made. Invasive ventilators are almost all dual limb, meaning that there is an inspiratory limb used to deliver a flow of gas to the patient and an expiratory limb through which the patient exhales. Flow through the expiratory limb is regulated by a ventilator-controlled valve. Since there is a

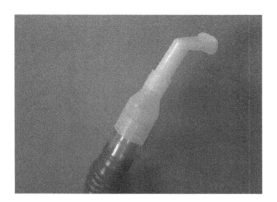

Figure 30.5 Example of a mouthpiece interface that can be used by a patient for "on-demand" ventilation. (*Source:* Michael Duff, RRT, Department of Respiratory Care, Children's Hospital of Philadelphia, Philadelphia, PA 19104)

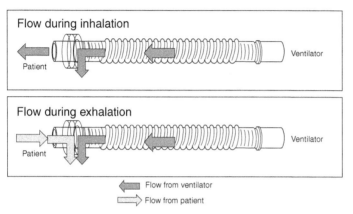

Figure 30.6 Flow in a single limb circuit with an intentional leak valve during different phases of respiration. When using a vented non-invasive mask, the intentional leak is at the mask and a separate valve is not needed. (*Source:* Courtesy of Richard Lin, modified from diagrams from Philips Respironics)

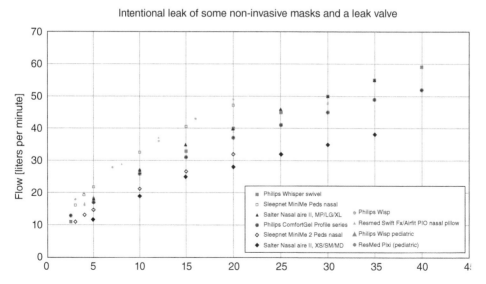

Figure 30.7 Graph showing intentional leak flow required to achieve pressures with different non-invasive interfaces (and a commonly used intentional leak valve). This does not account for any non-intentional leak from leak around the interface (compiled from manufacturer mask and valve specifications). (*Source:* Courtesy of Richard Lin)

defined path through which the patient will exhale, there is no need for a controlled leak with this type of circuit. In fact, the presence of any leak will make it more difficult to ventilate the patient, and therefore, non-vented styles of NIV interfaces are necessary. A vented interface has too much leak to be used with a dual limb circuit, leading to insensitivity for triggering and loss of support.

The Practice of Non-invasive Ventilation

Once an interface is identified and a strategy of ventilation is selected, the final step is putting the plan into action. Care needs to be taken, especially with younger patients, to allow them to accommodate the mask initially by placing the mask on their face without headgear, then with the headgear in place, with the ventilator circuit attached, and then with the BIPAP unit on and delivering breaths. Communication with the patient when awake allows for the opportunity to assess the level of comfort with ventilation pressures and timing. However, once in bed, trying to fall asleep, some patients may have trouble with the sensation of air blowing on or in their nose. For this situation, most ventilators have a "ramp" feature to slowly increase the pressures up to the prescribed pressures over a period of time. This allows a patient to fall asleep as the NIV is initiating and can improve tolerance.

Traditional CPAP and BIPAP machines are only approved for patients weighing 30 kgs or more, and they do not have a backup battery system, which makes them inappropriate for patients requiring continuous ventilation. However, newer machines, like the Trilogy from Phillips and Astral from Resmed, are approved for 5 kgs and up. The Trilogy Evo, which is the newest version of the Trilogy is approved for patients 2.5 kg and up. However, one should remember that the variety of non-invasive interfaces for even 5 kg patients is limited. These newer devices come with car chargers and battery systems for portability and power outages. Thus, these systems are appropriate for continuous use. Should a patient only need ventilatory support at night, then one of the traditional BIPAP units could be used.

There are various machines from several manufacturers with different capabilities. The team will usually look for the right fit that best meets the clinical needs of the patient. Most manufacturers have traditional settings for CPAP and BIPAP auto-titrating features, heated humidifiers, and limited alarm features. The Astral, Trilogy, and similar NIV machines have greater capabilities for patient needs and a better alarm package. These machines offer traditional CPAP, BIPAP, volume ventilation, pressure ventilation, and MPV.

All new CPAP, BIPAP, and NIV machines have a memory to track usage and data. These devices can get their data downloaded via modem, Bluetooth, SD card, or on-site interface. These features help the team monitor and adjust settings as needed in the home setting. There are several options to choose from, so communication with the discharging team is imperative.

Monitoring gas exchange is critical in determining the proper BIPAP support for a patient. Since the ultimate purpose is ensuring proper gas exchange (oxygen [O_2] delivery and carbon dioxide [CO_2] removal), both CO_2 and CO_2 need to be measured continuously. Because of the nasal flow from BIPAP or CPAP, nasal end tidal CO_2 will not work properly. However, transcutaneous CO_2 can provide a good trend of capillary CO_2. These monitors require a fair amount of maintenance for them to have reliable readings and are typically only used in the hospital or sleep lab setting. They only provide a trend and not breath-to-breath CO_2 analysis.

Once gas exchange is optimized, it is important to ensure that work of breathing is minimized. This can be assessed by how synchronously the chest wall and abdomen are moving during respiration, or the level of thoracoabdominal asynchrony. This can be assessed qualitatively by assessing the patient or objectively during a sleep study by using thoracic and abdominal inductance bands.

If there is a problem with patient tolerance, gas exchange, or work of breathing, it is important to go through a comprehensive assessment in order to identify the problem. First, ensure that the nasal mask is seated properly on the nose and that there is no air leak around the periphery, and if there is, try reseating the mask or trying another interface (mask or cannula). Second, ensure that the mouth is closed and there is no oral air leak or if there is a leak, consider using a chin strap to keep the mouth closed or changing to an oronasal or full-face mask. Third, ensure that there is no non-intentional leak in the ventilator circuit and that all connections are intact.

Finally, if there is poor patient–ventilator synchrony, then there may be adjustments that can be made to the ventilator settings. This may include increasing the triggering sensitivity to make the ventilator more sensitive to patient effort, or changing how the breath ends by making the duration shorter or longer. There may be benefit in adjusting the size of the breath (which is determined by the pressure difference IPAP-EPAP), or adjusting the distending pressure (EPAP) to ensure that the breath is delivered to a fully open upper and lower airway. There are times when it may not be possible for the non-invasive ventilator to sense respiratory effort, particularly in patients who have poor muscular strength. In those cases, it may be possible to pick a breath size and respiratory rate that is adequate to meet the patient's minute ventilation needs and be able to achieve that minute ventilation without complete patient–ventilator synchrony.

Extended troubleshooting can be needed in the scenario where the NIV-dependent patient has an intercurrent illness, such as patients who are on NIV because of muscle weakness. These patients may need admission to an intensive care unit to receive treatments of increased support or increased frequency to overcome their acute illness. These treatments can include increased settings on the non-invasive ventilator or possibly intubation for invasive mechanical ventilation, enhanced clearance therapies or frequencies of existing therapies, and intravenous or inhaled antibiotic therapy as appropriate. Eventually, these patients transition to the pulmonary unit, where support is weaned conservatively paying close attention to heart rate and work of breathing.

When weaning ventilatory support, it is important to follow vital signs, gas exchange parameters, and subjective assessment of work of breathing and patient comfort. For patients with respiratory muscle weakness, they may not exhibit an increased work of breathing with worsening respiratory failure, so experience and insight in performing an assessment is critical. Gas exchange can be followed by continuous pulse oximetry and transcutaneous CO_2 values, whereas end tidal CO_2 monitoring is not feasible because of the nasal interface. Sustained mild hypoxemia and elevated CO_2 values indicate hypoventilation, and there may need to discuss limiting decreases of support or trials off support. Oxygen therapy to treat hypoxemia may actually mask hypoventilation with a tiring sprinting patient, and therefore oxygen must be used cautiously. Airway clearance therapies including bronchodilators, hypertonic saline, intrapulmonary percussive ventilation, and cough assist may be required as adjuncts and may need to be done more frequently than baseline. A decrease in the frequency of episodes of hypoxemia during lengthening of trials on lower support or off support will be evidence to the team that the patient is improving. Trials may start as short as 30 min twice daily and will then gradually lengthen. The weaning strategy of giving a patient time-limited trials on less support is useful as it gives them a chance to recover from the trial period during which they have to do more work of breathing.

Deciding on when an NIV patient can be discharged home from a hospital admission or from an emergency department visit often involves soliciting the input of the Pulmonary team who cares for the patient. They will be the ones who will have the best insight into how compliant and capable the patient and family are and will be responsible for continuing management as an outpatient. Input from caregivers who help care for the patient at home and the home respiratory company is also helpful in understanding whether a regimen of increased care, if required, can be carried out in the home setting.

Further Reading

1 Amaddeo, A., Frapin, A., and Fauroux, B. (2016). Review long-term non-invasive ventilation in children. *The Lancet Respiratory* 12: 1–10.
2 Bach, J.R. and Martinez, D. (2011). Duchenne muscular dystrophy: continuous noninvasive ventilatory support prolongs survival. *Respir Care* 56 (6): 744–750.
3 Eagle, M., Baudouin, S.V., Chandler, C. et al. (2002 Dec). Survival in Duchenne muscular dystrophy: improvements in life expectancy since 1967 and the impact of home nocturnal ventilation. *Neuromuscular Disorders* 12 (10): 926–929.
4 Finkel, R.S., Mercuri, E., Meyer, O.H. et al. (2018). Diagnosis and management of spinal muscular atrophy: part 2: pulmonary and acute care; medications, supplements and immunizations; other organ systems; and ethics. *Neuromuscular Disorders* 28 (3): 197–207.
5 Sawnani, H., Thampratankul, L., Szczesniak, R.D. et al. (2015). Sleep disordered breathing in young boys with Duchenne muscular dystrophy. *The Journal of Pediatrics* 166 (3): 640–641.
6 Birnkrant, D.J., Bushby, K., Bann, C.M. et al. (2018). Diagnosis and management of Duchenne muscular dystrophy, part 2: respiratory, cardiac, bone health, and orthopaedic management. *The Lancet Neurology* 17 (4): 347–361.

31

Tracheostomy Tubes

Joanne Stow[1], Allison E. Boyd[1], and Jerry Cabrera[2]

[1] *Division of Otolaryngology, Department of Surgery, Children's Hospital of Philadelphia, Philadelphia, PA, USA*
[2] *Smith's Medical, Gary, IN, USA*

Introduction

A five-year-old child with a tracheostomy is brought into your emergency department in respiratory distress. He is tachypneic and retracting with pulse oximeter readings in the mid-80s. He is making sounds around his tracheostomy tube. Parents deny any sick contacts. He is not febrile. He was weaned off ventilator support six months ago. Could his distress be related to a problem with his tracheostomy tube? Absolutely.

There are several reasons that a patient may need to have a tracheostomy tube. The major indications are to bypass an inadequate upper airway, to provide a pathway for ventilator support in the home, or to assist with pulmonary clearance (see Table 31.1). The patient may need this artificial airway for an entire lifetime, or it may be temporary. The patient may be undergoing a staged airway reconstruction or may be in the process of working toward decannulation. The patient's airway may be anatomically normal or grossly abnormal. It is important to know why the patient has the tracheostomy tube, the details regarding the tube itself, and the child's current airway to help guide the clinician's airway assessment and need for intervention (see Table 31.2).

This chapter reviews important questions to ask and physical findings to note when first assessing the patient with a tracheostomy tube (see Table 31.3). We will review the anatomy of tracheostomy tubes, discuss the different materials they are made of, describe some of the features these tubes can have, and talk about how they can be custom-designed to accommodate patient anatomy. We will also talk about routine tracheostomy tube selection, care, and maintenance, as well as the steps for performing a tracheostomy tube change and discuss troubleshooting and management in case of an emergency. We review the emergency supplies and equipment that must always accompany a patient with a tracheostomy tube. Finally, we will briefly discuss the use of speaking valves and capping, and touch upon the process of successful decannulation and "graduation" from a tracheostomy tube.

Emergency Management of the Hi-Tech Patient in Acute and Critical Care, First Edition. Edited by
Ioannis Koutroulis, Nicholas Tsarouhas, Richard J. Lin, Jill C. Posner, Michael Seneff, and Robert Shesser.
© 2021 John Wiley & Sons Ltd. Published 2021 by John Wiley & Sons Ltd.

Table 31.1 Examples of indications for a tracheostomy.

Need for chronic ventilatory support	Need to bypass extrathoracic airway obstruction	Need to promote sufficient pulmonary clearance
• Respiratory pump failure – Hypotonia – Guillain-Barre syndrome – Degenerative neurologic or neuromuscular conditions: spinal muscle atrophy (SMA), amyotrophic lateral sclerosis (ALS), and muscular dystrophy – Diaphragmatic paresis – Spinal cord injury • Respiratory control failure – Hypoxic ischemic encephalopathy – Central hypoventilation syndrome: congenital or acquired • Circulatory failure – Left heart failure • Respiratory failure – Tracheomalacia – Bronchomalacia – Restrictive lung disease due to thoracic insufficiency, severe scoliosis/kyphosis – Pulmonary hypoplasia – Chronic lung disease of prematurity (bronchopulmonary dysplasia) – Acute respiratory distress syndrome	• Lymphatic or vascular malformation • Craniofacial anomalies: micrognathia, glossoptosis, midface hypoplasia, and hemifacial microsomia • Facial trauma • Pharyngeal hypotonia • Airway tumor • Bilateral vocal cord paralysis • Glottic stenosis • Subglottic stenosis	• Hypoxic ischemic encephalopathy • Intractable seizure disorder • Hypotonia • Cerebral palsy • Impaired gag or swallow • Guillain-Barre syndrome • Degenerative neurologic or neuromuscular conditions: SMA, ALS, myasthenia gravis, and muscular dystrophy

Tracheostomy Tube Basics

Tracheostomy tubes are commonly called "trach" tubes. Most modern tracheostomies are made of a plastic polymer such as polyvinylchloride (PVC) or polyurethane (PU), or of silicone. Stainless steel tubes used to be commonplace but are less frequently used and very rare in the pediatric population today. The inner diameter (ID) in millimeters is used most often to designate the size of the tube, analogous to the convention for endotracheal tubes. The tube parts (Figure 31.1) consist of the connector, the flange or faceplate, and the shaft of the tube. The connector is an ISO (International Organization for Standardization) standard with 15 mm outer diameter. All tracheostomy tubes have a distal shaft which extends through the tracheal stoma into the trachea. The flange or faceplate has holes or slots on the sides through which the securement device around the neck is anchored. The ID and outer diameter (OD) are usually listed on the tube flange or faceplate (Figure 31.2). Some trach tubes also have the length of the tube printed on the flange or faceplate, while others only have the length listed on the packaging. Most pediatric tracheostomy tubes are

Table 31.2 Airway-related questions for the clinician to ask.

Why does the patient have a tracheostomy?

Is the patient's airway anatomy normal?

Is the patient able to be mask ventilated or intubated from above? If not, what is the plan to secure their airway in the event of decannulation/emergency?

What is the model and size of the tracheostomy tube? Is it a custom-designed tube?

Did you bring a spare trach (same size) with you today?

Did you bring your emergency equipment? [as a public service reminder-recommended items include "go" bag of supplies, oxygen (tank or concentrator), suction machine, pulse oximeter, ventilator (if applicable)]

If trach has a cuff:

   Inflated: Yes/No

   Inflation volume: What is the usual inflation volume? What is it currently inflated with?

   Type of cuff: air, water, or foam

Any difficulty with trach tube changes?

When was the last trach tube change? How often is it usually changed?

Any change in baseline respiratory secretions?

Any changes in baseline respiratory support? More work of breathing or increased need for supplemental oxygen?

Any recent airway surgeries?

Who is the physician that manages the tracheostomy?

Is the patient currently being actively treated for any trach-related issue?

Table 31.3 Initial physical assessment pertaining to tracheostomy.

Tracheostomy stoma site	Erythema, drainage, odor, bleeding, (moist) granulation, (dry) keloids, swelling, crepitus, tenderness, rash, unusual stoma size or shape (should roughly match the diameter of the trach tube). Evaluate markings on the tracheostomy flanges to compare specifications of the tracheostomy tube in situ to what the family/caregiver has reported.
Neck	Tightness of the securement device (typically Velcro ties), erythema, pressure injuries, blisters, rashes, odor
Respiratory effort, phonation	Retractions, air leak around the tracheostomy stoma, air leak through nose/mouth, ability to phonate
Respiratory secretions	Color, amount (change in frequency of suctioning), thickness, odor, bleeding

---

so called "single cannula," meaning that the tube has no removable lining. Many adult tracheostomy tubes are so called "double cannula," because they do have a removable inner lining; these will be discussed more in depth in the following text.

Some tracheostomy tubes also have a proximal shaft which provides additional length between the connector and the flange, allowing the connection to the ventilator circuit to be away from the patient's neck.

If the trach has a cuff, it is usually located near the distal end of the shaft. A cuffed tracheostomy tube has an inflation line which runs from the cuff up along the shaft and extends through the flange. The pilot balloon is as distensible as or more distensible than the cuff itself and acts as an external indicator of whether the cuff is inflated or not.

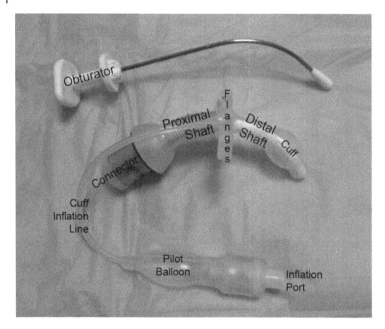

Figure 31.1 Tracheostomy anatomy. Pictured is a Bivona FlexTend TTS tracheostomy tube illustrating parts that can be found in tubes which have a cuff and a proximal shaft.
(*Source:* Courtesy of Michael Duff, RRT, Department of Respiratory Care, The Children's Hospital of Philadelphia, Philadelphia.)

All trach tubes come with an obturator (Figure 31.3), which is a guide made of metal or stiffer plastic and extends the full length of the distal (and proximal, if applicable) shaft and has a blunt tip at the end. It is inserted into the tracheostomy tube before the tube is inserted into the patient. The obturator serves two purposes: (i) stiffen the distal shaft of the tube and (ii) round out the tip of the shaft. This makes it easier to insert the tube through the stoma and guide the tube through the tract to the trachea. With a single cannula trach, the obturator is placed into the tube prior to insertion and then removed after the insertion is completed. With a double cannula trach (which will be discussed in more detail in the following text), the obturator takes the place of the inner cannula during insertion and is replaced with the inner cannula after the insertion.

The curvature of the neonatal and pediatric tubes is less acute than adult tube curvature and is standard amongst all manufacturers.

Tracheostomy Tube Sizing

The size specification is typically done using the ISO 5366 standard, which uses the ID in millimeters, ranging from 2.5 to 11 mm in 0.5 mm increments. The other modifier frequently used for the size specification is the patient age category: neonatal or pediatric. If there is not an age category listed, it is implied to be an "adult" trach. This age category specification determines the curvature and distal shaft length (and proximal shaft length, if applicable) associated with the ID. For the same ID, a pediatric tube is longer than a neonatal and an adult tube is longer than a pediatric (Figure 31.4). Neonatal trach tube sizes start at 2.5 mm ID and increase in 0.5 mm increments up to 4.0 mm. Pediatric trach tube sizes start at 2.5 mm ID and increase in 0.5 mm increments up to 6.0 mm. Adult trach tubes

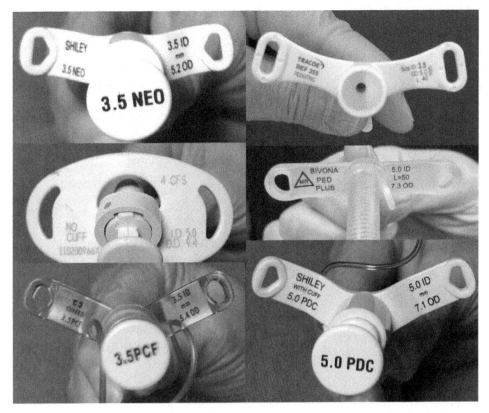

Figure 31.2 Examples of labelling on tracheostomy flanges. Note that usually the ID and OD, and sometimes the distal shaft length, are on the right flange. Other information, such as the manufacturer, style name, reorder information, age category, presence of cuff, and MRI compatibility, are on the left flange. (*Source:* Courtesy of Michael Duff, RRT, Department of Respiratory Care, The Children's Hospital of Philadelphia, Philadelphia.)

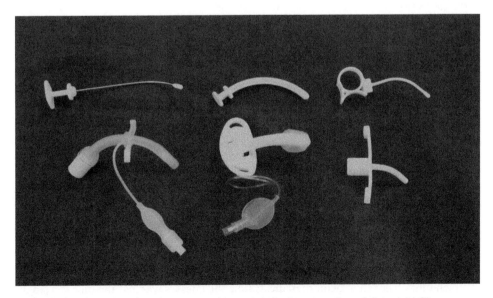

Figure 31.3 Examples of tracheostomy tubes and their obturators. From left to right, Bivona FlexTend TTS, Shiley CFS, and TRACOE mini. (*Source:* Courtesy of Michael Duff, RRT, Department of Respiratory Care, The Children's Hospital of Philadelphia, Philadelphia.)

Relationship of tracheostomy outer diameter and length for a specified inner diameter

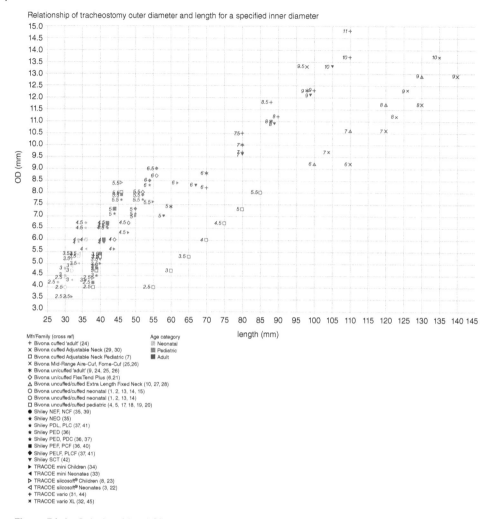

Mfr/Family (cross ref)
+ Bivona cuffed 'adult' (24)
✕ Bivona cuffed Adjustable Neck (29, 30)
☐ Bivona cuffed Adjustable Neck Pediatric (7)
✕ Bivona Mid-Range Aire-Cuf, Fome-Cuf (25,26)
◇ Bivona un/cuffed FlexTend Plus (6,21)
△ Bivona uncuffed/cuffed Extra Length Fixed Neck (10, 27, 28)
○ Bivona uncuffed/cuffed neonatal (1, 2, 13, 14, 15)
○ Bivona uncuffed/cuffed neonatal (1, 2, 13, 14)
☐ Bivona uncuffed/cuffed pediatric (4, 5, 17, 18, 19, 20)
● Shiley NEF, NCF (35, 39)
★ Shiley NEO (35)
★ Shiley PDL, PLC (37, 41)
★ Shiley PED (36)
★ Shiley PED, PDC (36, 37)
■ Shiley PEF, PCF (36, 40)
◆ Shiley PELF, PLCF (37, 41)
▼ Shiley SCT (42)
▶ TRACOE mini Children (34)
◀ TRACOE mini Neonates (33)
▷ TRACOE silcosoft® Children (8, 23)
◁ TRACOE silcosoft® Neonates (3, 22)
+ TRACOE vario (31, 44)
✕ TRACOE vario XL (32, 45)

Age category
▨ Neonatal
▨ Pediatric
■ Adult

Figure 31.4 Relationship of OD and length for single cannula tracheostomies of different IDs and manufacturers. This graph illustrates the following: (1) the variation of OD (vertical axis) for a given ID depends on the manufacturer and is mainly due to differences in the materials used to make the tracheostomy tube, with silicone trachs (hollow symbols) tending to be thicker than PVC (filled symbols); and (2) how age category affects the trach length (horizontal axis) for a given ID. Note the overlap in IDs available in the different categories. (*Source*: Courtesy of Richard Lin)

sizes start at 5.0 mm ID. As the ID increases, the length also increases. The overlap in IDs between neonatal and pediatric and adult tubes provide more options to choose a tube that best fits a patient's body habitus and anatomy.

Although the specification of the tube is based on the ID, the factor that may determine how well the tracheostomy fits into the patient is the outer diameter (OD) of the tube. The factors that affect the OD of the tube for a given ID have mainly to do with the material of which the trach tube is manufactured. Silicone trach tubes tend to be thicker than PVC or PU trach tubes. The other factor that affects tube thickness is whether the tube is a single cannula or double cannula, as we will discuss further in the following text. The tracheostomy stoma is frequently the narrowest part of the path from stoma to trachea, and is most often the place that OD becomes an issue. Some tracheostomy tubes may have additional

Table 31.4 Recommendations for tracheostomy size based on age and weight.

Age range/weight	Suggested tracheostomy size (ID in mm)
Preterm infants <2.5 kg	2.0–3.0
Neonates 2.5–5 kg	3.0–3.5
Infants 5–8 kg	3.5–4.5
Children 8–10 kg	4.0–5.0
Children 10–15 kg	4.5–5.5
Children 15–20 kg	5.0–6.0
Children 20–35 kg	6.0–7.5
Women	7.0–9.0
Men	8.0–10.5

components such as cuff inflation line or subglottic suction line which may add to the outer dimension of the tube.

Choosing a tracheostomy tube size can be done using the same formula for endotracheal tube selection. The most common formulas used are (age + 16) / 4 or (age/4)+4 for an uncuffed tube, and ½ size smaller for a cuffed tube. Table 31.4 shows some recommendations for tracheostomy tube sizes based on a patient's age and weight. The tube is not intended to fill the entire trachea but is chosen to occupy enough space in the airway such that the patient is able to get adequate respiratory support. There are other factors that may influence the size selected for a child.

Reasons to consider a smaller tube for age:

- Prematurity
- Small, syndromic child
- Known history of complete tracheal rings
- In process of preparing for trach decannulation

Reasons to consider a larger tube for age:

- Long history of ventilator support
- High pressure/high volume ventilator support
- Tracheomegaly
- High body mass index

Some manufacturers still use the Jackson sizing designation (used for an older style of tracheostomy tube) for their tracheostomy tubes; in this case, the number associated with the size does not correspond to the ID. As a rule of thumb, the Jackson size plus four gives the approximate OD of the tube in millimeters. This is more commonly seen with the Medtronic adult Shiley tracheostomy tubes.

There are many manufacturers of tracheostomy tubes. We focus here on tubes from three manufacturers that are commonly used at our institution as well as the neighboring adult institution. Tables 31.5 and 31.6 compares some of the available sizes and dimensions as well as some of the features that they offer.

Covidien (Shiley brand) and Tracoe produce plastic polymer tubes. Smiths-Medical (Bivona, Portex) and Tracoe produce silicone tracheostomy tubes for children.

Table 31.5 Single cannula trach tubes.

cuffed	Mfr	material	age designation	inner diameter range [mm]	outer diameter range [mm]	distal length range [mm]	proximal length range [mm]	Cross reference	Mfr designation, comments
uncuffed	Bivona	silicone	neonatal	2.5–4.0	4.0–6.0	30–36		1	Bivona uncuffed neonatal (V- or straight-flange)
uncuffed	Bivona	silicone	neonatal	2.5–4.0	4.0–6.0	30–36	20	2	Bivona uncuffed neonatal FlexTend (V- or straight-flange)
uncuffed	Tracoe	silicone	neonatal	2.5–4.0	4.4–6.0	30–36	15–22	3	TRACOE silcosoft® for Neonates and Infants
uncuffed	Bivona	silicone	pediatric	2.5–5.5	4.0–8.0	38–46		4	Bivona uncuffed pediatric (V- or straight-flange)
uncuffed	Bivona	silicone	pediatric	2.5–5.5	4.0–8.0	38–46	20–30	5	Bivona uncuffed pediatric FlexTend (V- or straight-flange)
uncuffed	Bivona	silicone	pediatric	4.0–6.0	6.0–8.0	44–56	30	6	Bivona uncuffed pediatric FlexTend Plus (V- or straight-flange)
uncuffed	Bivona	silicone	pediatric	2.5–5.5	4.0–8.0	56–86	flange-dependent	7	Adjustable hyperflex (V-flange)
uncuffed	Tracoe	silicone	pediatric	2.5–5.5	4.4–8.4	38–46	20–30	8	TRACOE silcosoft® for Children
uncuffed	Bivona	silicone	"adult"	5.0–9.0	7.4–12.3	60–98		9	Bivona Uncuffed
uncuffed	Bivona	silicone	"adult"	6.0–9.0	9.2–12.9	100–130		10	Bivona Uncuffed Extra Length Fixed Neck Flange Hyperflex
uncuffed	Tracoe	silicone	"adult"	6.0–11.0	8.2–14.8	70–110	flange-dependent	11	TRACOE vario; adjustable shaft, adjustable flange
uncuffed	Tracoe	silicone	"adult"	7.0–10.0	9.7–13.7	104–135	flange-dependent	12	TRACOE vario; adjustable shaft, adjustable flange

cuffed	Bivona	silicone	neonatal	2.5–4.0	4.0–6.0	30–36		13	Bivona TTS cuffed neonatal (V- or straight-flange)
cuffed	Bivona	silicone	neonatal	2.5–4.0	4.0–6.0	30–36		14	Bivona Aire-cuf neonatal (V- or straight-flange)
cuffed	Bivona	silicone	neonatal	3.0–4.0	4.7–6.0	32–36		15	Bivona Fome cuf neonatal (V-flange)
cuffed	Bivona	silicone	neonatal	2.5–4.0	4.0–6.0	30–36	20	16	Bivona FlexTend with TTS cuff neonatal (V- or straight-flange)
cuffed	Bivona	silicone	pediatric	2.5–5.5	4.0–8.0	38–46		17	Bivona TTS cuffed pediatric (V- or straight-flange)
cuffed	Bivona	silicone	pediatric	2.5–5.5	4.0–8.0	38–46		18	Bivona Aire cuf pediatric (V- or straight-flange)
cuffed	Bivona	silicone	pediatric	2.5–5.5	4.0–8.0	38–46		19	Bivona Fome-cuf pediatric (V-flange)
cuffed	Bivona	silicone	pediatric	2.5–5.5	4.0–8.0	38–46	20–30	20	Bivona FlexTend with TTS cuff pediatric (V- or straight-flange)
cuffed	Bivona	silicone	pediatric	4.0–6.0	6.0–8.0	44–56	30	21	Bivona FlexTend Plus with TTS cuff pediatric (V- or straight-flange)
cuffed	Tracoe	silicone	neonatal	2.5–4.0	4.4–6.0	30–36	15–22	22	TRACOE silcosoft® for Neonates and Infants; water cuff
cuffed	Tracoe	silicone	pediatric	2.5–5.5	4.4–8.4	38–46	20–30	23	TRACOE silcosoft® for Children; water cuff,customizable: multiple lengths availabe for a given ID
cuffed	Bivona	silicone	"adult"	5.0–9.0	7.4–12.3	60–98		24	Bivona® TTS™ Cuffed

(Continued)

Table 31.5 (Continued)

cuffed	Mfr	material	age designation	inner diameter range [mm]	outer diameter range [mm]	distal length range [mm]	proximal length range [mm]	Cross reference	Mfr designation, comments
cuffed	Bivona	silicone	"adult"	5.0–9.5	7.4–13.3	60–98		25	Bivona® Mid-Range Aire-Cuf® (can also come with talk attachment)
cuffed	Bivona	silicone	"adult"	5.0–9.5	7.3–13.3	60–98		26	Bivona® Fome-Cuf® (can also come with talk attachment up to 9.0 ID)
cuffed	Bivona	silicone	"adult"	6.0–9.0	9.2–12.9	100–130		27	Bivona® TTS™ Extra Length Fixed Neck Flange Hyperflex™
cuffed	Bivona	silicone	"adult"	6.0–9.0	9.2–12.9	100–130		28	Bivona® Mid-Range Aire-Cuf® Extra Length Fixed Neck Flange Hyperflex™
cuffed	Bivona	silicone	"adult"	6.0–9.0	9.2–12.9	110–140	flange-dependent	29	Bivona® TTS™ Adjustable Neck Flange Hyperflex™
cuffed	Bivona	silicone	"adult"	6.0–9.0	9.2–12.9	110–140	flange-dependent	30	Bivona® Mid-Range Aire-Cuf® Adjustable Neck Flange Hyperflex™
cuffed	Tracoe	silicone	"adult"	6.0–11.0	8.2–14.8	70–110	flange-dependent	31	TRACOE vario; adjustable shaft, adjustable flange; subglottic suction available
cuffed	Tracoe	silicone	"adult"	7.0–10.0	9.7–13.7	104–135	flange-dependent	32	TRACOE vario; adjustable shaft, adjustable flange; subglottic suction available
uncuffed	Tracoe	PVC	neonatal	2.5–4.0	3.6–5.6	30–36		33	TRACOE mini
uncuffed	Tracoe	PVC	pediatric	2.5–6.0	3.6–8.4	32–62		34	TRACOE mini; customizable: multiple lengths avaiable for a given ID, choice of 3 angles

				ID (mm)	OD (mm)	Length (mm)		No.	Notes
uncuffed	Shiley	PVC	neonatal	2.5–4.5	4.2–6.7	28–36		35	Shiley™ NEF (NEO is retired predicate version, OD is roughly 0.2 mm smaller, starts at 3 mm ID)
uncuffed	Shiley	PVC	pediatric	2.5–5.5	4.2–7.9	38–46		36	Shiley™ PEF (PED is retired predicate version, OD is roughly 0.2 mm smaller; starts at 3 mm ID)
uncuffed	Shiley	PVC	pediatric	5.0–6.5	7.3–9.0	50–56		37	Shiley™ PELF (PDL is retired predicate version, OD is roughly 0.2 mm smaller)
uncuffed	Tracoe	PVC	"adult"	6.0–11.0	8.2–14.8	70–110	flange-dependent	38	TRACOE vario; adjustable shaft, adjustable flange; fenestration available
cuffed	Shiley	PVC	neonatal	2.5–4.5	4.2–6.7	28–36		39	Shiley™ NCF
cuffed	Shiley	PVC	pediatric	2.5–5.5	4.2–7.9	38–46		40	Shiley™ PCF
cuffed	Shiley	PVC	pediatric	5.0–6.5	7.3–9.0	50–56		41	Shiley™ PLCF (PLC is retired predicate version, OD is roughly 0.2 mm smaller)
cuffed	Shiley	PVC	"adult"	5.0–10.0	7.0–13.3	58–105		42	Shiley™ SCT
cuffed	Shiley	PVC	"adult"					43	Shiley™ Adult Flexible Evac, Jackson 4–10, nominal outer cannula ID 6-5-10
cuffed	Tracoe	PVC	"adult"	6.0–11.0	8.2–14.8	70–110	flange-dependent	44	TRACOE vario; adjustable shaft, adjustable flange; subglottic suction available
cuffed	Tracoe	PVC	"adult"	7.0–10.0	9.7–13.7	104–135	flange-dependent	45	TRACOE vario; adjustable shaft, adjustable flange; subglottic suction available

Table 31.6 Double cannula trach tubes.

fenestration	cuff	Mfr	Material	Inner cannula type (disposable vs reusable)	Inner cannula inner diameter range [mm]	Outer cannula outer diameter range [mm]	distal length range [mm]	Mfr designation, comments
unfenestrated	uncuffed	Portex	PVC	disposable	5.0–9.0	9.2–14.0	64.5–87.5	Blue Line Ultra (nominal 6.0-10.0)
unfenestrated	uncuffed	Portex	PVC	disposable	5.0–9.0	8.2–13.7	62.4–79.7	Uncuffed Flex D.I.C. (nominal 6.0-10.0)
unfenestrated	uncuffed	Portex	PVC	disposable	5.0–9.0	8.5–14.0	62.4–79.7	Uncuffed D.I.C. (nominal 6.0-10.0)
unfenestrated	uncuffed	Shiley	PVC	either	5.5–9.0	9.4–13.8	62–79	Flexible Adult Cuffless; Jackson 4-10, nominal outer cannula ID 6-5-10
unfenestrated	uncuffed	Shiley	PVC	disposable	5.0–8.0	9.6–13.3	90–105	XLT extended length, proximal (XLTUP) or distal (XLTUD) options
unfenestrated	uncuffed	Tracoe	PU	reusable	4.0–10.0	7.2–13.8	49–80	Twist
unfenestrated	cuffed	Portex	PVC	disposable	5.0–9.0	9.2–14.0	64.5–87.5	Suctionaid (nominal 6.0-10.0); with subglottic suction
unfenestrated	cuffed	Portex	PVC	disposable	5.0–9.0	9.2–14.0	64.5–87.5	Blue Line Ultra Cuffed (nominal 6.0-10.0)
unfenestrated	cuffed	Portex	PVC	disposable	5.0–9.0	8.2–13.7	62.4–79.7	Cuffed Flex D.I.C. (nominal 6.0-10.0)
unfenestrated	cuffed	Portex	PVC	disposable	5.0–9.0	8.5–14.0	62.4–79.7	Cuffed D.I.C. (nominal 6.0-10.0)
unfenestrated	cuffed	Shiley	PVC	either	5.5–9.0	9.4–13.8	62–79	Flexible Adult Cuffed; Jackson 4-10, nominal outer cannula ID 6-5-10
unfenestrated	cuffed	Shiley	PVC	either	5.5–9.0	9.4–13.8	62–79	Shiley™ Adult Flexible Evac, Jackson 4-10, nominal outer cannula ID 6-5-10

Fenestration	Cuff	Manufacturer	Material	Type	Size	Range 1	Range 2	Description
unfenestrated	cuffed	Shiley	PVC	disposable	5.0–8.0	9.6–13.3	90–105	XLT extended length, proximal (XLTCP) or distal (XLTCD) options
unfenestrated	cuffed	Tracoe	PU	reusable	4.0–10.0	7.2–13.8	49–80	Twist; available with subglottic suction OR air supply line for speaking
fenestrated	uncuffed	Portex	PVC	disposable	5.0–9.0	9.2–14.0	64.5–87.5	Blue Line Ultra Uncuffed Fenestrated (nominal 6.0-10.0)
fenestrated	uncuffed	Portex	PVC	disposable	5.0–9.0	8.5–14.0	62.4–79.7	Uncuffed Fenestrated D.I.C. (nominal 6.0-10.0)
fenestrated	uncuffed	Shiley	PVC	reusable	5.0–8.9	9.4–13.8	65–81	DCFN; Jackson 4, 6, 8, 10
fenestrated	uncuffed	Shiley	PVC	disposable	5.0–8.9	9.4–13.8	62–79	CFN; Jackson 4, 6, 8, 10
fenestrated	uncuffed	Tracoe	PU	reusable	4.0–10.0	7.2–13.8	49–80	Twist
fenestrated	uncuffed	Tracoe	PU	reusable	7.0–10.0	9.8–12.8	85–92	Twist plus; fenestrations on inner and outer curve
fenestrated	cuffed	Portex	PVC	disposable	5.0–9.0	9.2–14.0	64.5–87.5	Blue Line Ultra Cuffed Fenestrated (nominal 6.0-10.0)
fenestrated	cuffed	Portex	PVC	disposable	5.0–9.0	8.5–14.0	62.4–79.7	Cuffed Fenestrated D.I.C. (nominal 6.0-10.0)
fenestrated	cuffed	Shiley	PVC	reusable	5.0–8.9	9.4–13.8	65–81	FEN; Jackson 4, 6, 8, 10
fenestrated	cuffed	Shiley	PVC	disposable	5.0–8.9	9.4–13.8	62–79	DFEN; Jackson 4, 6, 8, 10
fenestrated	cuffed	Tracoe	PU	reusable	4.0–10.0	7.2–13.8	49–80	Twist; available with subglottic suction
fenestrated	cuffed	Tracoe	PU	reusable	7.0–10.0	9.8–12.8	85–92	Twist plus; fenestrations on inner and outer curve; available with subglottic suction

Shiley Tracheostomy Tubes

Shiley tracheostomy tubes were one of the earliest neonatal and pediatric tubes on the market. The tubes are made of a rigid PVC material which softens at body temperature. This material is less costly than silicone, but the tubes are not reusable. As discussed in the preceding text, since the walls of these trach tubes are thinner, they have a smaller OD for a given ID as compared to a silicone tube. These trach tubes are easier to insert than silicone tubes because of the rigidity of the material. There is one length available in each neonatal and pediatric tube in sizes 2.5 mm (ID) through 4.5 mm. There are two lengths available in pediatric tubes in sizes 5.0 mm through 6.5 mm. Medtronic can customize the tracheostomy by altering parameters such as the flange angle, length, curvature, and fenestration location if needed. Shiley tubes may be cuffed or uncuffed. Cuffs on Shiley tubes are also plastic, and the bulkiness of the cuff adds several millimeters to the OD. Therefore, a cuffed Shiley tube may be more difficult to insert and remove.

Medtronic has recently altered the shape of the cuff (Taperguard), which decreases the pressure exerted on the walls of the trachea from the earlier models. In the newer versions of the neonatal and pediatric trach tubes, the flanges are now made of a softer material than previous models and are transparent, allowing easier visualization of the peristomal skin. The flanges are still in a slightly V-shaped configuration, with a slightly more acute angle for pediatric versions as compared to the neonatal ones. The shaft is still made with PVC, but is a softer version, which improves comfort although with a thicker wall and slightly larger OD (by roughly 0.2 mm). The connector is flush to the flanges, and, for many younger children who have short necks, this can cause the chin to rest against the connector and increase the risk of irritation or accidental disconnects from ventilator tubing.

Shiley also has both single cannula and double cannula adult trach tubes available. The double cannula trach tubes have a face plate that maneuvers in the vertical plane. There are models with and without a cuff, with disposable or re-usable inner cannulas, and with fenestrations. The adult Shiley trach tubes have also recently been upgraded to a more flexible material and the number of options have been expanded, but at the time of this writing these are only available on the European market.

Tracoe Tracheostomy Tubes

Tracoe neonatal and pediatric tracheostomy tubes (so called "mini") are also made of PVC, which is less costly than silicone. The tubes can be cleaned and reused. The flanges are slightly V-shaped, and the connector is flush to the flanges. Tracoe mini tubes are available in sizes of 2.5–6.0 mm. The company "customizes" these tubes by making a wide variety of lengths available for each ID. All Tracoe mini tubes are uncuffed. Tracoe also makes a neonatal and pediatric tracheostomy tube made of flexible wire-reinforced silicone (the "silcosoft" line), which can be uncuffed or have a water-filled cuff. These tracheostomy tubes can also have a proximal shaft.

Tracoe has also product lines for adults. Their "vario" line consists of single cannula tracheostomy tubes made from PVC and can have multiple features, including an adjustable flange, adjustable shaft length, an air cuff, and subglottic suction. Their "twist" line consists of double cannula tracheostomy tubes made from PU, which allows them to be thinner but maintain strength. This allows them to have a smaller OD for a given ID. The tubes can be fenestrated, cuffed, and can also have subglottic suction or a talk port.

Bivona and Portex Tracheostomy Tubes by Smiths-Medical

Bivona tracheostomy tubes are made of silicone. Silicone material is softer and more pliant than PVC or PU plastics. These tubes are more expensive than Shiley and Tracoe products, but may be sterilized and reused up to five times for pediatric sizes, and up to ten times for adult sizes. The flanges can be V-shaped or straight across. Some models have a "FlexTend" option, which is a flexible proximal limb that extends outward from the trach flange so that the ventilator tubing connector is away from the chin. Bivona tubes are available in sizes 2.5–6.0 mm. There is one length available in neonatal and pediatric tubes in sizes 2.5–4.0 mm, and there are two lengths available in pediatric tube in sizes 2.5–6.0 mm. Smiths-Medical tubes can be cuffed or uncuffed. Cuff options are air-filled, water-filled, or a foam cuff. Smiths-Medical tracheostomy tubes can be customized for length, curvature, flange shape, and cuff.

Some models of the silicone trachs are reinforced with stainless steel wire, which can affect MRI compatibility. The models with stainless steel wire are MRI compatible up to 3 T. However, the wire compromises the clarity of the MRI images if the study area is near the trach tube location. The package insert gives detailed information regarding product use in MRI studies. The Smith-Medical company customer support line can also be called for further guidance (1-800-258 5361).

Smiths Medical also makes the Portex Blue Line family of double cannula adult tracheostomy tubes, which have a PVC construction. Features of this family include the ability to have fenestrations, air-filled cuffs, and subglottic suction ports.

Tracheostomy Cuffs

The primary purpose of a tracheostomy cuff is to improve ventilation support by minimizing (not eliminating) the leak around the trach tube. The amount of leak around a tracheostomy tube cuff may vary slightly depending upon the patient's position because the trachea is not a rigid structure. Historically, a cuff was also thought to help decrease aspiration of oral secretions for some patients although the cuff can also become a potential site for secretions to accumulate. As discussed below, a subglottic suction port can help mitigate that issue. A tracheostomy cuff can be left deflated once a patient no longer requires ventilatory support. Patients who require ventilator support overnight and remain off the ventilator during the day may have the cuff deflated while awake and inflated overnight.

Cuff deflation increases opportunity for vocalization around the trach tube for some children and can provide benefits for swallowing as well. Cuff deflation MUST be done before using devices such as a cap or speaking valve since these devices require the ability for air to flow around the tracheostomy tube and through the native airway.

Tracheostomy cuff volume should be assessed at least every 12 hours. Care must be taken to avoid overinflation of the tracheostomy cuff. Overinflation is defined as the complete loss of air leak around the tracheostomy tube. Cuff overinflation will cause distension of the tracheal wall over time and erosion of the tracheal mucosa at the level of the cuff.

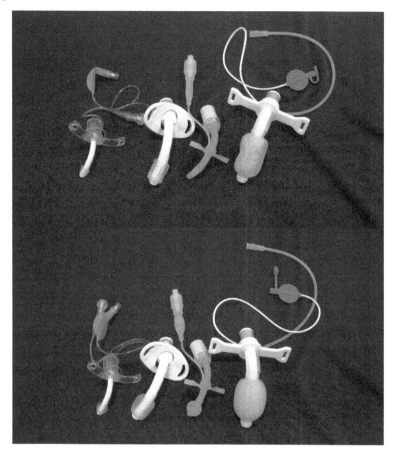

Figure 31.5 Examples of tracheostomy cuffs: From left to right: air (Shiley™ TaperGuard™), air, water (Bivona® TTS™), foam (Bivona® Fome-Cuf®). In the upper image, the cuffs are deflated; in the lower image, the cuffs are inflated. (*Source:* Courtesy of Michael Duff, RRT, Department of Respiratory Care, The Children's Hospital of Philadelphia, Philadelphia.)

Distention of the trachea leads to increased leak and loss of ventilator support. Progressive mucosal ulceration can lead to a rare, but fatal, erosion through the tracheal wall into the innominate artery which causes massive hemorrhage.

There are three types of tracheostomy tube cuffs: air-filled, water-filled, and a foam cuff (Figure 31.5). The purpose for the cuff remains the same, no matter what type of cuff a tracheostomy tube has. A plastic trach always has an air-filled cuff. Silicone tracheostomy tube cuffs can have any of these three types.

Air-Filled Cuff

Both silicone and plastic tracheostomy tubes may have air-filled cuffs (such as the Bivona® Aire-Cuf® or Shiley™ TaperGuard™). Inflation pressure is assessed using a manometer. To avoid overinflation, the amount of pressure that an air-filled cuff exerts on the trachea should ideally be maintained below 20–25 cm H_2O and not exceed 30 mm H_2O (Hess).

An alternative metric to minimize the risk of over-inflation is to use the minimal leak technique. To use this method, the practitioner places a stethoscope over the larynx and slowly inflates the cuff with air until the leak stops, then removes a small amount of air so that a slight leak heard at the peak inflating pressure during a patient's ventilatory cycle. The rationale behind this approach is that, if air is able to escape past the cuff, then the pressure on the mucosal tissue of the trachea cannot be that elevated.

An air cuff remains slightly boggy even when deflated due to its plastic material, and this can make tracheostomy tubes more difficult to insert and remove. Trach tubes with air cuffs can be made easier to insert by lubricating the cuff well, manually massaging the cuff to squeeze out as much air as possible, and to withdraw air from the cuff using a syringe that has a greater volume than the cuff. Sometimes a vasoconstrictor agent like oxymetazoline can be applied to the stoma prior to the tracheostomy change to maximize its size to make the change easier.

Water-Filled Cuff

Only silicone trach tubes have water-filled cuffs, which are also made from silicone (such as the Bivona® TTS™ cuff). Minimal leak technique is used to determine cuff inflation volumes. A manometer cannot be used to assess cuff pressure on a water-filled cuff. A water-filled cuff that is deflated completely is very snug to the shaft of the tube, making tubes with these cuffs the easiest to insert and remove. It is not unusual for a water-filled cuff to inflate asymmetrically such that the cuff is "lopsided." This typically is not an issue for the patient unless they have some asymmetry in their airway anatomy. It can usually be addressed by massaging the cuff, deflating the cuff, and then reinflating it again.

Foam Cuff

A foam cuff (such as Bivona® Fome-Cuf®) is rare. It is typically used for non-verbal patients who have been on ventilation for a long period of time and have developed a distended area within the trachea from chronic use of a cuff. The foam cuff is, by its nature, self-inflating. Unlike other cuffs, these must be actively deflated with a syringe to allow insertion into the patient. The cuff is allowed to self-inflate by opening the valve on the inflation line. The cuff inflation can be augmented by connecting the inflation line to the inspiratory side of the ventilator circuit (before gas enters the active humidifier). When the ventilator delivers a breath, the cuff inflates more and has more of a seal. When the ventilator cycles to the exhalation phase, the cuff pressure also decreases, and therefore the cuff is less inflated. This synchronized cuff inflation plus the large contact surface of a foam cuff tends to create less stress on the tracheal walls over time. There is no need to assess cuff inflation on a foam cuff as it will not exceed the inflation pressure supplied by the ventilator. The other attractive features of a foam cuff are its ability to conform to an irregular surface (such as an irregular tracheostomy stoma) and to self-center, which makes it an ideal cuff if a patient has an asymmetric airway. A foam cuff remains slightly distended even when deflated, which can make tracheostomy changes more difficult. Insertion of the foam cuff requires use of a three-way stopcock, which is used to deflate cuff as much as possible and to keep the cuff deflated while the tracheostomy tube is being inserted.

Adult tracheostomy features

Inner cannulas

Some adult tracheostomy tubes have a removable inner sleeve or "cannula," which extends the full length of the shaft and can be removed and replaced. This permits the inner surface of the tracheostomy to be cleaned without having to change the entire tracheostomy tube. Depending on the model, this inner cannula may be single-use or reusable. Tracheostomy tubes with this feature are called "double" cannula. The double cannula inherently makes the tracheostomy "thicker," since it causes the OD to be larger for a given ID. For example, a 6.0 mm ID Shiley single cannula tracheostomy has an OD of 8.3 mm. The equivalent double cannula version with the same ID has an OD of 10.1 mm. This makes the double cannula feature practical only for adult tracheostomy tubes. The smallest inner cannula is 5.5 mm for Shiley and 4.0 mm for Tracoe. Neonatal and pediatric tracheostomy tubes are "single" cannula.

Fenestrations

Another feature associated with double cannula tracheostomy tubes is the ability to have fenestrations in the outer cannula in the distal part of the curve. The fenestrations are holes through the wall of the cannula, which allow the tracheostomy to stay in place and serve as a conduit from the distal trachea to the extrathoracic airway, allowing the patient to breathe freely without needing to remove the tracheostomy or deflate the cuff. To allow these fenestrations to be used, the inner cannula in the tracheostomy must also have fenestrations and the connector to the inner cannula is typically capped, and the cuff, if present, is deflated. Since the fenestrations allow the patient to pass air through their extrathoracic airway and across their vocal cords, it allows them to vocalize. To allow the patient to receive respiratory support and clearance therapies, the fenestrated inner cannula is replaced with a non-fenestrated one. Fenestrated tracheostomies are not without issues, however. One is that the location of the fenestrae may be positioned so that they can be occluded by the posterior tracheal wall. Another is that the inner cannula may cause posterior displacement of the outer cannula and can promote the formation of granulation, which can grow through and occlude the fenestrae. This can cause bleeding or resistance to insertion and removal of the inner cannula and may also cause the tracheostomy to become difficult to remove. Lastly, there can be trauma to the posterior tracheal wall when a patient is suctioned through a fenestrated tracheostomy with a fenestrated inner cannula. There are patients who this tracheostomy serves well; however, one must be aware of the potential pitfalls.

Subglottic suction and talk ports

Analagous to the feature on endotracheal tubes, some tracheostomy tubes have a subglottic suction port. This type of suction port is used only with cuffed trach tubes. The inlet of a subglottic suction port is positioned just above the cuff to help manage secretions that pool above the tracheostomy cuff by providing a mechanism for suction and removal. This is most helpful for patients who have lost airway protective reflexes and aspirate their oral secretions, helping mitigate risk to the lungs from aspiration. This type of suction port can also help decrease the volume of secretions that drain from the tracheostomy stoma, which may be helpful in healing the stoma if there is an issue with dehiscence or granulation. Tracoe (in their Twist and vario lines), Shiley (in their Evac line), and Smiths Medical (in their Portex Suctionaid line) have subglottic lines as an option. The subglottic suction line is connected to an intermittent high-magnitude suction or continuous low-magnitude suction. These suction lines are around 2–2.8 mm in inner diameter and can frequently become clogged with mucoid secretions and need routine maintenance to keep them clear by flushing with either water or air.

Talk ports are used for patients who require an inflated cuff for secretion control or for ensuring adequate respiratory support. Patients with an inflated cuff generally have less of an ability to vocalize since they are unable to move air across their vocal cords. This lack of exhaled air flow can be mitigated with the use of a talk port. This port is connected to a gas source (with a maximum flow of 8–10 lpm) with a flow diverter in line. The patient can occlude the diverter with their thumb and direct flow through the talk port, which is above the cuff. This directs gas flow towards the glottis, which the patient can use to phonate. In some ways, the talk port and subglottic suction port are the same, but the direction of flow is different. Tracoe (in their vario line) and Smiths Medical (in their Aire Cuf and Fome Cuf line) have talk ports as an option in their tracheostomy tubes. Ideally, this gas source is humidified to prevent drying of extrathoracic airway mucosal tissue.

Evaluation of Tracheostomy Tube Positioning

Chest Radiograph

Chest radiograph can be used to evaluate the position of the tracheostomy tube in the airway. On chest radiograph, the distal tracheostomy tube tip should ideally be located at T2–T3. However, the appearance of tube length on X-ray can be affected by a number of factors. The trach may appear artificially high if the securement device is loose or if the ventilator tubing is being pulled at the time the film is taken (Figure 31.6). Also, the

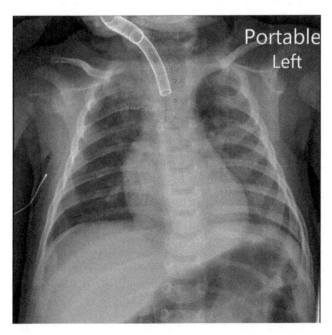

Figure 31.6 Chest X-ray showing tracheostomy placement, noting both vertebral body landmarks as well as a measurement from the tip of the tracheostomy to the carina. (*Source:* Courtesy of Richard Lin)

position of the tip may also change if the X-ray beam is not directly anterior–posterior, making the film slightly lordotic or anti-lordotic. Referencing the tip to the patient's carina may be more reliable since the reference and device are in the same plane. Typically a distance of at least one cm above the carina is desirable.

Tracheoscopy

Tracheoscopy is a procedure that involves passing a flexible endoscope (laryngoscope or bronchoscope) through the tracheostomy tube. This procedure is usually performed by an otolaryngologist. A tracheoscopy can evaluate for tube position within the trachea, distance of tube to carina, inflammation, tracheomalacia, obstruction due to backwalling or intratracheal granulation, and mucus plugging. Tracheoscopy can also help define how the position of the tracheostomy tube changes with changes in the patient's head and neck position.

Routine Tracheostomy Care

Tracheostomy Site Care

Routine tracheostomy stoma assessment and care is essential for the prevention of injury or infection that may occur with an artificial airway in place. The stoma site should be cleaned twice daily with water or a mild soapy solution and dried. If a dressing is used at the site, it should be changed twice daily after the stoma is cleaned. The site will typically have a small amount of clear to white mucous drainage. A patient with absent or ineffective gag or swallow may have copious oral secretions that drain out at the stoma and require more frequent dressing changes. It is important to note changes to the stoma appearance as well as the amount, color, consistency, and odor of secretions at the stoma.

Trach Stoma Dressings

Most patients use a dressing at the tracheostomy site to absorb drainage and provide skin protection. A variety of products are commonly used, and selection may be based on the volume of drainage or skin integrity at the stoma (insert chart – mepilex regular, mepilex lite, fenestrated gauze, fenestrated fome, and mepilex ag). Some patients have minimal stomal drainage and prefer no dressing at the trach site.

Securement Devices

The tracheostomy tube can be secured around the neck with a variety of commercially available devices. One- or two-piece cloth straps with Velcro fasteners are most commonly used. Other common securement devices may be made of absorbent material, cotton, neoprene, or beaded chain. They can be disposable or reusable. The device should be secured, but not so snugly as to cause breakdown due to pressure – a gap of one to two finger breadth is recommended between the neck and the device. Each patient should have additional securement devices in their emergency supply bag. Some patients may have a template to help guide the length to cut a securement device to best fit their neck.

It is important that the device remains clean and dry. The skin around the neck should be washed and dried daily and inspected for breakdown or rashes. The securement device is usually changed daily or every other day to prevent skin breakdown or infections due to moisture. The patient may also use additional dressings under the securement device to prevent rashes and pressure injuries.

Tracheostomy Tube Suctioning

Suction Catheter Size

Suction catheter size is based on the ID (size) of the tracheostomy tube. The size in French is roughly twice the number of the diameter. For example, a 8 French suction catheter is used with a 4.0 trach tube.

Suction Catheter Depth

The tip of the suction catheter should extend just past the tip of the tracheostomy tube; this measurement should be documented and adhered to in order to prevent suction trauma to the tracheal mucosa.

Suction Frequency

The tracheostomy tube should be suctioned when there is evidence of visual or audible secretions in the airway. Suctioning should also be considered if the patient has a sudden hypoxemia or an acute increase in work of breathing. The tracheostomy tube does not need to be suctioned on a scheduled basis. An inline suction catheter device is strongly recommended for patients with a lot of secretions on constant ventilator support to avoid de-recruitment and atelectasis from frequent loss of the support during open suctioning. To minimize the loss of respiratory support, suctioning should be limited to sessions of 5–10 seconds.

The use of saline lavage is not routinely recommended; instead, humidification should be used for patients receiving mechanical ventilation and for patients with thick secretions.

Tracheostomy Emergencies

It is helpful to have a stepwise approach to dealing with tracheostomy emergencies (Figure 31.7).

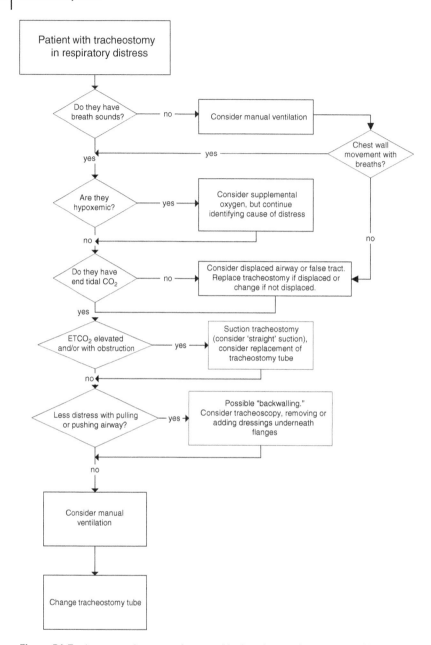

Figure 31.7 A systematic approach to troubleshooting tracheostomy problems.

Mucus Plugging

Mucus plugging is usually a gradual loss of airway diameter due to thick mucus adhering to inner lumen of the tracheostomy tube. If the obstruction is prolonged or becomes totally occlusive, it can lead to an acute event which could progress to a cardiopulmonary arrest. The initial presenting symptoms include increased work of breathing, slightly lower pulse oximeter readings, and irritability. Breath sounds may be decreased. It may or may not be difficult to pass the suction catheter. Sometimes, the child may have an increased air leak or phonate more around the trach tube. Factors that increase the risk of mucus plugging include lengthy periods of time off humidification, dehydration, increased secretions due to a respiratory illness, a prolonged length of time since last trach tube change, or inadequate pulmonary clearance. Some actions to take are as follows:

- Increase oxygen support if pulse ox is <92%.
- Assess breath sounds. If any wheezing, administer bronchodilator.
- Suction the trach tube and re-assess breath sounds.
- If no improvement in breath sounds or work of breathing, change the tracheostomy tube to rule out partial obstruction. *Caution: if the child has eaten in the past hour, there is an increased risk of vomiting during the tracheostomy tube change.*
- Set up supplies on a clean surface. Confirm that the replacement tracheostomy tube is the same size and length as the child's current tube. If trach has a cuff, inflate cuff prior to insertion to check for leak and to ensure that cuff inflates equally around the tube. Attach securement device to the flanges and lubricate tip with sterile water dissolvable lubricant.
- Perform a two-person trach change: Place the child on a shoulder roll to better expose the trach site. The child's head needs to remain in contact with the bed. In older patients with head control, the tracheostomy change is sometimes done with them sitting up. If there is a gastrostomy tube or nasogastric tube in place, unclamp the tube to allow it to vent. One caregiver prepares the new tracheostomy tube for insertion, making sure it is the appropriate size, that the external surface is lightly lubricated, and that, if applicable, the cuff functions appropriately. One person is designated the 'remover' and the other the 'inserter.' The remover holds the current tracheostomy tube in place while the inserter deflates the cuff and removes the securement. The remover removes the tracheostomy tube, and the inserter inserts the new tracheostomy tube, and removes the obturator. The remover disconnects the ventilator circuit from the old tube and reconnects it to the new tube, assesses breath sounds after placement, and inflates the cuff (if present). The inserter continues to hold the tube (acting as the tracheostomy securement) until the remover finishes securing it.

You may or may not see mucus plugging within the old tube. It may still have been the problem, and the plug may have been dislodged during the tube removal and is eventually resorbed by the body or is expectorated. Suction the new tracheostomy tube to make sure that the airway is clear.

Accidental decannulation

Displacement of the tracheostomy tube is an insidious, but not uncommon, cause of respiratory distress. It should be high in the differential diagnoses for a patient with a tracheostomy who has acute onset of increased work of breathing and should be among the first etiologies to exclude. Depending on whether the patient has extrathoracic airway obstruction or is ventilator dependent, hypoxemia or distress may not occur immediately. Sometimes the initial sign of decannulation is the patient's newfound ability to vocalize, indicating that they are passing air through their native airway instead of their tracheostomy tube. Even patients who are on mechanical ventilation may not trigger a ventilator alarm with decannulation if the distal shaft of the airway is kinked, if the tip of the tracheostomy is partially occluded by skin or mucosa, or if the patient is young and has a tracheostomy with a small ID.

The major step for diagnosing decannulation is to suspect it. Diagnosing is usually straightforward as it usually consists of making sure the tracheostomy is properly placed, although with dressings at the stoma it may not be clear, particularly if the trach tube is still in the stoma but not in proper placement. Capnometry can be diagnostic as decannulation will always lead to loss of end-tidal CO_2, and continuous capnometry can be helpful for early diagnosis.

The intervention consists of reinserting the displaced tracheostomy and then doing a planned tracheostomy change to make sure that the patient gets a clean trach tube. If there is only a partial decannulation and the airway cannot be re-established with manipulation or removal and reinsertion, then an emergent tracheostomy change may be needed.

False tract

A false tract is a potential passage, typically anterior to the trachea, that the tracheostomy tube slips into on insertion during a tracheostomy change or in the process of a partial decannulation. As with accidental decannulation, there may be acute onset of increased work of breathing and respiratory distress. If continuous capnometry in use, there will be a loss of end-tidal CO2. There will be resistance to air movement and lack of chest wall movement with manual ventilation breaths.

It is important to recognize the possibility that the tracheostomy has slipped into a false tract. Typically, this is apparent because the tracheostomy tube is unable to be inserted as deeply as normal.

Steps to address the tracheostomy slipping into a false tract are to remove the tracheostomy, reinsert the obturator into the tube, and reattempt insertion of the tube, trying to find the correct pathway of travel into the trachea. If that is unsuccessful, then an attempt should be made with the emergency tracheostomy tube (often selected to be made of PVC and is typically 1/2 size smaller (0.5 mm) for children and one size (1.0 mm) for adults). This frequently works because it is easier for the smaller tube to go into the correct passage, particularly since it is frequently made of a stiffer material.

If a tracheostomy tube cannot be inserted, then the patient may need to be supported with bag-valve-mask ventilation from above (with occlusion of the stoma).

Some experienced practitioners try replacing the obturator with a suction catheter and then 'finding' the airway passage with the suction catheter, then inserting the tracheostomy tube over the suction catheter in a fashion similar to Seldinger technique.

An ENT surgeon can navigate around a false tract by putting a tracheoscope through a tracheostomy tube and then inserting the scope through the stoma and finding the trachea by visualization, advancing the tracheostomy tube over the scope.

Inability to Insert Same-Size Tracheostomy Tube

Inability to replace a tracheostomy tube may be due to technical issues like inadequate neck extension and inability to visualize the stoma, or it could be due to patient issues like anxiety and crying, leading to tightening of the stomal aperture. Other situations where this scenario arises includes obstructive granulomas at the trach site or the delayed reinsertion of a tracheostomy tube in a patient who has decannulated (and thus the stoma has had a chance to close). Another cause may be that the patient's primary tracheostomy tube is one with an air-filled cuff. The approach needed will depend somewhat on the reason that replacement is difficult, and the rapidity of intervention will depend on how dependent the patient is on the artificial airway. The vast majority of time there is an issue with insertion of a tracheostomy tube, it is because of resistance at the narrowest part of the pathway from stoma to trachea, which is usually the tracheostomy stoma. Some of the steps to troubleshoot this include:

- Attempt reinsertion with an obturator, especially if one was not used on the first attempt. As discussed earlier, the obturator stiffens the tracheostomy tube and also smooths out the tip of the trach tube, which can make it easier to insert.
- Try to reposition patient by extending neck to get better exposure of the stoma. Sometimes there are other approaches that may work, such as inserting the tracheostomy tube using an approach from the side instead of following a path collinear with the trachea.
- If the issue appears to be an air-cuffed tracheostomy tube, maneuvers such as trying to deflate the cuff with a smaller syringe or simultaneous external pressure to deflate the cuff may help.
- If obstructive granulation is an issue, then treating the granulation ahead of a scheduled tracheostomy change may be warranted. Vasoconstrictors, such as topical oxymetazoline, may also be helpful.
- If the difficulty is because the stoma is closing since the patient is crying, often being patient and waiting to insert when they inhale can be helpful.
- If the difficulty is because of a delayed reinsertion, then an attempt with a smaller tracheostomy tube (such as the emergency tube) may be warranted. The patient may need dilation of the stoma the next time they have a tracheostomy change.
- If another attempt with an obturator fails, then use the emergency tracheostomy tube.
- If the emergency tracheostomy fails, then consider calling for help before trying again.
- Consider mask ventilation if possible (i.e., patient does not have high-grade extrathoracic airway obstruction).

Further Reading

1 Holzman, R.S. (2016). Airway Management. In: *Smith's Anesthesia for Infants and Children*, vol. 18 (eds. P.J. Davis and F.P. Cladis), 349–369. Philadelphia, PA: Elsevier. Print.

2 Fahl, A. (2020). Tracheostomy tubes and tube care. In: *Tracheotomy and Airway, A Practical Guide*, vol. 19 (eds. E. Klemm and A. Nowak), 233–247. Switzerland: Springer.

3 Hess, D. (2005). Tracheostomy tubes and related appliances. *Respir Care* 50 (4): 497–510.

4 Mitchell, R.B., Hussey, H.M., Setzgen, G. et al. (2013). Clinical consensus statement: tracheostomy care. *Otolaryngology–Head and Neck Surgery* 148 (1): 6–20.

5 Caparros, A.C.S. and Forbes, A. (2014). Mechanical ventilation and the role of saline instillation in suctioning adult intensive care unit patients an evidence-based practice review. *Dimensions of Critical Care Nursing* 33 (4): 246–253.

6 Björling, G., Axelsson, S., Johansson, U-B. et al. (2007). Clinical use and material wear of polymeric tracheostomy tubes. *Laryngoscope* 117(9):1552–1559. doi: 10.1097/MLG.0b013e 31806911e3.

7 Tweedie, D.J., Cooke, J., Stephenson, K.A., et al. (2018) Paediatric tracheostomy tubes: recent developments and our current practice. *J Laryngol Otol.* 132:961–968.

Index

Note: Page numbers in *italic* refer to figures, page numbers in **bold** refer to tables.

Emergency Management of the Hi-Tech Patient in Acute and Critical Care, First Edition. Edited by
Ioannis Koutroulis, Nicholas Tsarouhas, Richard J. Lin, Jill C. Posner, Michael Seneff, and Robert Shesser.
© 2021 John Wiley & Sons Ltd. Published 2021 by John Wiley & Sons Ltd.